ACUTE ENDOCRINOLOGY

For other titles published in this series, go to www.springer.com/series/7680

ACUTE ENDOCRINOLOGY

FROM CAUSE TO CONSEQUENCE

Edited by

GREET VAN DEN BERGHE, MD, PhD

Catholic University of Leuven, Department of Intensive Care Medicine, Leuven, Belgium

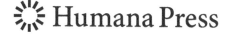 Humana Press

Greet Van den Berghe
Catholic University of Leuven
Department of Intensive
Care Medicine, Leuven
Belgium
greet.vandenberghe@med.kuleuven.be

ISBN 978-1-60327-176-9   ISBN 978-1-60327-177-6 (eBook)
DOI 10.1007/978-1-60327-177-6

Library of Congress Control Number: 2008933363

Printed on acid-free paper

springer.com

Preface

Until recently, endocrinology and critical care medicine were two specialties in medicine that were rather uncomfortable with each other and hence quite isolated. Fortunately, these two 'alien' disciplines have joined forces in successful attempts to perform high quality research in order to clarify the unknown. By integrating endocrinology in critical care medicine, or vice-versa depending on the specialty of the observer, new experimental and clinical data on the complex endocrine and metabolic derangements accompanying non-endocrine severe illnesses came available which generated important novel insights with relevant clinical implications. In addition, the state of the art diagnosis and management of primary endocrine diseases that represent life-threatening situations leading to ICU admission has been updated. This issue of Contemporary Endocrinology aims at compiling the new findings. The book indeed covers both areas of 'Acute Endocrinology' that are often taking care of at very distant sites within hospitals. The first part deals with the classical life-threatening illnesses caused by primary endocrine diseases such as thyrotoxicosis, hypothyroidism, acute adrenal crisis, acute calcium disorders, pheochromocytoma, severe hyper- and hypoglycemia . The second part looks at endocrinology from the ICU side, starting with a general overview of the dynamic neuroendocrine and metabolic stress responses in the condition of intensive care-dependent, non-endocrine critical illness. Alterations within several of the endocrine axes briefly touched upon in the overview chapter are then further discussed in detail in the following chapters: critical illness induced alterations within the growth hormone axis, the thyroid axis and the pituitary adrenal axis, changes in catecholamines, glucose control, and salt and water metabolism. This last chapter on salt and water disturbances bridges both the endocrine and non-endocrine causes and their specific approaches.

I am confident that this book provides a unique and up-to-date overview of the state of the art knowledge of interest to the most alien of disciplines in medicine and stimulates further interdisciplinary research in this important and exciting field.

Greet Van den Berghe, MD, PhD

Contents

Contributors

MIKAEL ALVES, MD, *Faculté de Médecine, Hôpital Raymond Poincaré (AP-HP), Paris Ile de France Ouest (Université de Versailles Saint Quentin), Garches, France*

DJILLALI ANNANE, MD, PhD, *Faculté de Médecine, Hôpital Raymond Poincaré (AP-HP), Paris Ile de France Ouest (Université de Versailles Saint Quentin), Garches, France*

PIERRE ASFAR, MD, PhD, *Département de Réanimation Médicale, CHU Angers, Université d'Angers, Angers, France*

XAVI BORRAT, MD, *Department of Intensive Care Medicine, Hospital Clinic, Barcelona, Spain*

ROGER BOUILLON, MD, PhD, *Laboratory of Experimental Medicine and Endocrinology (Legendo), Catholic University of Leuven, Leuven, Belgium*

KENNETH D. BURMAN, MD, PhD, *Endocrine Section, Washington Hospital Center, Georgetown University School of Medicine, Washington DC, USA*

ENRICO CALZIA, MD, PhD, *Sektion Anästhesiologische Pathophysiologie und Verfahrensentwicklung, Universitätsklinikum, Ulm, Germany*

SHERN L. CHEW, MD, PhD, *Division of Endocrinology, St Bartholomew's Hospital, West Smithfield, London, UK*

JOSEPH N. FISHER, MD, *Division of Endocrinology, Department of Medicine, University of Tennessee, Health Science Center, Memphis, TN, USA*

PHILLIP GORDON, MD, *National Institute of Diabetes and Digestive and Kidney Disease, National Institutes of Health, Bethesda, MD, USA*

JEAN-MARC GUETTIER, MD, *National Institute of Diabetes and Digestive and Kidney Disease, National Institutes of Health, Bethesda, MD, USA*

KEN K. Y. HO, MD, PhD, *Department of Endocrinology, St Vincent's Hospital and Pituitary Research Unit, Garvan Institute of Medical Research, Sydney, New South Wales, Australia*

ABBAS E. KITABCHI, MD, PhD, *Division of Endocrinology, Department of Medicine, University of Tennessee, Health Science Center, Memphis, TN, USA*

LIES LANGOUCHE, PhD, *Department of Intensive Care Medicine, University Hospital Gasthuisberg, Catholic University of Leuven, Leuven, Belgium*

PAUL LEE, MD, *Department of Endocrinology, St Vincent's Hospital and Pituitary Research Unit, Garvan Institute of Medical Research, Sydney, New South Wales, Australia*

ix

LIESE MEBIS, MSc, *Department of Intensive Care Medicine, University Hospital Gasthuisberg, Catholic University of Leuven, Leuven, Belgium*

DIETER MESOTTEN, MD, PhD, *Department of Intensive Care Medicine, University Hospital Gasthuisberg, Catholic University of Leuven, Leuven, Belgium*

SUZANNE MYERS ADLER, MD, *Division of Endocrinology and Metabolism, Washington Hospital Center, Georgetown University School of Medicine, Washington DC, USA*

POWLIMI J. NADKARNI, MD, *Endocrine Section, Washington Hospital Center, Georgetown University School of Medicine, Washington DC, USA*

PETER RADERMACHER, MD, PhD, *Sektion Anästhesiologische Pathophysiologie und Verfahrensentwicklung, Universitätsklinikum, Ulm, Germany*

UMASUTHAN SRIRANGALINGAM, MD, *Department of Endocrinology, St Bartholomew's Hospital, West Smithfield, London, UK*

SOPHIE J. VAN CROMPHAUT, MD, PhD, *Department of Intensive Care Medicine, University Hospital Gasthuisberg, Catholic University of Leuven, Leuven, Belgium*

GREET VAN DEN BERGHE, MD, PhD, *Department of Intensive Care Medicine, University Hospital Gasthuisberg, Catholic University of Leuven, Leuven, Belgium*

ILSE VANHOREBEEK, PhD, *Department of Intensive Care Medicine, University Hospital Gasthuisberg, Catholic University of Leuven, Leuven, Belgium*

JOSEPH VERBALIS, MD, PhD, *Division of Endocrinology and Metabolism, Georgetown University Medical Center, Washington DC, USA*

LEONARD WARTOFSKY, MD, PhD, *Division of Endocrinology and Metabolism, Washington Hospital Center, Georgetown University School of Medicine, Washington DC, USA*

I ENDOCRINE DISEASES CAUSING POTENTIALLY LIFE-THREATENING EMERGENCIES

1 Thyrotoxicosis

Powlimi J. Nadkarni, MD and Kenneth D. Burman, MD

CONTENTS

INTRODUCTION

Thyrotoxicosis refers to a state of excess thyroid hormones in the circulation resulting in signs and symptoms of thyroid over-activity. The sources of thyrotoxicosis can originate either from the thyroid gland or from an extra-thyroidal source. The term hyperthyroidism refers to thyrotoxicosis resulting from direct production of excess thyroid hormone by the thyroid gland itself *(1)*. The severity of thyrotoxicosis can range from subclinical laboratory abnormalities to overt thyroid storm depending on the degree of thyroid hormone elevation, etiology, age of the patient, and extra-thyroidal manifestations *(1)*. In the United States, the prevalence of thyrotoxicosis is estimated to be 1.2%, of which 0.7% is secondary to subclinical hyperthyroidism *(1,2)*. The most common cause of endogenous thyrotoxicosis is Graves' disease. Other common causes include toxic multinodular goiter, solitary toxic adenoma, subacute and postpartum

From: *Contemporary Endocrinology: Acute Cause to Consequence*
Edited by: G. Van den Berghe, DOI: 10.1007/978-1-60327-177-6_1,
© Humana Press, New York, NY

thyroiditis, and iodine exposure. More unusual etiologies are thyroid-stimulating hormone (TSH) secreting pituitary adenomas, trophoblastic tumors secreting HCG, and struma ovarii. Box 1 reviews the causes of thyrotoxicosis.

Box 1: Causes of Thyrotoxicosis

Thyroidal (Hyperthyroidism):
Graves' disease
Toxic multinodular goiter
Solitary toxic adenoma
Thyroiditis

   – Subacute
   – Painless/silent
   – Postpartum

Iodine-induced

   – Amiodarone-induced

Trophoblastic tumors

   – Hydatidiform mole
   – Choriocarcinoma

Hypersecretion of TSH

   – TSH secreting pituitary adenoma

Pituitary resistance to thyroid hormone

Extra-thyroidal:
Thyrotoxicosis factitia
Ectopic thyroid tissue

   – Struma ovarii
   – Metastatic functioning differentiated thyroid cancer

CAUSES OF THYROTOXICOSIS

Graves' Disease

EPIDEMIOLOGY

Graves' disease (also known as von Basedow's disease in Europe) was first described in 1835 by Robert Graves, who identified the triad of goiter, palpitations, and exophthalmos. It is now well-recognized that hyperthyroidism due to Graves' disease is caused by antibodies that stimulate the thyroid gland TSH receptor to produce excess thyroid hormone resulting in the signs and symptoms of thyrotoxicosis. Graves' disease is the most common etiology of endogenous hyperthyroidism worldwide accounting for sixty to eighty percent of patients with hyperthyroidism *(3)*. It is a common autoimmune disorder in the United States with an annual incidence around 0.5 per 1000 *(4)*. It is more prevalent among women than men and most commonly occurs between about the age twenty and fifty *(3,4)*.

PATHOGENESIS

The underlying mechanism behind Graves' disease is an autoimmune reaction from auto-antibodies that bind to the TSH receptor in the thyroid gland. There is a simultaneous and variable production of thyrotropin stimulatory and inhibitory antibodies resulting in differences in the severity of presentation *(3)*. Thyroid stimulatory antibodies have dual function causing not only hyperfunction of the thyroid gland, but also hypertrophy and hyperplasia of the thyroid follicles resulting in the characteristic diffuse goiter *(3,5)*. On pathologic examination, lymphocytic infiltration is also seen. Female gender is a strongly associated predisposing factor linked to the development of Graves' disease with a female to male incidence ratio of 7 to 10:1 *(6)*. Other postulated etiologies include a combination of genetic, viral, stress-induced, and environmental (medications, radiation exposure) factors *(1,3)*. Smoking, although weakly associated with Graves' disease, is a significant risk factor for the development of Graves' ophthalmopathy *(7)*.

CLINICAL MANIFESTATIONS

The classic triad of Graves' disease is a presentation of diffuse goiter, signs and symptoms of thyrotoxicosis, and ophthalmopathy. Occasionally, an infiltrative dermopathy (i.e., pretibial myxedema) can also accompany the symptoms *(1)*. The severity of symptoms often depends on the degree of thyrotoxicosis but the majority of patients present with nervousness, fatigue, hand tremor, heat intolerance, weight loss despite a good appetite, a rapid heartbeat or palpitations *(3)*. The major symptoms and signs of hyperthyroidism and specifically those manifesting during Graves' disease are listed in Box 2. Extra-thyroidal manifestations of Graves' disease include Graves' eye disease and Graves' skin disease. Fifty percent of patients initially present with clinically evident eye disease and of those, eye disease is manifested within a year (prior to or following) of the diagnosis of hyperthyroidism *(3)*. In contrast, dermopathy occurs in only one to two percent of patients with Graves' disease, generally co-existent with severe ophthalmopathy *(3)*. The physical findings of ophthalmopathy and dermopathy in the setting of a patient with hyperthyroidism and diffuse goiter are adequate to confirm the clinical diagnosis of Graves' disease. Testing for serum thyroid antibodies (i.e., thyroid stimulating immunoglobulins) and a radionuclide scan (i.e., ^{123}I) showing diffuse trapping of isotope with an elevated percent uptake can provide further diagnostic aids in making the diagnosis.

Box 2: Major Symptoms and Signs of Hyperthyroidism and of Graves' Disease and Conditions Associated with Graves' Disease

MANIFESTATIONS OF HYPERTHYROIDISM

Symptoms:

- Hyperactivity, irritability, altered mood, insomnia, inability to concentrate
- Heat intolerance, increased sweating
- Palpitations
- Fatigue, weakness
- Dyspnea
- Weight loss with increased appetite (weight gain in 10% of patients)
- Pruritis
- Increased stool frequency
- Thirst and polyuria
- Oligomenorrhea or amenorrhea, loss of libido

Signs:

- Sinus tachycardia, atrial fibrillation
- Fine tremor, hyperkinesis, hyperreflexia
- Warm, moist skin
- Palmar erythema, onycholysis
- Hair loss
- Muscle weakness and wasting
- Rare: Congestive (high-output) heart failure, chorea, periodic paralysis (primarily in Asian men), psychosis

Manifestations of Graves' disease

- Diffuse goiter
- Ophthalmopathy (grittiness and discomfort in the eye, retrobulbar pressure or pain, eyelid lag or retraction, periorbital edema, chemosis, scleral injection, exophthalmos (proptosis), extraocular-muscle dysfunction, exposure keratitis, optic neuropathy)
- Localized dermopathy (usually in the pretibial area but can occur elsewhere such as in the preradial area and face)
- Lymphoid hyperplasia, including thymic hyperplasia
- Thyroid acropachy

Conditions associated with Graves' disease

- Type 1 diabetes mellitus
- Addison's disease
- Vitiligo
- Pernicious anemia
- Alopecia areata
- Myasthenia gravis
- Celiac disease
- Other autoimmune disorders associated with the HLA-DR3 haplotype

Adapted From: Weetman AP. Graves' Disease. NEJM 2000; 343(17):1236–1248

Copyright © 2000 Massachusetts Medical Society. All rights reserved (3).

EXTRA-THYROIDAL MANIFESTATIONS

Orbitopathy. Approximately fifty percent of patients have clinically evident ophthalmopathy manifesting most frequently as eyelid retraction, lid-lag, and periorbital edema *(3)*. Only three to five percent have severe eye disease defined as affecting vision or quality of life *(3,8)*. Eye disease can be unilateral (5–15%) or bilateral (85–95%); when bilateral, ocular disease is usually asymmetric *(9)*. Orbital sonograms and/or CT scans (without intravenous radiocontrast) can be helpful to identify and monitor specific manifestations and these techniques identify abnormalities in the orbit more frequently than is found clinically. Graves' ophthalmopathy generally manifests within eighteen months of pre sentation of the hyperthyroidism in a bimodal pattern, peaking in the fifth and seventh decades of life *(8)*. Although it is overall more common in females, it appears that the more severe forms of eye disease appear to have a higher prevalence in men and older patients. Cigarette smoking has been implicated with a higher frequency of ophthalmopathy, a higher degree of disease severity, and with a lower effectiveness of medical therapy *(8)*.

Dermopathy. Graves' dermopathy occurs in approximately one to two percent of patients with Graves' disease. It is most common over the anterolateral aspects of the shin (i.e., pretibial myxedema) but can occur in other locations as well after minimal trauma *(3)*. Once identified, prudent treatment with high-potency topical steroids and occlusive dressings may cause regression of the skin lesions; however if long-standing, it may be more difficult to treat *(1)*.

TREATMENT

Graves' hyperthyroidism is treated via antithyroid drugs, radioactive iodine ablation, or surgery. Specific treatment preferences vary with geographic area, clinical circumstance, and physician and patient preference. These different treatment modalities will be reviewed in further detail later in this chapter.

TOXIC MULTINODULAR GOITER

Multinodular goiter is the most common endocrine disorder worldwide, affecting 500 to 600 million people (10). Although it is often associated with iodine deficiency, even with iodine repletion, the prevalence of sporadic goiters remains about four to seven percent (11). Occasionally, hyperfunction of the initially nonfunctional 'non-toxic' nodules does occur leading to thyrotoxicosis and resultant 'toxic' multinodular goiter. Typically, thyrotoxicosis develops in patients after the age of 50 who have longstanding goiters. The prevalence is higher in women than men and can occur precipitously after exposure to medications or radiocontrast dye containing iodine (1). Thyrotoxicosis secondary to toxic multinodular goiter tends to be milder than that of Graves' disease and ophthalmopathy is absent (12). On laboratory evaluation, TSH is suppressed while T_3 and T_4 are normal or elevated (usually slightly). ^{123}I uptake and scanning reveals normal to increased uptake in a heterogeneous pattern with focal areas of uptake corresponding to autonomously functioning nodules (1). Radioactive iodine ablation or surgery is recommended as definitive treatment for toxic nodules of the thyroid (13). Radioiodine is the treatment of choice for most patients, although the doses tend to be larger than in Graves' disease because the glands tend to be larger with less ^{131}I uptake (1).

Caution must be made when treating a patient with toxic multinodular goiter with ^{131}I. There may be a transient enlargement of the thyroid gland in the days and weeks following the ^{131}I therapy. The ^{131}I therapy is less consistent in rendering the patient euthyroid or hypothyroid than in Graves' disease and the patient's thyroid function tests must be monitored closely to ensure that there is no sudden increase in serum T_4 and T_3 levels. Some patients may require a second or third dose of ^{131}I. The radioactive iodine uptake may need to be enhanced by the use of small doses of recombinant human TSH, but again this should be performed by experienced clinicians since the rhTSH may cause enlargement of the thyroid gland and the dose of rhTSH requires experienced judgment. Surgical thyroidectomy must also be performed by an experienced thyroid surgery team, and usually the patients are rendered euthyroid with antithyroid medications prior to surgery, but there is still a risk of sudden release of T_4 and T_3 and thyroid storm at surgery.

SOLITARY TOXIC ADENOMA (PLUMMER'S DISEASE)

Also known as hyperfunctioning solitary nodule, toxic nodule, or Plummer's Disease, solitary toxic adenoma is an autonomously functioning thyroid nodule in an otherwise basically normal thyroid gland. Like multinodular goiter, the nodule usually has been present for a number of years and eventually becomes hyperfunctioning. Patients typically present at the age of 30–40 years with a history of a longstanding growing lump in the neck *(1)*. Adenomas generally grow to 2.5–3 cm before becoming hyperfunctional *(1)*. Laboratory evaluation is consistent with hyperthyroidism and radioactive uptake and scan shows localized uptake in the toxic nodule. Definitive therapy is similar to a toxic multinodular goiter in that radioactive iodine ablation or surgery is recommended. In older patients radioiodine therapy may be the preferred treatment modality, while young patients or those with large nodules should undergo surgical excision *(12)*. It is difficult to give specific recommendations regarding therapy and it should be individualized and discussed with the patient. Other possible therapeutic options are ultrasound-guided laser thermal ablation or percutaneous ethanol injection *(14)*. Advantages to these procedures include avoiding surgery or exposure to radiation; disadvantages include multiple visits, discomfort due to the ethanol injection, and rarely, toxic necrosis of the larynx *(15)*. This technique is considered more experimental and is utilized mainly by a few specialized centers.

Thyroiditis

SUBACUTE THYROIDITIS (DE QUERVAIN'S THYROIDITIS)

Subacute thyroiditis is also termed painful subacute thyroiditis, de Quervain's thyroiditis, Giant-cell thyroiditis, subacute granulomatous thyroiditis, and pseudogranulomatous thyroiditis. It is the most common form of thyroid discomfort occurring in up to five percent of patients with thyroid disease *(16)*. There is a 5:1 female to male predilection during the ages of 20–60 years. Hypotheses for a viral etiology exist but remains to be established. Generally, it occurs several weeks following a viral illness with a prodrome of generalized myalgias, pharyngitis, low-grade fever, and fatigue. Patients then complain of neck pain, swelling, and symptoms of thyrotoxicosis *(21)*. On laboratory evaluation, TSH is suppressed with modest elevations of thyroid hormones (usually T_4 greater than T_3), along with marked elevation of the erythrocyte sedimentation rate and C-reactive protein *(17)*. Other useful markers include a mild elevation of the leukocyte count and normal or mildly elevated antithyroglobulin and antithyroperoxidase antibody titers. [123]I radioactive uptake is usually less than five percent during the hyperthyroid phase as the release of T_4 and T_3 suppresses TSH and then the radioactive iodine uptake.

Typically, the thyrotoxicosis is self-limiting and returns to normal in two to three months but can result in permanent hypothyroidism in up to five percent of patients *(18,19)*. Treatment for the hyperthyroid phase is aimed at symptomatic relief with non-steroidal anti-inflammatory agents or salicylates for pain control and beta-adrenergic blockade for tachycardia. In more moderate to severe cases of thyrotoxicosis, a short course of high dose glucocorticoids (prednisone 40 mg daily tapering over two to three weeks) may be beneficial *(21)*.

Subacute thyroiditis usually has a characteristic course with the patients presenting with hyperthyroidism, low radioactive iodine uptake, and neck discomfort (that can radiate). This phase lasts until the stores of T_4 and T_3 are depleted (usually four to six weeks) and then the patient passes through a euthyroid phase while his/her T_4 and T_3 decrease to below normal, and his/her TSH is elevated. In this phase, which also usually lasts four to six weeks, the patient's thyroid gland synthesizes thyroid hormone and gradually T_4 and T_3 stores are replenished and secreted, resulting in normal T_4, T_3, and TSH and restoration of the euthyroid state. Subacute thyroiditis usually does not recur.

PAINLESS/SILENT THYROIDITIS

Painless or silent thyroiditis is a destructive form of thyroiditis accounting for approximately one percent of all causes of thyrotoxicosis *(21)*. In this inflammatory condition, a triphasic thyroid hormone profile can be seen as preformed thyroid hormones are released into the circulation resulting in a transient thyrotoxicosis, followed by a transient euthyroid to hypothyroid transition, and then finally by euthyroidism. The thyrotoxicosis of this form of thyroiditis tends to be T_4 predominant reflecting the destruction of the thyroid gland releasing preformed thyroid hormone, as opposed to the T_3 toxicosis of Graves' disease or toxic nodular goiter *(21)*. It can occur in all ages, but peaks at 30–40 years of age with a 2:1 female to male ratio. The signs and symptoms of thyrotoxicosis are mild or silent and typically do not require treatment. On physical exam, a small, nontender, firm, diffuse goiter is present in fifty percent of patients *(20)*. Thyroid antibody titers are high and a low 24-hour uptake of ^{123}I is useful (less than five percent). The majority of patients have spontaneous recovery but some may have recurrence. Painless thyroiditis differs from subacute thyroiditis because of the lack of neck discomfort and because the transition from hyperthyroidism to hypothyroidism to euthyroidism is less consistent in course and timing than subacute thyroiditis.

POSTPARTUM THYROIDITIS

Also termed as subacute lymphocytic thyroiditis, postpartum thyroiditis is an inflammatory destructive condition of the thyroid gland where pre-formed thyroid hormones are released from the thyroid gland into the circulation. This is thought to be an autoimmune process and the pathology of the thyroid gland shows lymphocytic infiltration. As the name implies, the thyrotoxicosis generally occurs one to six months postpartum and is followed by a recovery phase resulting in hypothyroidism four to eight months after delivery and lasting for four to six months *(21)*. Spontaneous recovery occurs in eighty percent of women within a year however permanent hypothyroidism may eventually develop over subsequent years in up to twenty percent of women *(6,22)*. The diagnosis is made in the appropriate clinical situation when signs and symptoms of thyrotoxicosis are present in the postpartum period. On physical exam, a small nontender goiter is usually present. Laboratory evaluation is generally significant for high concentrations of thyroid antibodies (thyroid peroxidase antibodies and thyroglobulin antibodies) *(23)*. When the etiology of thyrotoxicosis is not clear, a 24-hour ^{123}I uptake and scan can be useful to distinguish postpartum thyroiditis from Graves' disease. Patients with postpartum thyroiditis should have a low (less than 5 percent) uptake *(21)*. In most cases of postpartum thyroiditis, the thyrotoxicosis is mild and does not warrant therapy. In more symptomatic cases, beta-blockade is required to alleviate the tachycardia. Antithyroid drug therapy is not indicated because the etiological factor is not overproduction of thyroid hormones *(21)*. Interestingly, postpartum thyroiditis tends to recur in an individual patient following subsequent pregnancies.

Iodine-Induced Thyrotoxicosis

JOD-BASEDOW EFFECT

Iodine-induced hyperthyroidism or the Jod-Basedow effect refers to the development of iodine-induced hyperthyroidism in subjects with endemic goiter due to iodine deficiency after the administration of supplemental iodine. This phenomenon occurs in a minority of the patients at risk but can rarely result in severe hyperthyroidism. The term 'Jod-Basedow' is also commonly used to refer to any cause of iodine induced hyperthyroidism even in an iodine sufficient area.

The Jod-Basedow effect also has relevance in areas of the world where dietary iodine is sufficient. In older adults who have a higher prevalence of nodular goiters, physicians must be aware of the possibility of inducing hyperthyroidism by the administration of large pharmacologic doses of iodine via medications (expectorants, amiodarone), diet (kelp, seaweed) or intravenous radiocontrast media *(1)*. Iodine exposure can be confirmed by demonstrating a low radioactive iodine uptake in conjunction with an increased urinary iodine excretion (greater than 1000 µg/day). Refer to Box 3 for the iodine content found in common medications *(24)*.

Box 3: Iodine Content of Some Iodine-Containing Medications and Radiographic Contrast Agents

Substance	Amount of iodine
Expectorants	
Iophen	25 mg/mL
Iodinated glycerol	15 mg/tablet
Calcidrine	152 mg/5 mL
Iodides	
Potassium iodide (saturated solution)	25 mg/drop
Pima syrup (potassium iodide [KI])	255 mg/mL
Lugol's solution (KI plus iodide)	5 mg/drop
Antiasthmatic drugs	
Elixophyllin-K1(theophylline) elixir	6.6 mg/mL
Antiarrhythmic drugs	
Amiodarone	75 mg/tablet
Antiamebic drugs	
Iodoquinol	134 mg/tablet
Topical antiseptic agents	
Povidone-iodine	10 mg/mL
Clioquinol cream	12 mg/gram
Douches	
Povidone-iodine	10 mg/mL
Radiographic contrast agents	
Iopanoic acid*	333 mg/tablet
Ipodate sodium*	308 mg/tablet
Intravenous preparations	140–380 mg/mL
Anti-cellulite therapy	
Cellasene	720 mcg/serving

* Not available in the United States.
From: Surks, MI in *UpToDate(24)*

AMIODARONE-INDUCED THYROTOXICOSIS

Amiodarone is an effective Class III anti-arrhythmic used in the prevention and treatment of both supraventricular and ventricular cardiac arrhythmias. Its mechanism of action is multifactorial, working by prolongation of the cardiac

action potential, as well as containing noncompetitive beta-adrenergic antagonist properties *(25,26)*. Unlike other classes of anti-arrhythmics, it also carries
a low incidence of proarrhythmia making it an extremely efficacious agent in
controlling arrhythmias and in the prevention of mortality *(26)*. Unfortunately,
its noncardiac effects, especially on the thyroid, can be significant.

The structure of amiodarone is similar to thyroxine and contains approximately 37% iodine by weight *(27)*. It contains 75 mg iodine per 200 mg tablet, of
which approximately 10% is deiodinated and released into the circulation as free
iodide *(27,28)*. With usual maintenance amiodarone doses of 200–600 mg/day,
this results in 50–100 times the daily requirement of iodine *(27)*. In addition, it
is a lipophillic agent with a half-life of 107 days having in long-lasting effects
even after discontinuation *(29)*.

The majority of patients who are administered amiodarone remain euthyroid; however, thyroid dysfunction does occur in 14–18% of patients taking
amiodarone *(27,30)*. Thyroid dysfunction secondary to amiodarone can either
be manifested as hypothyroidism or hyperthyroidism. The development of
amiodarone-induced hypothyroidism (AIH) versus amiodarone-induced thyrotoxicosis (AIT) tends to correlate with daily iodine intake. AIH is more prevalent
in iodine-sufficient areas of the world; whereas AIT is more prevalent in iodine-
deficient regions *(30)*.

Amiodarone-induced thyrotoxicosis (AIT) is more common in males, most
likely attributable to the higher prevalence of amiodarone use in men, and can
occur at any time after exposure to amiodarone *(27)*. It can be subdivided into
two types based on the etiology of the hyperthyroidism. It is important to distinguish between the two types because the treatment is different for each type.

Type 1 AIT: Type 1 AIT usually occurs in patients with pre-existent or
'latent' underlying thyroid disease, most commonly non-toxic multinodular goiter or Graves' disease. The thyroid disease is exacerbated by amiodarone, which
causes an iodine-induced increased synthesis and release of thyroid hormones
resulting in hyperthyroidism.

Type 2 AIT: Type 2 AIT is a destructive form of thyroiditis induced by
amiodarone. These patients do not have underlying thyroid disease but develop
hyperthyroidism after preformed thyroid hormones are released into the circulation once released from damaged thyroid follicular cells. Once thyroid hormone stores are depleted, the patient can return to a euthyroid state or become
hypothyroid.

The treatment of AIT differs based on the type; so, it is important to try to
differentiate the etiology. Unfortunately, distinguishing between the two types
is frequently a diagnostic challenge. Laboratory data tends to be of limited
value as thyroid function testing indicates a hyperthyroid state in both types,
thyroid auto-antibodies tend to be negative in both, and serum IL-6 values

(an inflammatory marker which may be elevated in Type 2 disease) have not yet proven to be very useful in iodine-replete areas of the world *(28,30)*. Nuclear imaging testing with radioactive iodine uptake have also proven to give poor yield in distinguishing Type 1 from Type 2 AIT *(28)*. Data from Italy has suggested that thyroid ultrasonography in conjunction with color flow Doppler studies may be the best diagnostic tool in differentiating the two types of AIT but these studies have yet to be replicated in iodine-replete regions of the world. Thyroid ultrasonography allows for rapid identification of nodular or goiterous thyroid tissue and color flow Doppler studies show normal or increased blood flow in Type 1 AIT contrasting with decreased blood flow in Type 2 AIT *(31)*.

Treatment of AIT is aimed at correcting the underlying etiology. Discontinuation of amiodarone is generally recommended; however, the long half-life as well as the necessity for treatment of life-threatening arrhythmias often precludes this from happening. The decision of whether to continue amiodarone should be made on cardiovascular morbidity and mortality data as applied to the patient in question. Several studies have shown that not only is amiodarone effective while patients are also taking thionamide therapy, there is also no difference in outcomes if amiodarone is stopped or continued *(32,33,34)*.

In Type 1 AIT, beta-blockers and anti-thyroid drugs have been the mainstay of treatment. High doses of methimazole (40–80 mg/day) or propylthiouracil (400–800 mg/day) are recommended due to high intrathyroidal iodine stores *(30)*. In cases of severe thyrotoxicosis, potassium perchlorate has also been shown to be a useful adjuvant therapy, although it is no longer readily available in the United States *(35)*. Complications from potassium perchlorate use include aplastic anemia and nephrotic syndrome *(36)*. However, multiple studies have shown side effects to be minimized with a limited treatment course of no longer than one month, and a total dose no greater than 1 gram/day *(35,37,38)*. In severe cases of thyrotoxicosis, refractory to medical therapy or when discontinuation of amiodarone is not a viable option due to life-threatening arrhythmia, surgical therapy via total thyroidectomy is another possibility. The main indications for surgery are failure of medical therapy, worsening cardiac disease, or preparation for cardiac transplantation *(39)*. Although these patients are high risk for perioperative morbidity and mortality given their hyperthyroid state and pre-existing cardiac status, thyroidectomy does result in immediate reversal of the hyperthyroid state and resolution of symptoms *(40)*.

In Type 2 AIT, the etiology is a 'destructive form' of thyroiditis so the mainstay of therapy is glucocorticoids. The hyperthyroid state is self-limiting and can last for one to three months, until the thyroid hormone stores are depleted, but resolves more quickly with glucocorticoid therapy *(27)*. Daily prednisone at a dose of 40–60 mg/day can result in rapid improvement of thyroid hormone levels, often occurring as soon as one week; however, it is recommended to maintain high levels of glucocorticoids for one to two months because rapid tapering can result in exacerbation of the hyperthyroidism *(30,35)*.

In addition to pure Type 1 and Type 2 AIT, there also appears to be a 'mixed' AIT that does not respond to targeted therapy. In these cases, it is reasonable to initiate triple therapy with thionamides, potassium perchlorate, and glucocorticoids *(27,30)*. Our clinical assessment is that it is frequently difficult to identify the specific subtype of disease and it is most prudent to treat as if there was 'mixed' AIT.

Gestational Trophoblastic Tumors

Human chorionic gonadotropin (HCG) is a glycoprotein hormone made by the placenta that is responsible for maintaining the corpus luteum during pregnancy. Structurally, it contains an alpha-subunit and a beta-subunit. The alpha-subunit is common to the pituitary glycoprotein hormones, HCG, TSH, LH, and FSH. In both animal and human models, it has been shown that high concentrations of HCG have thyroid stimulating activity by binding and activating the TSH receptor *(41)*. The incidence of hyperthyroidism in trophoblastic disease can be as high as 25–60% because HCG levels typically exceed 100,000–300,000 mIU/mL *(42)*. HCG levels greater than 200,000 mIU/mL are generally needed to cause hyperthyroidism *(41)*.

HYDATIDIFORM MOLE

Hydatidiform moles are cytogenetically inappropriate gestational tumors arising from trophoblastic embryonic tissue. Complete hydatidiform moles are female with 45 paternally derived chromosomes. Partial hydatidiform moles are triploid and contain some recognizable embryonic and fetal tissues *(41)*. The incidence of molar pregnancies in the United States is 1 in 1500 pregnancies and in the United Kingdom 1 in 1000. It is several times more prevalent in Asian and Latin American countries *(43)*. Patients with hydatidiform moles express large amounts of HCG and can have signs and symptoms of thyrotoxicosis ranging from subclinical hyperthyroidism to overt thyrotoxicosis in proportion to the amount of HCG secreted. Symptomatic relief can be provided with beta-adrenergic blockade but definitive therapy is achieved with surgical resection of the tumor. When possible, correction of the underlying problem with restoration of the HCG to normal levels will correct the hyperthyroidism. Rarely is definitive therapy such as a thyroidectomy required. Propylthionracil (PTU) or methimazole can be used to render a patient euthyroid as well.

CHORIOCARCINOMA

Choriocarcinoma is a malignant tumor containing cytotrophoblast and syncytiotrophoblast without chorionic villi that can originate from normal conception or from a molar pregnancy and invades the myometrium *(41)*. It occurs in about 1 in 50,000 pregnancies. Because of its low prevalence, the incidence of thyrotoxicosis in choriocarcinoma has only been reported in a limited number of case reports. Signs and symptoms of thyrotoxicosis are proportional to the elevation of HCG and medical treatment with methotrexate and other anti-neoplastic agents can reduce HCG levels and ameliorate the thyrotoxicosis.

Hypersecretion of TSH

TSH SECRETING PITUITARY ADENOMA

TSH secreting pituitary adenomas are a rare cause of thyrotoxicosis with a prevalence of about one per million in the general population *(44)*. The hallmark of TSH-secreting tumors is 'inappropriate secretion of TSH' in the presence of high levels of free thyroid hormones (FT_4 and FT_3) *(44,45)*. Historically, these tumors were diagnosed as invasive macroadenomas, but with the advent of ultrasensitive immunometric assays and improved radiologic techniques, they are now being diagnosed at a much earlier stage *(44)*. Clinically, features of hyperthyroidism are present, although may be milder than expected and a goiter is almost always present *(46)*. High concentrations of circulating thyroid hormones in the presence of detectable TSH levels characterize the hyperthyroidism secondary to TSH-secreting pituitary adenomas *(44)*. It is emphasized that even a detectable or normal serum TSH level is considered inappropriate in the context of a clinically hyperthyroid patient with an elevated FT_4 and TT_3. The TSH in these patients may be abnormally glycosylated resulting in relatively more biologic activity than normal TSH as evidenced by the finding of elevated T_4 and T_3 despite a low normal or normal TSH level (albeit inappropriate for the hyperthyroidism) *(47)*.

Once inappropriate secretion of TSH is identified, further laboratory testing and pituitary imaging is necessary to fulfill the diagnostic criteria of TSH secreting pituitary adenoma. Characteristically, there is an elevated circulating free alpha-subunit level, as well as alpha-subunit/TSH molar ratio *(44)*. The alpha-subunit/TSH molar ratio is calculated using the following formula: (alpha-subunit in micrograms per L divided by TSH in milliunits per L) $\times$ 10 *(45)*. A molar ratio greater than 1.0 in the appropriate clinical context is generally indicative of a TSH secreting pituitary adenoma. Although rarely performed now, dynamic testing via either T_3 suppression testing or thyrotropin-releasing hormone (TRH) stimulation testing can further aid in the diagnosis. In patients with a TSH secreting pituitary tumor, complete inhibition of TSH secretion after a T_3 suppression test (80–100 μg/day per 8–10 days) is unusual and is probably the most sensitive and specific test to diagnose TSH secreting pituitary adenomas, although it is strictly contraindicated in elderly patients or in those with coronary disease *(46)*. Because of the potential for causing cardiac arrhythmias, the T_3 suppression test is rarely used. TSH stimulation after TRH injection (200–500 µg, iv) fails to stimulate TSH secretion or shows a delayed response in 92% patients and can also aid in the diagnosis *(48)*. Unfortunately, however, TRH is not currently commercially available. Therefore, in clinical practice the diagnosis is usually made by the proper clinical context and finding an abnormally high alpha subunit to TSH molar ratio and a pituitary adenoma on MRI or CT. A thorough evaluation for other pituitary hormone abnormalities is also performed.

Treatment is aimed at removing the pituitary adenoma via surgery and radiation therapy. Adjuvant medical therapy with somatostatin therapy can also be useful for long-term management but remains to be established as tools for primary management *(46)*.

PITUITARY RESISTANCE TO THYROID HORMONE

Resistance to thyroid hormone (RTH) is another rare cause of thyrotoxicosis with an estimated incidence of 1:50,000. Most patients with RTH, however, are either euthyroid or hypothyroid, with a smaller percentage exhibiting hyperthyroidism. There have been over 600 cases in 200 families described in the literature with an autosomal dominant mode of transmission *(49,50)*. Similar to patients with TSH secreting pituitary adenomas, these patients present with persistent elevation of circulating thyroid hormone levels in association with elevated or inappropriately normal TSH levels. Patients with RTH can be classified into two subcategories: generalized resistance to thyroid hormone (GRTH) and pituitary resistance to thyroid hormone (PRTH). The majority of patients have GRTH, where both the pituitary and peripheral tissues are resistant to the effects of T_3. Because the resistance to thyroid hormone is present in a generalized pattern, the elevated circulating thyroid hormone levels cannot bind properly to the nuclear T_3 receptor and as a result do not cause clinical hyperthyroidism. In contrast, PRTH patients have only pituitary resistance to thyroid hormone and normal peripheral tissue sensitivity. These patients manifest the classical signs and symptoms of hyperthyroidism *(51)*.

Evaluation of these patients should attempt to distinguish RTH from TSH secreting pituitary adenoma. Patients with RTH generally have an alpha-subunit/TSH molar ratio about 1.0 or <1.0, a normal or exaggerated TRH-stimulated TSH, and a normal pituitary MRI *(44,45)*. A family history of similar thyroid abnormalities can be helpful. In over 95% of the patients, the underlying pathophysiology can be attributed to a mutation of the TRβ gene *(51)*. This gene can be sequenced to unequivocally confirm the diagnosis. Currently, no specific treatment is available to fully correct the defect and treatment should be aimed at mitigating the symptoms.

THYROTOXICOSIS FACTITIA

Thyrotoxicosis factitia is a clinical syndrome caused by an excess of exogenous thyroid hormone, whether intentional or not. It may occur in patients (usually with hypothyroidism) who are being over-replaced with levothyroxine or in patients who are ingesting thyroid hormones. It should be considered or investigated in the presence of thyrotoxicosis of unknown etiology, after other causes have been ruled out. The clinical scenario is typically of a young to middle-aged individual who has an underlying psychiatric disturbance, although older adults should not be excluded. The diagnosis of thyrotoxicosis factitia should be considered when there is unexplained thyrotoxicosis with the following parameters: elevated serum total and/or free thyroid hormone levels, undetectable serum thyrotropin levels, low/undetectable serum thyroglobulin concentrations, normal radioactive iodine uptake (RAIU), absence of a goiter, and the absence of circulating anti-thyroid antibodies (52).

Treatment consists of decreasing the dose or withdrawing thyroid hormone as well as evaluating for an underlying psychiatric disorder (53). Occasionally patients may be ingesting products, such as weight loss preparations, that contain active thyroid hormone or active analogues (i.e., tiratricol or Triac) (54). Patients may not realize these preparations have the capacity to cause hyperthyroidism and patients should be questioned about ingestion of over the counter preparations.

Ectopic Thyroid Tissue

Struma Ovarii

Struma ovarii is a rare cause of thyrotoxicosis where an ovarian tumor contains thyroid tissue. The incidence is low with only 0.3–1% of all ovarian tumors manifesting features of struma ovarii. Ovarian teratomas have a slightly higher predilection toward developing into struma ovarii with an incidence of 2–4% (55,56). Women with struma ovarii typically present with abdominal fullness and signs and symptoms of hyperthyroidism that can range from mild to overt. The diagnosis can be made with whole body radioactive iodine uptake imaging revealing uptake in the pelvis with very low uptake in the neck area (57). Temporizing treatment with thionamides can be attempted before definitive therapy with surgical resection of the tumor (58).

Metastatic Functioning Differentiated Thyroid Tissue

Thyrotoxicosis secondary to functioning metastases of differentiated thyroid cancer is an extremely rare clinical situation. There have only been 47 published reports in the literature dating from 1946 to 2005 (59). The clinical picture is similar to thyrotoxicosis from Graves' disease, except in the setting of thyroid cancer with evidence of bulky, widespread metastatic disease *(60)*. Pathology is typically consistent with well-differentiated follicular carcinoma and the metastases tend to be in the usual locations (bone, lung, and mediastinum) *(60)*. A review of the literature indicates that gender of the patient, age at onset, time elapsed until onset of metastases, and the 10-year survival rate are comparable for metastatic follicular carcinoma, with or without coexisting thyrotoxicosis *(61)*. A radioactive iodine scan will demonstrate thyroid tissue in metastatic locations. Laboratory evaluation is consistent with a hyperthyroid state with the occasional presence of an isolated T_3 toxicosis *(59,60)*. The treatment is directed at targeting both the thyroid cancer and the symptoms of thyrotoxicosis. Thyroidectomy (if not previously performed) followed by ^{131}I ablation with dosimetric doses, if the metastases are radioavid, allows for the most effective therapeutic option *(60)*.

OTHER FORMS OF THYROTOXICOSIS

Subclinical Hyperthyroidism

The constellation of laboratory findings of an undetectable to low serum thyrotropin concentration, with normal serum triiodothyronine and thyroxine concentrations is known as subclinical hyperthyroidism *(62)*. This is a common clinical situation with a prevalence of 0.7–3.2% in the general population, depending on the TSH cutoff used to describe it (perhaps even higher with advancing age) and is generally caused by the same diseases that cause overt hyperthyroidism *(64,63)*. From a pathophysiologic standpoint, these patients have excess thyroid hormone secretion that is sufficient to raise the serum T_4 and T_3 levels to higher than is appropriate for that individual patient (albeit still within the broad 'normal range'), resulting in a decrease in serum TSH levels. It is important to evaluate these patients clinically and to obtain repeat FT_4, T_3, and TSH concentrations over a several week period to document stability of these abnormalities. In many cases, measurement of serum thyroid antibodies (TPO, Tg, and TSI), a thyroid sonogram, and a RAIU and scan may be useful. Subclinical hyperthyroidism has been associated with an increased risk of atrial fibrillation and mortality, decreased bone mineral density in postmenopausal women, and mild hyperthyroid symptoms *(64)*.

Treatment of subclinical hyperthyroidism remains controversial, given the lack of prospective randomized controlled trials showing clinical benefit with restoration of the euthyroid state *(64,65)*. Recommendations from a Consensus Panel from 2004 suggest little evidence for clinical benefit from treatment of subclinical thyroid disease (serum TSH 0.1–0.45 μU/mL) and recommend against routine treatment of patients with TSH levels in these ranges, but does recommend therapy for patients with a serum TSH consistently less than

). More recent literature from 2007 suggest that treatment may be /lder individuals whose serum TSH levels are less than 0.1 μU/mL igh-risk patients, even when the serum TSH is between 0.1 μU/mL and ... er limit of the normal range *(64)*. Treatment strategies vary from frequent monitoring of thyroid function tests to medical treatment with small doses of thionamides (methimazole 5–10 mg daily or propylthiouracil 50 mg one to three times daily), to more aggressive radioactive iodine ablation. The appropriate treatment modality depends on the individual context and discussion between the physician and the patient.

Thyroid Storm

Thyroid storm is an uncommon but serious complication of a thyrotoxic state generally occurring in patients with underlying untreated thyrotoxicosis exacerbated by a precipitating event such as surgery or iodine exposure *(1)*. Because of the associated high mortality, early recognition of thyroid storm is critically important, and treatment is aimed at improving both the thyrotoxic state as well as abrogating the mitigating event. The diagnosis of thyrotoxic crisis relies upon the clinical picture, which forms the basis for certain diagnostic criteria *(66)*. The clinical picture of thyroid storm or severe thyrotoxicosis is frequently one of the severe hypermetabolism showing evidence of high fever, tachycardia, arrhythmias, heart failure, hypotension, gastrointestinal symptoms, and neurological manifestations including apathy, coma, and stupor *(1)*. Drs. Burch and Wartofsky have formulated a rating system to help determine the likelihood a patient is in thyroid storm or has severe thyrotoxicosis *(66)*. Despite early diagnosis and treatment, the mortality of thyroid storm remains high. Once recognized, the treatment of impending or established thyroid storm is aimed at a combination of supportive care, correction of the precipitating event, as well as targeting every therapeutically accessible point in the thyroid hormone synthetic, secretory, and peripheral action pathways *(66)*.

Inhibition of new thyroid hormone synthesis is achieved with thionamide drugs (propylthiouracil or methimazole); inhibition of thyroid hormone release via iodine or lithium carbonate therapy; and inhibition of T_4 to T_3 conversion in peripheral tissues by agents such as propylthiouracil (PTU), corticosteroids, non-selective beta-adrenergic blockade (specifically, propranolol), and iopanoic acid (which is no longer commercially available) *(66,67,68)*. In resistant cases, removal of excess circulating thyroid hormone can be accomplished by plasmapheresis or charcoal plasmaperfusion *(66,67,68)*. Initial medical management of thyrotoxicosis depends on the severity of the thyrotoxicosis but generally consists of beta-adrenergic blockade, thionamide therapy, and corticosteroids. Once effective blockade of the synthetic hormone pathway has been established with thionamides, iodine therapy or lithium may be added within hours to provide inhibition of thyroidal release into the circulation *(67,68)*. Close systematic monitoring of these patients, usually in an intensive care unit setting, is important.

TREATMENT OF THYROTOXICOSIS

Anti-thyroid Drugs

Anti-thyroid drugs are a class of medications known as thionamides whose mechanism of action is to inhibit thyroid hormone synthesis by interfering with thyroid peroxidase-mediated iodination of tyrosine residues in thyroglobulin, thereby blocking the production of thyroxine and triiodothyronine. In the United States, Europe, and Asia, propylthiouracil and methimazole are widely used. In the United Kingdom and other British commonwealths, carbimazole, an analogue of methimazole, is also used *(69,79)*. In addition to blocking thyroid hormone synthesis, propylthiouracil has an additive effect of blocking peripheral conversion of thyroxine to triiodothyronine both in the thyroid gland and in peripheral tissues, but this is considered to be of minor clinical significance.

The recommended starting dose of propylthiouracil is 100–300 mg in three divided doses and of methimazole is 10–30 mg daily. Maintenance doses of 5–10 mg of methimazole or 50–100 mg of propylthiouracil twice daily maintain the euthyroid state in most patients *(79)*. The dosage of these medications will depend on the clinical context and the severity of the hyperthyroidism. Both drugs are thought to be equally effective at improving the thyrotoxic state but have practical considerations when considering individual therapy. Propylthiouracil is preferred during pregnancy because methimazole has been associated with the development of a rare scalp abnormality called aplasia cutis. Methimazole is usually easier for patient compliance due to its once daily dosing. Antithyroid drug therapy may also be used as a temporizing measure (e.g., in patients who are severely thyrotoxic, elderly, or with cardiac problems) prior to definitive therapy with radioactive iodine or surgery. Generally, propylthiouracil and methimazole are discontinued for two to three days prior to radioactive testing and treatment *(79)*. All patients should be euthyroid prior to surgery except in very unusual circumstances.

REMISSION

If medical therapy of Graves' disease is initiated, in some patients it will be decided to have a trial of 12–18 months of therapy with antithyroid drugs with frequent monitoring of thyroid function tests for evidence of relapse. After an arbitrary time period of 12–18 months, the medications can be tapered to determine if the patient is in remission *(70)*. If relapse occurs, it commonly happens within the first three to six months of discontinuing medication *(71)*. Risk factors for remission include severe hyperthyroidism, large goiters, high T_3 to T_4 ratios, and high anti-thyroid antibody titers *(69)*. Lifelong monitoring for thyroid function should continue regardless of course. Spontaneous remission is not anticipated for toxic adenomas and toxic multinodular goiters, therefore long term antithyroid drug therapy is usually not recommended and definitive therapy, perhaps after rendering the patient euthyroid with antithyroid agents, with radioactive iodine or surgery is recommended *(79)*.

SIDE EFFECTS

The side effect profile of thionamides ranges in severity from minor to life-threatening. Minor side effects including cutaneous reactions (urticarial or macular rashes), arthralgias, and gastrointestinal upset occur in up to five percent of patients with equal frequency for both drugs *(72)*. These side effects resolve with discontinuation or switching of the medication, however cross-reactivity can occur in up to fifty percent of cases *(69)*.

It has been suggested that thionamide therapy has been associated with a drug-induced lupus like syndrome often presenting with a vasculitic rash, fever, joint symptoms, and granulocytopenia. While there is likely an underlying immunological mechanism involved, the absence of the consistent presence of antinuclear antibodies and other required criteria precludes the diagnosis of a true drug-induced systemic lupus erythematosis *(73,74)*. These symptoms generally improve with discontinuation of the drug but in moderate to severe cases, it may be prudent to pursue treatment with corticosteroids (prednisone 0.5–1 mg/kg) depending on the severity of the disease.

Agranulocytosis is a rare, but serious complication of antithyroid drugs occurring in 0.37 percent of patients receiving propylthiouracil and 0.35 percent of patients receiving methimazole *(75)*. It generally occurs within weeks of starting medication and patients present with fever and a sore throat. However, it can occur at any time during therapy. The agranulocytosis can be either an idiosyncratic reaction that cannot be predicted or occasionally patients will have a gradual lowering of their white blood cells (WBC) and absolute neutrophil count (ANC) that presages even lower values. For this reason, it is recommended that patients have serial complete blood count (CBCs) prior to and during antithyroid agent therapy since routine monitoring of the WBC count has been shown to be an effective predictor of agranulocytosis *(76)*. When agranulocytosis occurs (or when the ANC has decreased significantly), the antithyroid medication should be stopped immediately and a white cell count with differential should be immediately drawn. An ANC less than 1,500 mm is usually an indication to indefinitely stop therapy and alternative medication (i.e., methimazole or PTU) should not be prescribed due to the high risk of cross-reactivity *(69,79)*. Depending on the clinical circumstances and the ANC value, the patient should be evaluated clinically and consultation with a hematologist should occur. White cell growth factors may be given to some of these patients.

Another even rarer complication of thionamide therapy is potentially fatal hepatotoxicity, which can occur in 0.1 to 0.2 percent of patients (72). Medication should immediately be stopped and supportive therapy be started for liver injury. Routine evaluation of CBC and complete metabolic panel (CMP) as well as thyroid function tests should be performed prior to starting antithyroid agents and serially while patients are taking these medications.

SPECIAL CONSIDERATIONS DURING PREGNANCY AND LACTATION

Both propylthiouracil and methimazole can cross the placenta and are Class D agents, but because of its slightly better side effect profile, propylthiouracil is the antithyroid drug of choice during pregnancy. Methimazole has been associated with fetal anomalies such as aplasia cutis and choanal and esophageal atresia in rare instances (69). When propylthiouracil is unavailable or not tolerated, methimazole may be considered as a substitute. Due to the risk of fetal hypothyroidism, both agents should be titrated to the lowest effective dose to minimize fetal thyroid injury.

Radioactive Iodine Ablation

Radioactive iodine ablation with ^{131}I has been used as definitive treatment for thyrotoxicosis since 1942. It is considered to be an efficacious, cost-effective, and safe therapy for treatment of thyrotoxicosis. It has long been thought that treatment of hyperthyroidism completely reverses the long-term sequelae, but recent studies have reported increased cardiovascular morbidity, especially due to cerebrovascular disease and arrhythmias, as well as fracture risk, persisting for up to thirty five years after treatment with radioactive iodine (77,78). It is at this time too premature to determine whether the effects on morbidity are secondary to radioactive iodine therapy or to the history of hyperthyroidism itself, although it likely relates to the latter (77). Regardless, given the possible long-standing consequences, it seems prudent not only to treat hyperthyroidism, but also to monitor patients with a history of hyperthyroidism life-long for sequelae.

A dose should be selected to cure hyperthyroidism and cause hypothyroidism within a three to six-month timeframe with the expectation for lifelong thyroid hormone replacement with periodic monitoring after treatment (79).

Two different generally accepted dose calculation strategies exist: (1) Fixed dose (typically 185–555 MBq or 5–15 mCi) or (2) Calculated dose based on thyroid gland size and percentage uptake at 24 hours. Larger initial doses with the expectation of subsequent hypothyroidism are more reliable in controlling thyrotoxicosis and avoiding remission (79). Radioiodine is strictly contraindicated during pregnancy and breastfeeding at any dose due to the risk of fetal thyroid ablation and fetal hypothyroidism and strict pregnancy testing should be done immediately prior to any dosage of radioiodine.

CALCULATING DOSE TO ADMINISTER

A formula based on gland size and uptake provides a reliable and high probability for cure with a single dose of ^{131}I and less than ten percent chance of retreatment *(79)*.

Formula: administered dose = (Z × size of gland (g) × 100) / (percentage uptake at 24 hours)

Z = desired number of becquerels or microcuries administered per gram (generally 3.7–7.4 MBq or 100–200 μCi).

FAILURE OF THERAPY

Occasionally, a patient may not respond to the initial dose of ^{131}I and may require retreatment. In these circumstances, it is recommended to delay retreatment until six months after the initial dose due to the potential for late response to radioablation *(79)*.

SIDE EFFECTS AND COMPLICATIONS

Short-term risks after ^{131}I therapy include a self-limiting radiation thyroiditis, which can be relieved with anti-inflammatory medications or corticosteroids. Acute release of thyroid hormone can also occur causing a transient worsening of thyrotoxicosis. This is also self-limiting but usually can be ameliorated with short-term use of anti-thyroid drugs *(79)*. Rarely this release of hormones may cause a clinically important rise in thyroid hormones and this possibility should be considered in all patients.

Long-term concerns include risk of subsequent cancers and infertility. No studies have shown increased risk for either malignancy or infertility with the doses of ^{131}I used to treat thyrotoxicosis; however, it is advised to avoid pregnancy for six to twelve months post-treatment *(79)*.

SURGERY

Another option for definitive treatment is surgery. Indications for surgery include a coexisting nonfunctional nodule suggestive of cancer on fine-needle aspiration biopsy *(79)*. Other circumstances which may warrant surgery for thyrotoxicosis include amiodarone-induced thyrotoxicosis, pregnancy, severe Graves' eye disease, or a patient's choice. A subtotal thyroidectomy by an experienced thyroid surgeon should be performed with care to avoid complications of hypoparathyroidism and superior recurrent laryngeal nerve injury. Patients should be counseled that the likelihood of hypothyroidism is nearly inevitable following thyroidectomy and should expect lifelong thyroid hormone replacement *(79)*. Patients should be rendered euthyroid prior to surgery but all patients are at risk for an exacerbation of thyroid hormone release and worsening of their hyperthyroidism. Careful intra-operative and post-operative monitoring is important.

REFERENCES

1. Davies TF, Larsen PR. Thyrotoxicosis. In: Larsen PR, ed. William's Textbook of Endocrinology, 10th edition. Philadelphia: WB Saunders Co, 2002:374–421.
2. Turnbridge WMG, Evered DC, Hall R. The spectrum of thyroid disease in a community. *Clin Endocrinol* (Oxf) 1977; 7:483–93.
3. Weetman AP. Graves' Disease. *NEJM* 2000; 343(17):1236–1248.
4. Vanderpump MPJ, Tunbridge WMG. The epidemiology of autoimmune thyroid disease. In: Volpe R, ed. Autoimmune endocrinopathies. Vol 15 of Contemporary Endocrinology. Totowa, NJ: Humana Press, 1999; 141–162.
5. LiVolsi VA. Pathology. In: Braverman LE, Utiger RD, eds. Werner and Ingbar's The Thyroid. 8th ed. Philadelphia: Lippincott Williams and Wilkins, 2000:488–511.
6. Nayak B, Hodak SB. Hyperthyroidism. *Endocrinol Metab Clin N Am* 2007; 36(3):617–656.
7. Bartalena L, Bogazzi F, Tanda ML, Manetti L, Dell'Unto E, Martino E. Cigarette smoking and the thyroid. *Eur J Endocrinol* 1995; 133:507–512.
8. Wiersinga WM, Bartalena L. Epidemiology and Prevention of Graves' Ophthalmopathy. *Thyroid* 2002; 12(10):855–860.
9. Burch HB, Wartofsky L. Graves' ophthalmopathy: Current concepts regarding pathogenesis and management. *Endocr Rev* 1993; 14:747–793.
10. Matovinovic J. Endemic goiter and cretinism at the dawn of the third millennium. *Annu Rev Nutr* 1983; 3:341–412.
11. Daniels GH. Thyroid nodules and nodular thyroids: a clinical overview. *Compr Ther* 1996; 22:239–250.
12. Day TA, Chu A, Hoang KG. Multinodular Goiter. *Otolaryngol Clin N Am* 2003; 36:35–54.
13. Okamoto T, Iihara M, Obara T. Management of Hyperthyroidism Due to Graves' and Nodular Diseases. *World J Surg* 2000; 24:957–961.
14. Pacella CM, Bizzarri G, Spiezia S et al. Thyroid tissue: US-guided percutaneous laser thermal ablation. *Radiology* 2004; 232:272–280.
15. Mauz PS, Maassen MM, Braun B et al. How safe is percutaneous ethanol injection for treatment of thyroid nodule? Report of a case of severe toxic necrosis of the larynx and adjacent skin. *Acta Otolaryngol* 2004; 124:1226–1230.
16. Greene JN. Subacute thyroiditis, *Am J Med* 1971; 51:97–108.
17. Pearce EN, Marino E, Bogazzi F, et al. The prevalence of elevated serum C-reactive protein levels in inflammatory and noninflammatory thyroid disease. *Thyroid* 2003; 13(7):643–648.
18. Farwell AP, Braverman LE. Inflammatory thyroid disorders. *Otolaryngol Clin North Am* 1999; 4:541–556.
19. Kitchener MI, Chapman IM. Subacute thyroiditis: a review of 105 cases. *Clin Nucl Med* 1989; 14:439–442.

20. Woolf PD. Transient painless thyroiditis with hyperthyroidism: a variant of lymphocytic thyroiditis? *Endocr Rev* 1980; 1:411–420.

21. Pearce EN, Farwell AP, Braverman LE. Thyroiditis. *NEJM* 2003; 348:2646–2655.

22. Premawardhana LD, Parkes AB, Ammari F, et al. Postpartum thyroiditis and long-term thyroid status: prognostic influence of thyroid peroxidase antibodies and ultrasound echogenicity. *J Clin Endocrinol Metab* 2000; 85:71–75.

23. Roti E, Emerson CH. Postpartum Thyroiditis. *J Clin Endocrinol Metab* 1992; 74:3–5.

24. Surks, MI. Iodine and Thyroid Function. In: UpToDate, Rose, BD (Ed), UpToDate, Waltham, MA, 2007.

25. Chaudhry, GM, Haffajee, CI. Antiarrhythmic agents and proarrhythmia. *Crit Care Med* 2000; 28:N158–N164.

26. Hohnloser, SH. Proarrhythmia with Class III Antiarrhythmic Drugs: Types, Risks, and Management. *Am J Cardiol* 1997; 80(8A):82G–89G.

27. Martino, E, Bartalena L, Bogazzi F, et al. The Effects of Amiodarone on the Thyroid. *Endocr Rev* 2001; 22:240–254.

28. Daniels, G. Amiodarone-Induced Thryotoxicosis. *JCEM* 2001; 86:3–8.

29. Zipes, DP, Prystowsky EN, Heger JS. Amiodarone: electrophysiologic actions, pharmacokinetics and clinical effects. *J Am Coll Cardiol* 1984; 3:1059–1071.

30. Basaria, S, Cooper, DS. Amiodarone and the thyroid. *Am J Med* 2005; 118:705–714.

31. Bogazzi, F, Bartalena L, Brogioni S, et al. Color flow Doppler sonography rapidly differentiates type 1 and type II amiodarone-induced thyrotoxicosis. *Thyroid* 1997; 7:541–545.

32. Osman, F, Franklyn JA, Sheppard MC, Gammage MD. Successful Treatment of Amiodarone-Induced Thyrotoxicosis. *Circulation* 2002; 105:1275–1277.

33. Sato K, Yamazaki K, Kanaji Y, et al. Amiodarone-induced thyrotoxicosis associated with thryotropin receptor antibody. *Thyroid* 1998; 8:1123–1126.

34. Reichert L, de Rooy H. Treatment of amiodarone induced hyperthyroidism with potassium perchlorate and methimazole during amiodarone treatment. *BMJ* 1989; 298:1547–1548.

35. Bartalena L, Brogioni S, Grasso L, et al. Treatment of amiodarone-induced thyrotoxicosis, a difficult challenge: results of a prospective study. *J Clin Endocrinol Metab* 1996; 81(8):2940–2933.

36. Soldin OP, Braverman LE, Lamm SH. Perchlorate clinical pharmacology and human health: a review. *Ther Drug Monit* 2001; 23:316–331.

37. Martino E, Aghini-Lombardi F, Mariotti S. Treatment of amiodarone-associated thryotoxicosis by simultaneous administration of potassium perchlorate and methimazole. *J Endocrinol Invest* 1986; 9:201–207.

38. Ergodan MF, Gulec S, Tutar E, et al. A stepwise approach to the treatment of amiodarone-induced thyrotoxicosis. *Thyroid* 2003; 13:205–209.

39. Gough J, Gough IR. Total thyroidectomy for amiodarone-associated thyrotoxicosis in patients with severe cardiac disease. *World J Surg* 2006; 30:1957–1961.

40. Houghton SG, Farley DR, Brennan MD, et al. Surgical management of amiodarone-associated thyrotoxicosis: Mayo Clinic Experience. *World J Surg* 2004; 28:1083–1087.

41. Hershman JM. Human Chorionic Gonadotropin and the Thyroid: Hyperemesis Gravidarum and Trophoblastic Tumors. *Thyroid* 1999; 9(7):653–657.

42. Goodarzi MO, Van Herle AJ. Thyrotoxicosis in a Male Patient Associated with Excess Human Chorionic Gonadotropin Production by Germ Cell Tumor. *Thyroid* 2000; 10(7): 611–619.

43. Fisher PM, Hancock BW. Gestational trophoblastic disease and their treatment. *Cancer Treatment Rev* 1997; 23:1–16.

44. Beck-Peccoz P, Brucker-Davis F, Persani L, et al. Thyrotropin-Secreting Pituitary Tumors. *Endocr Rev* 1996; 17(6):610–638.

45. Brucker-Davis F, Oldfield EH, Skarulis MC, et al. Thyrotropin-Secreting Pituitary Tumors: Diagnostic Criteria, Thyroid Hormone Sensitivity, and Treatment Outcome in 25 Patients Followed at the National Institutes of Health. *J Clin Endocrinol Metab* 1999; 84(2): 476–486.

46. Beck-Peccoz P, Persani L. Medical Management of Thyrotropin-Secreting Pituitary Adenomas. *Pituitary* 2002; 5:83–88.

47. Beck-Peccoz P, Piscitelli G, Amr S, et al. Endocrine, biochemical, and morphological studies of a pituitary adenoma secreting growth hormone, thyrotropin (TSH), and alpha-subunit: evidence for secretion of TSH with increased bioactivity. *JCEM* 1986; 62(4):704–11.

48. Socin HV, Chanson P, Delemer B, et al. The changing spectrum of TSH-secreting pituitary adenomas: diagnosis and management in 43 patients. *Eur J Endocrinol* 2003; 148:433–442.

49. Refetoff S, Weiss RA, Usala SJ. The syndromes of resistance to thyroid hormone. *Endocr Rev* 1993; 14:348–399.

50. Brucker-Davis F, Skarulis MC, Grace MB, et al. Genetic and Clinical Features of 42 kindreds with resistance to thyroid hormone. The National Institutes of Health Prospective Study. *Annals of Int Med* 1995; 123:572–583.

51. Olattegu T, Vanderpump M. Thyroid Hormone resistance. *Ann Clin Biochem* 2006; 43: 431–440.

52. Bogazzi F, Bartelena L, Scarcello G, et al. The age of patients with thyrotoxicosis factitia in Italy from 1973 to 1996. *J Endocrinol Invest* 1999; 22(2):128–133.

53. Daniels GH. Hyperthyroidism: multiple possibilities in the female patient. 1999; 44(1):6–11.

54. Bauer BA, Elkin PL, Erickson D, et al. Symptomatic Hyperthyroidism in a Patient Taking the Dietary Supplement Tiratricol: *Case Report. Mayo Clin Proc* 2002; 77(6):587–590.

55. Ayan A, Yanik F, Tuncer R, et al. Struma ovarii. *Int J Gynecol Obstet* 1993; 118(2):112–113.

56. Grandet PJ, Remi MH. Struma ovarii with hyperthyroidism. *Clin Nucl Med* 2000; 25(10):763–765.

57. Joja I, Asakawa T, Mitsumori A, et al. I-123 uptake in nonfunctional struma ovarii. *Clin Nuc Med* 1998; 23:10–12.

58. Nahn PA, Robinson E, Strassman M. Conservative therapy for malignant struma ovarii: a case report. *J Reprod Med* 2002; 47:943–945.

59. Tardy M, Tavernier E, Sautot G, et al. A case of hyperthyroidism due to functioning metastasis of differentiated thyroid carcinoma: Discussion and literature review. *Ann Endocrinol* 2007; 68(1):39–44.

60. Paul SJ, Sisson JC. Thyrotoxicosis caused by thyroid cancer. *Endocrinol Metab Clin North Am* 1990; 19(3):593–612.

61. Salvatori M, Saletnich I, Rufini V, et al. Severe Thyrotoxicosis Due to Functioning Pulmonay Metastases of Well-Differentiated Thyroid Cancer. *J Nucl Med* 1998; 39(7):1202–1207.

62. Toft AD. Subclinical Hyperthyroidism. *NEJM* 2001; 345(7):512–516.

63. Hallowell JG, Staehling NW, Flanders WD, et al. Serum TSH, T4, and thyroid antibodies in the United States population (1988–1994): National Institutes of Health and Nutrition Examination Survey (NHANES III). *JCEM* 2002; 87(2):489–499.

64. Cooper DS. Approach to the patient with subclinical hyperthyroidism. *JCEM* 2007; 92(1): 3–9.

65. Surks MI, Ortiz E, Daniels GH, et al. Subclinical thyroid disease: scientific review and guidelines for diagnosis and management. *JAMA* 2004; 291(2):228–238.

66. Burch HB, Wartofsky L. Life-Threatening Thyrotoxicosis: Thyroid Storm. *Endocrinol Metab Clin North Am* 1993; 22(2):263–277.

67. Boehm TM, McLain J, Burman KD, et al. Iodine treatment of iodine-induced thyrotoxicosis. *J Endocrinol Invest* 1980; 4:418–424.

68. Boehm TM, Burman KD, Barnes S, et al. Lithium and iodine combination therapy for thyrotoxicosis. *Acta Endocrinologica* 1980; 94:174–183.

69. Cooper, DS. Antithyroid Drugs. *NEJM* 2005; 352:905–917.

70. Abraham P, Avenell A, Watson WA, et al. Antithyroid drug regimen for treating Graves' hyperthyroidism. *Cochrane Database Syst Rev* 2004; 2:CD003420.

71. Vitti P, Rago T, Chiovato L, et al. Clinical features of patients with Graves' disease undergoing remission after antithyroid drug treatment. *Thyroid* 1997; 7:369–375.

72. Cooper DS. The side effects of antithyroid drugs. *Endocrinologist* 1999; 9:457–476.

73. Wing SS, Fantus GI. Adverse Immunologic Effects of Antithyroid Drugs. *CMAJ* 1987; 136:121–127.

74. Wiik A. Clinical and laboratory characteristics of drug-induced vaculitic syndromes. *Arthritis Res Therapy* 2005; 7:191–192.

75. Tajiri J, Noguchi S. Antithyroid drug-induced agranulocytosis: special reference to normal white blood cell count agranulocytosis. *Thyroid* 2004; 14:459–462.

76. Tajiri J, Noguchi S, Murakami T, et al. Antithyroid drug-induced agranulocytosis. The usefulness of routine white blood cell count monitoring. *Arch Int Med* 1990; 150(3):621–624.

77. Metso S, Auvinen A, Salmi J, et al. Increased long-term cardiovascular morbidity among patients treated with radioactive iodine for hyperthyroidism. *Clin Endocrinol* 2007; Epub: 1–8.

78. Franklyn JA, Maisonneuve P, Sheppard MC, et al. Mortality after the Treatment of Hyperthyroidism with Radioactive Iodine. *NEJM* 1998; 338:712–718.

79. Iagaru A, McDougall IR. Treatment of Thyrotoxicosis. *J Nucl Med* 2007; 48:379–389.

2

Myxedema Coma

Suzanne Myers Adler, MD
and Leonard Wartofsky, MD

CONTENTS

INTRODUCTION

Myxedema coma is the most severe form of hypothyroidism and, although rare today, still carries a high mortality rate without prompt diagnosis and aggressive treatment. Myxedema coma continues to be a medical emergency that presents with deteriorating mental status, hypothermia, and multiple organ system abnormalities. Because myxedema coma may have a variable clinical presentation, the diagnosis may be challenging, and patients may not necessarily present with classic findings of either myxedema (defined as hypothyroid-induced swelling of the skin and soft tissue), or indeed even coma. Two of the twelve patients first reported with hypothyroidism in 1879 likely died of myxedema coma (1), and myxedema coma remains important to recognize today due to its high associated mortality of 50–60% despite early diagnosis and customary therapy.

From: *Contemporary Endocrinology: Acute Cause to Consequence*
Edited by: G. Van den Berghe, DOI: 10.1007/978-1-60327-177-6_2,
© Humana Press, New York, NY

EPIDEMIOLOGY

Estimates of the prevalence of hypothyroidism vary among countries likely due to the true differences in its prevalence in different geographic areas and because there is no internationally standardized definition of hypothyroidism. Conclusions from the majority of studies are consistent with the results from the Whickam, England study that found a four-fold greater prevalence of hypothyroidism in women than men with 7.5% of women and 2.8% of men having a TSH >6 mIU/L *(2)*. In addition, a follow-up analysis of a dozen studies from various countries estimated the overall prevalence of hypothyroidism to be 5% *(3)*. Fortunately, the prevalence of myxedema coma is much less common with perhaps 300 cases reported in the literature *(4–8)*. Because of the gender disparity in the frequency of hypothyroidism, myxedema coma is more common in women than men. And because hypothyroidism is most common in the later decades of life, most women presenting with myxedema coma will be elderly.

CLINICAL PRESENTATION

Precipitating Factors

The majority of patients with myxedema coma present with hypothermia during the winter months. One hypothesis for the observed seasonal tendency of myxedema coma holds that decreased endogenous heat production from marked hypothyroidism is compounded by a diminished capacity to sense temperature in the elderly *(9)*. Very cold weather appears to actually lower the threshold for vulnerability such that an otherwise stable hypothyroid individual will slip into coma after cold exposure. However, the propensity for coma may be augmented by concomitant illness such as pneumonia, sepsis, cardiovascular compromise, or stroke thereby complicating a patient's clinical presentation.

An infection from any cause may be a primary initiating event or may occur secondarily such as pneumonia following aspiration in a comatose patient (Table 1). Metabolic abnormalities such as retention of carbon dioxide, hypoxia, hyponatremia, and hypoglycemia are associated with myxedema coma and may contribute to the development of coma in hypothyroid patients as they are known to do so even in euthyroid individuals. Not uncommonly, myxedema coma may slowly develop after admission to the hospital for some other diagnosis such as fracture. With failure to make a diagnosis of severe hypothyroidism and appropriately treat it, patients may incur adverse outcomes related to their overall slowed metabolic state. For example, drug metabolism is slowed in hypothyroidism and the clinical expression of the hypothyroid state may be worsened by a relative overdose of sedatives or hypnotics, narcotics, and analgesics that can suppress respiratory drive and worsen any already underlying CO_2 retention

Table 1
Myxedema Coma: Exacerbating and Precipitating Factors

Hypothermia
Cerebrovascular accidents
Congestive heart failure
Myocardial infarction
Infections
Gastrointestinal bleeding
Burns
Trauma
Medications
  Amiodarone
  Anesthetics
  Barbiturates
  Beta-blockers
  Diuretics
  Lithium carbonate
  Narcotics
  Phenothiazines
  Phenytoin
  Rifampin
  Sedatives
  Tranquilizers
Metabolic disturbances exacerbating myxedema coma
  Hypoglycemia
  Hyponatremia
  Acidosis
  Hypoxemia
  Hypercapnia
  Hypercalcemia

caused by severe hypothyroidism. Association of myxedema coma with lithium therapy *(10,11)* and amiodarone therapy *(12)* have also been reported. Whatever the precipitating cause, the course typically is lethargy progressing to stupor and then coma, with respiratory failure and hypothermia, all of which may be hastened by the administration of the medications such as those described above that depress respiration and other brain functions.

A medical history may not be attainable at the time of presentation. Although patients may not have a history of hypothyroidism until they present with myxedema coma, often at times there is a history of antecedent thyroid disease, radioiodine therapy or thyroidectomy, or thyroid hormone therapy that was inappropriately discontinued. In perhaps 5% of cases of myxedema coma, the underlying etiology of hypothyroidism is pituitary or hypothalamic disease rather than primary thyroid failure. Although central hypothyroidism as a precipitating factor is rare, there have been reports of myxedema coma in individuals with both primary thyroid failure and pituitary origin (13,14). One case occurred as long as six years following severe obstetric hemorrhage and the development of post-necrotic pituitary atrophy, or Sheehan syndrome, in conjunction with chronic autoimmune thyroiditis. One series from a hospital survey in Germany (15) reported 24 patients (20 women, 4 men; mean age 73 years) with myxedema coma (although the authors reclassified 12 patients as having severe hypothyroidism but not coma) with the following clinical profile: 23 patients had underlying hypothyroidism, 9 of whom had previously diagnosed disease and 1 patient had central hypothyroidism. Findings on presentation included hypoxemia in 80%, hypercapnia in 54%, and hypothermia with a temperature <94°F in 88%. Six patients (25%) died despite treatment with thyroid hormone. Since the clinical presentation of myxedema coma can be quite variable, it is important to maintain a high index of suspicion, particularly if presented with an elderly female patient with signs and symptoms compatible with hypothyroidism who is beginning to manifest mental status changes and some of the typical findings described below.

Physical Examination and Laboratory Findings

Patients commonly demonstrate the characteristic features of severe hypothyroidism such as dry skin, sparse hair, hoarseness, macroglossia, periorbital edema, nonpitting edema of the hands and feet, delayed deep tendon relexes, and altered mentation. In the absence of a history of thyroid disease, it is essential to carefully examine the patient for a surgical scar on the neck that may indicate a former thyroidectomy or lobectomy. Physical examination may therefore reveal no palpable thyroid tissue or there may be a goiter present. Bradycardia is common and hypotension is an ominous finding when present that can be exacerbated by low cardiac output and low blood volume (5).

Hypothermia deserves special mention as this sign has been the first clinical clue to the diagnosis of myxedema coma in many reported cases. As noted above (15), hypothermia is present in virtually all patients with myxedema coma and may be quite profound (<80°F). The ultimate response to therapy and survival has been shown to correlate with the degree of hypothermia with the worst prognosis in patients with a core body temperature <90°F.

Laboratory evaluation may reveal hypoglycemia caused by downregulation in metabolism and decreased gluconeogenesis; however, it is important to also consider concomitant adrenal insufficiency when hypoglycemia is present *(5,8)*. Severe hypothyroidism causes reduced renal free water clearance, fluid retention, and hypoosmolar hyponatremia. Decreased renal function as evidenced by serum creatinine elevations may be present. Elevated creatine kinase concentrations, in particular skeletal muscle fraction, and elevated lactate dehydrogenase levels are thought to result from abnormalities in membrane permeability. In addition, patients may demonstrate hyperlipidemia, anemia, and mild leukopenia *(5,14,16)*. The presence of anti-thyroid antibodies indicates underlying Hashimoto's disease and increased risk for severe hypothyroidism *(13)*.

Neuropsychiatric Manifestations

Similar to findings observed in patients with uncomplicated hypothyroidism, those with severe hypothyroidism may have a history of lethargy, slowed mentation, poor memory, cognitive dysfunction, depression, or even psychosis. However, their impaired state of consciousness often precludes patients from actually complaining of these symptoms. Up to 25% of individuals with myxedema coma may experience focal or generalized seizures, possibly related to hyponatremia, hypoglycemia, or hypoxemia due to reduced cerebral blood flow *(17)*.

Cardiovascular Manifestations

Patients with hypothyroid heart disease and those with myxedema coma may develop nonspecific electrocardiographic abnormalities, cardiomegaly, bradycardia, and reduced cardiac contractility. Although these findings may lead to low stroke volume, reduced cardiac output, and even edema, clinical congestive heart failure is not often seen except in patients with pre-existing heart disease *(18)*. It is uncommon for oxygen delivery to the tissues to be compromised, despite low cardiac output, given the overall reduced metabolic rate and associated reduction in oxygen demand. An enlarged cardiac silhouette may suggest ventricular dilatation or the presence of a pericardial effusion. In a recent case report, a patient was described with myxedema coma who presented with presyncope, prolongation of the QT interval, and polymorphic ventricular tachycardia also known as torsades de pointes *(19)*. Clinical presentation with recurrent pericardial effusion and loss of consciousness, but without the classic preceding symptoms of hypothyroidism, has also been documented *(13)*. Decreased intravascular volume in the setting of cardiovascular abnormalities may lead to hypotension, cardiovascular collapse, and shock. It is important to note that hypotension may be refractory to vasopressor therapy alone and if required, should be administered concomitantly with thyroid hormone.

Respiratory Manifestations

The arterial blood gas measurement in a patient with myxedema coma often reveals hypoxia, hypercapnia, and respiratory acidosis reflecting the underlying pathophysiology of this disease state. In severe hypothyroidism, decreased hypoxic respiratory drive and reduced ventilatory response to hypercapnia may occur *(20)*. However, respiratory dysfunction and hypoventilation may be exacerbated by impaired respiratory muscle function due to hypothyroidism-induced myopathy and neuropathy leading to diaphragmatic dysfunction, as well as by obesity-related disorders such as obstructive sleep apnea *(21–23)*. Respiratory depression may progress to alveolar hypoventilation and worsening hypoxia which can then lead ultimately to CO_2 narcosis and coma. Although many factors may contribute to the development of coma, the central depression in ventilatory drive and reduced response to CO_2 seem to be the principal factors *(24,25)*. The presence of pleural effusion, ascites, or factors that may reduce lung volume will worsen respiration, as will any reduction in the effective airway opening from macroglossia or nasopharyngeal or laryngeal edema. Irrespective of the cause of the respiratory depression and hypoventilation, most patients will require intubation and mechanically assisted ventilation. The need for assisted ventilation may be prolonged and recovery delayed despite initiation of thyroid hormone therapy because of the potential for complications in any critically ill patient with respiratory failure *(26)*.

Gastrointestinal Manifestations

Gastrointestinal symptoms in patients with myxedema coma include anorexia, nausea, abdominal pain, and constipation with fecal retention related to decreased gut motility. Physical exam may reveal abdominal distention with hypoactive bowel sounds related to reduced intestinal motility that may lead to paralytic ileus and megacolon. Absorption of oral medications may be compromised if gastric atony is present. Gastrointestinal bleeding is a rare complication of hypothyroidism *(27)*. Hypothyroidism-related neurogenic oropharyngeal dysphagia associated with delayed swallowing, aspiration, and risk of aspiration pneumonia has been described *(28)*.

Renal and Electrolyte Manifestations

Patients with myxedema coma may have bladder atony with urinary retention. Decreased glomerular filtration rate occurs and hyponatremia often is found and may be responsible for exacerbating lethargy and confusion. The mechanism by which hypothyroidism induces hyponatremia is not entirely understood *(29)*. Decreased delivery of water to the distal nephron *(30)*, increased proximal nephron free water reabsorption, impaired free water excretion, and baroreceptor-mediated activation of arginine vasopressin (AVP) secretion from low cardiac output may all lead to hyponatremia. However, evidence suggests that hyponatremia in severe hypothyroidism may be mediated by AVP-independent mechanisms. In one series of patients with untreated myxedema coma who underwent hypertonic saline infusion and then free-water loading, plasma AVP was appropriately suppressed (i.e., not inappropriately elevated) in those hyponatremic myxedema patients who demonstrated a degree of impaired urinary dilution during free water loading. This observation provides evidence that decreased free water excretion in myxedema is not due entirely to inappropriate plasma AVP elevation *(31)*. Urinary sodium excretion is normal or increased, and urinary osmolality is high relative to plama osmolality.

Manifestations of Coincident Infectious Disease

Patients who fail to survive myxedema coma commonly have been shown to have had unrecognized infection and sepsis. Because hypothermia is a consistent finding in myxedema coma, a temperature within the normal range is suggestive of an underlying infection. Associated signs of infection such as tachycardia and diaphoresis will also be absent. Patients may be mildy leukopenic or may have a normal white blood cell count with a left shift with increased band forms. Pneumonia may exacerbate or even cause hypoventilation, and a patient is at increased risk for aspiration pneumonitis caused by neurogenic dysphagia, semicoma, or seizures *(17,28)*. Clinicians should always consider the possibility of an underlying infection in these patients while maintaining a low threshold for the initiation of broad-coverage antibiotic therapy *(32)*.

DIAGNOSIS

Myxedema coma should lead the differential diagnosis in a patient with a history of, or physical findings consistent with hypothyroidism in the setting of stupor, confusion, or coma, particularly when hypothermia is present. Standard clinical thermometers do not measure temperatures lower than 34.4°C (94°F) and should therefore not be used in this setting given the likelihood of inaccurate results. When hypothermia is suspected, low-reading rectal thermometers or rectal thermistor probes should be used *(33)*. The clinical presentation in many patients may be sufficiently clear to make measurements of thyroid function tests necessary only for confirmation of the diagnosis. Given a reasonable index of suspicion, empiric thyroid hormone replacement should be immediately initiated while awaiting the results of these tests, including serum TSH and free thyroxine (free T4), which should only take several hours in most centers. Although a markedly elevated serum TSH might be expected in myxedema coma, patients with concomitant severe non-thyroidal illness may demonstrate a state akin to 'euthyroid sick' syndrome *(34, 35)* which may be termed 'hypothyroid sick' *(36)*. Here TSH secretion from pituitary thyrotrophs is decreased, and the serum levels of TSH may therefore not be as high as might be expected *(37)*. In those patients whose severe hypothyroidism is central in etiology, TSH will be low or normal. However, all patients with myxedema coma, whether central or primary in origin, will have decreased free T4 and triiodothyronine (T3) concentrations. In patients with the 'hypothyroid sick' syndrome, serum T3 levels may be unusually low (<25 ng/mL) *(36)*. Besides detecting electrolyte abnormalities, diagnostic evaluation should include laboratory assessment for concurrent adrenal insufficiency, myocardial infarction, and a thorough work-up for infection including at the very least blood cultures, urinalysis and urine culture, and chest radiograph.

TREATMENT

Once the diagnosis of myxedema coma is made or is even suspected, therapy should be initiated immediately because of the high mortality rate otherwise. However, in elderly patients, in particular those with underlying cardiac conditions, thyroid hormone therapy should be administered judiciously given the inherent risks. It is important to note that administering thyroid hormone therapy alone without treating all of the affiliated metabolic derangements would not likely lead to a successful recovery. All patients should therefore be admitted to the intensive care unit for close monitoring of pulmonary and cardiac abnormalities, volume status, and electrolyte abnormalities.

Ventilatory Support

Upon admission to the intensive care unit, physical examination, arterial blood gas measurement, and imaging should be performed to evaluate for pulmonary infiltrate or tracheal compression from macroglossia or laryngeal myxedema as described above. The initiation of mechanical ventilation via endotracheal tube or tracheostomy if needed should not be delayed in order to adequately treat or prevent hypoxia and hypercapnia. Intensive care protocol usually routinely measures arterial blood gas with changes in ventilatory settings, and extubation should not be attempted until the patient regains consciousness and is able to maintain the patency of their own airway and manage their respiratory secretions. Typically, mechanical ventilation will be required for 24–48 hours, but may be longer in those patients whose hypoventilation and coma result from drug-induced respiratory depression. Moreover, some patients with myxedema coma may require prolonged ventilatory support for several weeks *(26)*, especially those with underlying lung disease such as chronic obstructive pulmonary disease (COPD).

Hypothermia

Hypothermic patients should be covered with blankets, so-called passive external rewarming. Unfortunately, passive rewarming carries a low likelihood of restoring body temperature to normal unless the patient has intact thermoregulatory mechanisms and adequate energy stores to produce endogenous heat. Active external rewarming with the use of forced-air warming systems or warming blankets should be used only as a last resort to restore body temperature to normal; warming blankets should be used extremely cautiously given the risk of hypotension progressing to shock from vasodilatation secondary to decreased peripheral vascular resistance induced by warmth. A safer and effective approach to hypothermia than active external rewarming is minimally invasive central rewarming. The techniques include airway rewarming with humidified oxygen at 40°C (104°F) and intravenous fluids heated to 40°C to 45°C, and these modalities do not place the patient at risk for profound hypotension. Careful blood glucose monitoring is imperative as the majority of hypothermic patients have depleted their glycogen stores, and hypothermia may mask hypoglycemic symptoms *(33)*. To ultimately normalize core body temperature in myxedema coma, thyroid hormone administration is essential; however, restoration of body temperature by thyroid hormone may take several days.

Hypotension

Treatment of hypothermia with external warming should be initiated concurrently with intravenous hydration with 5% to 10% glucose in half-normal saline or with isotonic saline if hyponatremia is present. Stress dosage of intravenous hydrocortisone (100 mg every 8 hours) must be given if there is a suspicion of coexistent primary or secondary adrenal insufficiency. Vasopressors may be required for profound hypotension that is refractory to aggressive volume repletion until thyroid hormone action begins; however, many hypothermic patients may already be maximally vasoconstricted peripherally in order to raise core body temperature.

Hyponatremia

Appropriate treatment for hyponatremia depends upon the severity and acuity with which the hyponatremia developed. Hyponatremia contributes to the altered mental status in myxedema coma, particularly in those with serum sodium levels < 120 mEq/L. The administration of thyroid hormone ameliorates hyponatremia such that euvolemic, normotensive patients with myxedema coma with mild hyponatremia may be treated only with thyroid hormone administration and perhaps fluid restriction. However, hypotensive patients will require volume expansion with normal saline with careful monitoring of serum sodium every 2 to 4 hours with a goal increase in serum sodium levels of 0.5–1 mEq/L/h; this slow rate of serum sodium correction will minimize the risk of central pontine myelinolysis *(38)*. Hypotonic fluids should be avoided so as not to worsen hyponatremia. Depending upon the individual patient's extracellular fluid volume status, a cautious approach is to follow hourly fluid input and output and to adjust intravenous hydration such that the total input does not exceed output thus permitting some free water losses. A trial of hypertonic 3% saline may be warranted for those patients with acute symptomatic hyponatremia with serum sodium <120 mEq/L until serum sodium reaches a level >125 mEq/L *(29)*, keeping in mind the general rule that an infusion of 3% saline at a rate of 1 cc/kg body mass/h raises serum sodium by 1 mEq/h. Absent hypotension, the administration of intravenous furosemide at a dose of 40 to 120 mg may be considered to promote water diuresis if hypertonic saline is used *(39)*.

Glucocorticoid Therapy

Glucocorticoids are commonly administered in patients with myxedema coma based upon a risk of coexistent actual or relative adrenal insufficiency. Patients with myxedema coma due to pituitary or hypothalamic disease may have diminished (ACTH, corticotropin) secretion in addition to low TSH secretion. Patients with a history of Graves' disease or Hashimoto's thyroiditis may also have autoimmune primary adrenal insufficiency. Although serum cortisol will be normal in the majority of patients with myxedema coma, parameters suggestive of underlying adrenal insufficiency include hypotension, hyponatremia, hyperkalemia, hypercalcemia, lymphocytosis and eosinophilia, hypoglycemia, and azotemia. If they are to be administered, glucocorticoids should be given early in the course of therapy prior to thyroid hormone administration so that the increased metabolic demands induced by thyroid hormone do not precipitate adrenal crisis.

In addition to the risk of coexistent primary or secondary adrenal insufficiency, it is deemed prudent to administer glucocorticoids because there is a risk that thyroid hormone therapy may increase cortisol clearance and precipitate adrenal insufficiency. Hydrocortisone is usually given intravenously at a dose of 50 to 100 mg every 6–8 hours for several days, after which time it is tapered or discontinued on the basis of improvement in clinical response, plans for further diagnostic evaluation, and adequacy of intact pituitary-adrenal function.

Myxedema Coma and Surgery

The general perioperative management of patients with hypothyroidism has been reviewed recently *(40)*. Non-emergent surgery should be deferred in a patient with myxedema coma. However, in the event that a patient with myxedema coma requires an emergent surgical procedure, the same general principles apply *(41,42)* with particular attention to careful monitoring of intra-operative and postoperative respiratory *(43,44)* and cardiac status. Occasionally the diagnosis of myxedema coma may be made during the immediate postop-erative period *(45)* when again a major concern is close monitoring for main-tenance of the airway. Myxedema coma has also been reported during obstetric labor *(46)*.

Thyroid Hormone Therapy

Because the prompt administration of thyroid hormone is essential for sur-vival in myxedema coma, the clinician must balance the life-saving benefits of restoring low serum and tissue thyroid hormone levels to normal against the risks of precipitating myocardial infarction or atrial tachyarrhythmias. Given the high mortality of myxedema coma, there is a clear benefit to achieving effective tis-sue levels of thyroid hormones as quickly as possible. However, the regimen with which to treat remains controversial and relates to whether to administer levothyroxine (LT4), liothyronine (LT3), or both. There are no controlled clini-cal trials comparing various treatment regimens in myxedema coma due to the rarity of this disease entity, so it is not currently known what comprises the optimal therapeutic approach, and recommendations tend to be empirical at best *(36)*. In theory, the administration of T4 alone to a hypothyroid individual should suffice because T4 is converted to meet the physiologic demands for T3 by 5'-monodeiodinase. However, the rate of extrathyroidal conversion of T4 to T3 is diminished in sick hypothyroid patients *(34,35)*, which is a potential drawback to total reliance on generation of T3 from T4. Parameters that favor T3 ther-apy include greater biological activity of T3 than T4 and a much more rapid onset of action of T3 than T4, which could increase opportunities for survival *(39,41)*. In addition, evidence from animal studies in the baboon model sug-gests that T3 crosses the blood-brain barrier more rapidly and more completely than T4 *(47)* with potential implications for earlier improvement in neuropsy-chiatric symptoms in patients with myxedema coma after treatment with T3 as compared to T4.

Despite decreased 5'monodeiodinase activity in the sick hypothyroid patient, administration of T4 may provide a smoother and more even, albeit slower, onset of action than T3 with a decreased risk of cardiac adverse events in particular. Whereas the onset of action of T3 is more rapid as described above, serum and likely tissue levels of T3 are more variable between doses of T3 than of T4. Although modern laboratories now have reliable assays for both T4 and T3, the interpretation of T4 levels may be easier given that T4 levels do not vary as much as T3 levels between doses. In any case, close monitoring of TSH is helpful in gauging the impact of therapy and adjusting thyroid hormone dosage in order to bring tissue content of thyroid hormone to effective levels.

Regardless of whether T3 or T4 is the thyroid hormone administered, dosage, frequency, and route of administration are additional factors to address. In the comatose patient, intravenous administration of thyroid hormone is preferred over that via nasogastric tube given the risk of aspiration and unpredictable absorption with the latter. Parenteral T4 preparations are available in vials containing 100 and 500 mcg. An initial intravenous high-dose bolus (i.e., 300 to 600 mcg) has been utilized for decades in order to replace the total extrathyroidal stores of T4; this initial bolus has been thought to be advantageous to bring thyroid hormone to effective levels as quickly as possible. The latter dosage is based upon kinetic studies that estimate the total body thyroxine pool to be 500 mcg *(36)*. Serum T4 levels rapidly increase to above normal and then return to the normal reference range within 24 hours of the initial high bolus dose. In turn, as T4 is converted to T3, serum T3 levels also rise, and serum TSH concentrations begin to fall towards normal *(48)*. After the initial bolus dose, a maintenance dose of 50 to 100 mcg daily intravenously or orally is recommended *(49)*.

Although it has been commonly held that an intravenous bolus dose of levothyroxine followed by maintenance therapy is optimal *(48,49)* , other evidence suggests improved outcomes with lower dose thyroid hormone therapy *(50,51)*. To further investigate levothyroxine dosing regimens, Rodriguez et al. *(52)* conducted a prospective trial where patients were randomized to received either a 500 mcg loading dose of intravenous levothyroxine followed by 100 mcg daily maintenance dose or only the maintenance dose. The overall mortality rate was 36.4% with a lower mortality rate in the high dose group (16.7%) versus the low dose group (60%), although the difference was not statistically significant. Poorer outcome was associated with a decreased level of consciousness, lower Glasgow coma score, and increased severity of illness on entry as determined by an acute physiology and chronic health evaluation II (APACHE II) score >20.

Parenteral T3 is available in 10 mcg vials. When given as sole thyroid hormone replacement therapy, the usual bolus dose is 10 to 20 mcg followed by 10 mcg every 4 hours for the first 24 hours, then 10 mcg every 6 hours for a day or two, by which time the patient should have become alert enough to transition to oral thyroid hormone administration *(36)*. Although improvement in body temperature and oxygen consumption will occur in 8 to 14 hours or longer after intravenous T4, similar benefits will occur within only 2 to 3 hours following T3 administration with substantial clinical improvement within 24 hours *(53)*. However, this benefit is accompanied by a larger risk of adverse cardiac events including sudden death that is seen particularly with high (25 mcg) doses of T3

(41,54). In one retrospective series of 11 patients, those with fatal outcomes had received higher doses of thyroid hormone and had calculated levels of T3 that were almost twice as high as those who survived *(55)*. In another series of 8 patients with myxedema coma, the first 3 patient who received high-dose intravenous T3 died of pneumonia whereas the remaining 5 patients who received lower dose T3 or T4 survived despite pulmonary complications *(51)*. Among 87 cases of myxedema coma reported in the literature, the authors of the aforementioned series found older age, cardiac complications, and high dose thyroid hormone replacement (T4 dose ≥ 500 mcg/d or T3 dose ≥ 75 mcg/d) were the factors associated with mortality within 1 month of treatment for myxedema coma. From their findings, the authors concluded that a bolus dose of 500 mcg of T4 should be safe in younger patients (< 55 years) without cardiac disease, but lower doses should be considered in elderly patients *(51)* who may only require 100 to 170 mcg of T4 daily *(5)*. It is important to note that outcomes may be somewhat difficult to analyze given first, the small number of patients in reported series owing to the rarity of myxedema coma, and secondly, the high mortality rate of myxedema coma despite what is deemed to be appropriate therapy.

In contrast to either of the above two therapeutic approaches, we feel that a prudent but effective approach is to administer both T4 and T3. As in any other hypothyroid patient, dose adjustment is based upon clinical and laboratory results. T4 is given intravenously in a dose of 4 mcg/kg lean body weight (approximately 200 to 250 mcg), followed by 100 mcg 24 hours later and then 50 mcg daily either intravenously or orally when permitted. T3 is also given intravenously in an initial dose of 10 mcg with a dose of 5 to 10 mcg every 8 to 12 hours depending upon the age and cardiac status of the patient, and T3 may be discontinued when the patient is able to tolerate oral maintenance doses of T4. While this approach cannot claim to be the optimal or preferred manner of treatment with thyroid hormone, it does make physiologic sense in relation to both safety and efficacy. This is particularly true in the 'hypothyroid sick' patient with myxedema coma in whom conversion of T4 to T3 would be delayed by their systemic illness. Clearly, no general guide to treatment can take into account all of the clinical factors that might affect sensitivity to thyroid hormone including age, compromised cardiovascular function, neuropsychiatric status, and other coexisting comorbidities that may affect drug distribution and metabolism and therefore drug dosages. Consequently, patients should be carefully monitored prior to administering each dose of thyroid hormone. Most patients with myxedema coma should recover with vigorous treatment and aggressive supportive measures. However, overall improved outcomes will derive from the early diagnosis and treatment of hypothyroidism.

SUMMARY

Myxedema coma represents the most extreme form of hypothyroidism and still carries a high mortality rate despite therapy. Myxedema coma typically presents in elderly women during the winter months and may be precipitated by infection, stroke, cardiac events, other systemic illness, and certain medications. Associated signs include hypothermia, decreased mentation, hyponatremia, hypoxia, and hypercapnia. Comprehensive treatment including aggressive supportive care in the intensive care unit is essential and may require assisted mechanical ventilation, warming methods, corticosteroids, vasopressors, and antibiotics. Thyroid hormone is crucial to survival, but it remains unclear whether to administer thyroxine, triiodothyronine, or both.

REFERENCES

1. Report of a committee of the Clinical Society of London to investigate the subject of myxedema. *Trans Clin Soc* Suppl, 21. 1888. London.
2. Tunbridge W, Evered D, Hall R, et al. The spectrum of thyroid disease in a community: the Whickham survey. *Clin Endocrinol* 1977; 7: 481–493. Oxford.
3. Vanderpump M, Tunbridge W. The Thyroid. Philadephia: Lippincott-Raven Publishers, 1996.
4. Fliers E, Wiersinga WM. Myxedema coma. *Rev Endocr Metab Dis* 2003; 4: 137–141.
5. Wall CR. Myxedema coma: diagnosis and treatment. *Amer Fam Phys* 2000; 62: 2485–2490.
6. Summers VK. Myxedema coma. *BMJ* 1953; 2: 336.
7. Ringel MD. Management of hypothyroidism and hyperthyroidism in the intensive care unit. *Critical Care Clinics* 2001; 17: 59–74.
8. Nicoloff JT, LoPresti JS. Myxedema coma: a form of decompensated hypothyroidism. *Endocrinol Metab Clin North Am* 1993; 22: 279–290.
9. Ballester JM, Harchelroad FP. Hypothermia: an easy-to-miss, dangerous disorder in winter weather. *Geriatrics* 1999; 54: 51–57.
10. Santiago R, Rashkin MC. Lithium toxicity and myxedema coma in an elderly woman. *J Emerg Med* 1990; 8(1): 63–66.
11. Waldman SA, Park D. Myxedema coma associated with lithium therapy. *Am J Med* 1989; 87(3): 355–356.
12. Mazonson PD, Williams ML, Cantley LK, et al. Myxedema coma during long-term amiodarone therapy. *Amer J Med* 1984; 77: 751–754.
13. Benvenga S, Squadrito S, Saporito F, et al. Myxedema coma of both primary and secondary origin, with non-classic presentation and extremely elevated creatine kinase. *Horm Metab Res* 2000; 32: 364–366.
14. Cullen MJ, Mayne PD, Sliney I. Myxoedema coma. *Ir J Med Sci* 1979; 148: 201–206.
15. Reinhardt W, Mann K. [Incidence, clinical picture and treatment of hypothyroid coma. Results of a survey]. *Med Klin (Munich)* 1997; 92(9): 521–524.
16. Doran GR, Wilkinson JH. The origin of the elevated activities of creatine kinase and other enzymes in the sera of patients with myxoedema. *Clin Chim Acta* 1975; 62: 203–211.
17. Sanders V. Neurologic manifestations of myxedema. *N Engl J Med* 1962; 266: 547–552.

18. Klein I. Thyroid hormone and the cardiovascular system. *Am J Med* 1990; 88: 631–637.
19. Schenck JB, Rizvi AA, Lin T. Severe primary hypothyroidism manifesting with torsades de pointes. *Am J Med Sci* 2006; 331: 154–156.
20. Zwillich CW, Pierson DJ, Hofeldt FD, et al. Ventilatory control in myxedema and hypothyroidism. *N Engl J Med* 1975; 292: 662–665.
21. Martinez FJ, Bermudez-Gomez M, Celli BR. Hypothyroidism: a reversible cause of diaphragmatic dysfunction. 1989; 96: 1059.
22. Wilson WR, Bedell GM. The pulmonary abnormalities in myxedema. *J Clin Invest* 1960; 39: 42.
23. Massumi RA, Winnacker JL. Severe depression of the respiratory center in myxedema. *Am J Med* 1964; 36: 876.
24. Ladenson PW, Goldenheim PD, Ridgway EC. Prediction of reversal of blunted respiratory responsiveness in patients with hypothyroidism. *Am J Med* 1988; 84: 877–883.
25. Domm BM, Vassallo CL. Myxedema coma with respiratory failure. *Am Rev Respir Dis* 1973; 107(5): 842–845.
26. Yamamoto T. Delayed respiratory failure during the treatment of myxedema coma. *Endocrinol Jpn* 1984; 31(6): 769–775.
27. Fukunaga K. Refractory Gastrointestinal Bleeding Treated With Thyroid Hormone Replacement. *J Clin Gastroenterol* 2001; 33: 145–147.
28. Urquhart AD, Rea IM, Lawson LT, et al. A new complication of hypothyroid coma: neurogenic dysphagia: presentation, diagnosis, and treatment. *Thyroid* 2001; 11: 595–598.
29. Adler SM, Verbalis JG. Disorders of body water homeostasis in critical illness. *Endocrinol Metab Clin North Am* 2006; 35: 873–894.
30. DeRubertis FRJr, Michelis MF, Blum M, et al. Impaired water excretion in myxedema. *Am J Med* 1971; 51: 41–53.
31. Iwasaki Y, Oiso Y, Yamauchi K, et al. Osmoregulation of plasma vasopressin in myxedema. *J Clin Endocrinol Metab* 1990; 70: 534–539.
32. Lindberger K. Myxoedema coma. *Acta Med Scand* 1975; 198(1–2): 87–90.
33. McCullough L, Arora S. Diagnosis and treatment of hypothermia. *Am Fam Physician* 2004; 70: 2325–2332.
34. Wartofsky L, Burman KD. Alterations in thyroid function in patients with systemic illness: the euthyroid sick syndrome. *Endocr Rev* 1982; 3: 164–217.
35. Adler SM, Wartofsky L. The nonthyroidal illness syndrome. *Endocrinol Metab Clin North Am* 2007; 36: 657–672.
36. Wartofsky L. Myxedema coma. *Endocrinol Metab Clin North Am* 2006; 35(4): 687–698.
37. Hooper MJ. Diminished TSH secretion during acute non-thyroidal illness in untreated primary hypothyroidism. *Lancet* 1: 48–49.
38. Sterns RH, Riggs JE, Schochet SSJr. Osmotic demyelination syndrome following correction of hyponatremia. *N Engl J Med* 1986; 314: 1535–1542.
39. Pereira VG, Haron ES, Lima-Neto N, Medeiros-Neto GA. Management of myxedema coma: report on three successfully treated cases with nasogastric or intravenous administration of triiodothyronine. *J Endocrinol Invest* 1982; 5(5): 331–334.
40. Stathatos N, Wartofsky L. Perioperative management of patients with hypothyroidism. *Endocrinol Metab Clin North Am* 2003; 32: 503–518.
41. Mathes DD. Treatment of myxedema coma for emergency surgery. *Anesth Analg* 1998; 86(2): 450–451.
42. Bennett-Guerrero E, Kramer DC, Schwinn DA. Effect of chronic and acute thyroid hormone reduction on perioperative outcome. *Anesth Analg* 1997; 85: 30–36.

43. Benfari G, de.Vincentiis M. Postoperative airway obstruction: a complication of a previously undiagnosed hypothyroidism. *Otolaryngol-Head&Neck Surg* 2005; 132: 343–344.
44. Batniji RK, Butehorn HF, Cevera JJ, et al. Supraglottic myxedema presenting as acute upper airway obstruction. *Otolaryngol-Head&Neck Surg* 2006; 134: 348–350.
45. Fritsch N, Tran-Van D, Dardare E, et al. [The myxoedema coma exists, we met it]. Ann Fr Anesth Reanim e-pub ahead of print, article in French. 2007.
46. Turhan NO, Kockar MC, Inegol I. Myxedematous coma in a laboring woman suggested a pre-eclamptic coma: a case report. *Acta Obstet Gynecol Scand* 2004; 83(11): 1089–1091.
47. Chernow B, Burman KD, Johnson DL, McGuire RA, O'Brian JT, Wartofsky L et al. T3 may be a better agent than T4 in the critically ill hypothyroid patient: evaluation of transport across the blood-brain barrier in a primate model. *Crit Care Med* 1983; 11(2): 99–104.
48. Ridgway EC, McCammon JA, Benotti J, Maloof F. Acute metabolic responses of patients with myxedema to large doses of intravenous L-thyroxine. 1972; 77: 549–555.
49. Holvey DN, Goodner CJ, Nicoloff JT, Dowling JT. Treatment of myxedema coma with intravenous thyroxine. *Arch Intern Med* 1964; 113: 89–96.
50. Khaleeli A. Myxoedema coma. A review. *Pahlavi Med J* 1978; 9(2): 126–151.
51. Yamamoto T, Fukuyama J, Fujiyoshi A. Factors associated with mortality of myxedema coma: report of eight cases and literature survey. *Thyroid* 1999; 9(12): 1167–1174.
52. Rodriguez I, Fluiters E, Perez-Mendez LF, Luna R, Paramo C, Garcia-Mayor RV. Factors associated with mortality of patients with myxoedema coma: prospective study in 11 cases treated in a single institution. *J Endocrinol* 2004; 180(2): 347–350.
53. MacKerrow SD, Osborn LA, Levy H, et al. Myxedema-associated cardiogenic shock treated with intravenous triiodothyronine. *Ann Intern Med* 1992; 117: 1014–1015.
54. Catz B, Russell S. Myxedema, Shock and coma. Seven survival cases. *Arch Intern Med* 1961; 108: 407–417.
55. Hylander B, Rosenqvist U. Treatment of myxoedema coma–factors associated with fatal outcome. *Acta Endocrinol (Copenh)* 1985; 108(1): 65–71.

3 Acute Adrenal Crisis

Paul Lee and Ken KY Ho

INTRODUCTION

Acute adrenal crisis is a life threatening endocrine emergency, requiring prompt diagnosis and immediate treatment. The recognition of adrenal crisis can be a clinical challenge as its presentation may be non-specific, with symptoms and signs masked by the precipitant leading to the crisis itself.

Addison's disease, first described by Thomas Addison in 1855, has a prevalence of 35–120 per million *(1)*. Addison's disease presenting as acute adrenal crisis is uncommon. There is increasing recent recognition of relative adrenal insufficiency which can also present as an acute crisis in the setting of critical illness (especially sepsis), human-immunodeficiency virus (HIV) infection or adrenal suppression from glucocorticoid therapy.

The current review provides clinicians with a framework for the management of acute adrenal crisis, covering physiology, aetiology, and therapy. Management principles are outlined, focusing on immediate treatment, education, and prevention. A high index of clinical suspicion is paramount in the successful management of acute adrenal crisis.

From: *Contemporary Endocrinology: Acute Cause to Consequence*
Edited by: G. Van den Berghe, DOI: 10.1007/978-1-60327-177-6_3,
© Humana Press, New York, NY

ADRENAL PHYSIOLOGY

Adrenal insufficiency is primarily due to cortical hypofunction; however, animal studies have demonstrated an important interplay between the medullary adrenergic and glucocorticoid systems in the regulation of steroid hormone synthesis *(2)*. The integrity of the cardiovascular system is dependent on a complex interplay between adrenocortical hormones, and the adrenergic system, that serves to regulate fluid homeostasis and vascular tone.

Circulatory shock is the cardinal feature of acute adrenal crisis. It is due to both hypovolemia and sodium depletion from mineralocorticoid deficiency, and vascular collapse from glucocorticoid deficiency. The precipitant of the crisis itself frequently contributes to the hemodynamic stress in the form of sepsis, hemorrhage, or cardiac dysfunction (Fig. 1).

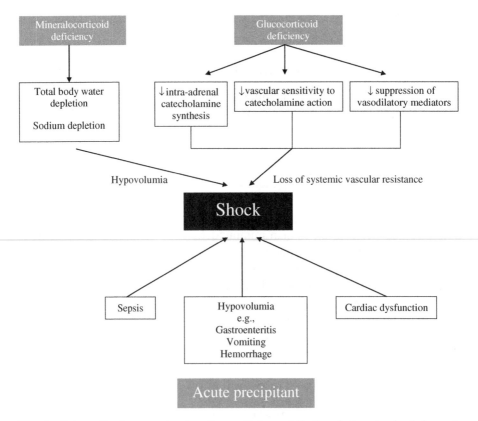

Fig. 1. Schematic diagram showing the multiple contributing factors to shock in acute adrenal crisis.

Water and sodium homeostasis: mineralocorticoid and anti-diuretic hormone

Aldosterone is regulated by the renin-angiotensin-aldosterone (RAA) system. The major trigger for renin release is a fall in perfusion pressure, from hemorrhage, hypotension, or a contraction of extracellular water volume after sodium loss. Aldosterone enhances sodium reabsorption in the distal convoluted tubule in exchange for potassium. Aldosterone insufficiency therefore results in inappropriate natriuresis and potassium retention. The loss of salt and water may be catastrophic during vomiting or diarrhoeal illness, with rapid deterioration to coma and death.

Anti-diuretic hormone (ADH) regulates free water excretion by increasing the permeability of the collecting tubule to water. Its secretion is stimulated by hyperosmolality and hypovolemia. In patients with chronic aldosterone insufficiency, sodium depletion impairs the counter-current mechanism essential to establish a hyperostomotic interstitium in the renal medulla, reducing ADH-medicated water reabsorption and accelerating volume depletion.

Although adrenocortical hormone (ACTH) acutely stimulates aldosterone release, it plays a minor role in the regulation of aldosterone secretion (3). Aldosterone deficiency is not a feature of secondary adrenal failure and explains why acute adrenal crisis is less frequently observed in secondary adrenal failure.

Glucocorticoid

Cortisol is required for the functioning of all tissues. It exerts important roles on cardiovascular function, appetite, and on the immune system, properties that are particularly relevant in understanding the pathophysiology of adrenal crisis.

CARDIOVASCULAR STABILITY

Vascular tone is maintained by 3 factors: adequate circulatory volume, cardiac contractility, and peripheral vascular tone. Glucocorticoids and catecholamines interact positively to maintain hemodynamic stability in human, by enhancing catecholamine action in vascular smooth muscle (4). A better understanding of the mechanism of their interactions has come from animal studies. Glucocorticoids potentiate the response of catecholamines by enhancing affinity to their receptors (5–8). The synthesis of major vasodilators by endothelium, including prostacyclin and nitric oxide, is suppressed by glucocorticoids (9–10). Glucocorticoids stimulate cardiac function by enhancing contractility. Animal (11) and human (12) studies showed cardiac contractility to be markedly impaired in glucocorticoid deficient state.

Glucocorticoids are also required for the normal functioning of chromaffin cells and their capacity to produce adrenaline. Activity of phenylethanolamine-N-methyltransferase (PNMT), a rate-limiting enzyme in adrenaline synthesis, has been shown (in animal studies) to be dependent on glucocorticoids transported via the intra-adrenal portal system *(8)*. This dependency is evident in patients with isolated glucocorticoid deficiency who manifest reduced synthesis of adrenaline both in resting and stressed clinical states *(13)*.

Glucocorticoid deficiency leads to circulatory collapse, reduced catecholamine synthesis, vascular desensitisation to circulating catecholamines, inappropriate vasodilation, and impaired cardiac contractility, which together with water and sodium repletion due to aldosterone deficiency, represents the hallmark of adrenal crisis.

APPETITE

Glucocorticoids play a central role in glucose metabolism, and regulate energy storage and utilisation through interaction with the sympathetic nervous system. An underappreciated effect of glucocorticoids is its potent orexigenic property *(14)*.

The appetite stimulating effect of glucocorticoids may involve mediation by the endocannabinoid system *(15)*. Both animal *(16)* and human *(17)* studies have demonstrated an increase in appetite and high-fat food ingestion in response to increased cortisol secretion from stress. The opposite occurs in glucocorticoid deficient states. Patients lose their appetite; weight loss and cachexia ensue as a consequence of advanced anorexia, impaired hepatic gluconeogenesis, and defective mobilisation of substrates from peripheral fat and muscle stores *(14)*. Glucocorticoids such as dexamethasone, are sometimes used as appetite stimulants in cachectic patients with advanced malignancy in the palliative care setting.

IMMUNITY

Glucocorticoids are a potent suppressor of the immune system. Endogenous glucocorticoids play an important role in the maintenance of host 'inflammatory' homeostasis.

The immune system is constitutively active *(18)*; immune cells, cytokines, and neuropeptides accumulate in injured tissue, forming micro-inflammatory foci that facilitate tissue healing and regeneration *(19)*. Glucocorticoids exert important actions on leukocyte traffic *(20)*, cytokines actions *(21)*, and adhesion molecule expression *(22)*. Equilibrium is maintained by the anti-inflammatory actions of glucocorticoids in areas of tissue damage to facilitate healing.

The absence of glucocorticoids result in an enhanced state of inflammation, causing an array of symptoms, which may be local or systemic. These symptoms are similar to those of patients with immune-mediated inflammatory disorders, such as arthralgia, myalgia, and lethargy. Low-grade pyrexia may arise from dysregulated production of inflammatory cytokines. Inflammation of the gastrointestinal tract, along with anorexia precipitated by the lack of glucoccorticoids may create a misleading clinical picture of abdominal pathology.

In essence, glucocorticoid sufficiency is central to the maintenance of cardiovascular stability, appetite regulation, and immune function. These three aspects of glucocorticoid function explain many of the manifestations of acute and chronic glucocorticoid deficiency.

AETIOLOGY OF ADRENAL INSUFFICIENCY

The evaluation of the cause of adrenal insufficiency in a particular patient depends on the clinical context. While some features are common to both primary and secondary adrenal insufficiency, an appreciation of the causes and associated clinical manifestations give important clues for the diagnosis of adrenal failure. The causes are diverse and so are the associated clinical manifestations (Table 1).

Primary adrenal failure

Hyperpigmentation is a cardinal sign of primary adrenal failure, regardless of its aetiology. It is universally found in long standing cases, arising from unrestrained secretion of ACTH and related peptides. It is evident in areas exposed to chronic friction (elbows and knees), to light (face and neck), areas that are normally pigmented (areolae and axillae), palmar creases, and buccal mucosa.

Once primary adrenal failure is suspected clinically, a common cause should be sought (Table 1). Patients with autoimmune adrenalitis more commonly present with chronic or subacute symptoms in the outpatient setting, while those with vascular, infective, neoplastic, or infiltrative causes are more commonly diagnosed in a hospitalised setting (Table 1).

AUTOIMMUNE ADRENALITIS

Autoimmune adrenalitis is the most common cause in Western countries, accounting for up to 70–90% of cases *(23)*. A clue pointing to autoimmune adrenalitis is an associated history of autoimmune disorders, including Graves' disease, Hashimoto's hypothyroidism, type 1 diabetes, pernicious anaemia, and vitiligo. At least 50% of patients with autoimmune adrenalitis have another autoimmune endocrine disorder *(24–26)*.

Table 1
Causes of adrenal insufficiency

Primary

Vascular	Adrenal infarction, hemorrhage (lupus anticoagulant or HITT)
Infiltrative	Lymproliferative disorder, metastatic disease, granulomatous disease e.g., sarcoidosis
Infective	Tuberculosis, meningococcal disease (presenting as adrenal hemorrhage), fungal infection, HIV infection
Autoimmune	Autoimmune adrenalitis, polyglandular autoimmune syndrome I and II
Traumatic	Abdominal blunt trauma or back trauma
Drugs	Ketoconazole (especially in patients with AIDS), etomidate
Congenital	Adrenoleukodystrophy, adrenal enzyme deficiencies

Secondary

Vascular	Pituitary infarction (Sheehan syndrome)
Neoplasm	Pituitary adenoma, metastasis
Infective	Tuberculosis and fungal infection
Infiltrative	Granulomatous disease (sarcoidosis, histiocytosis), hemochromatosis
Inflammatory	Lymphocytic hypophysitis
Traumatic	Brain injury
Radiation	Post-pituitary radiation
Drugs	Abrupt cessation of prolonged glucocorticoid therapy (including inhaled glucocorticoid)
Critical illness	Relative glucocorticoid deficiency
Others	ACTH deficiency

ADRENAL HEMORRHAGE AND INFARCTION

The adrenal glands are prone to vascular damage because of the lack of a direct arterial supply. The adrenal cortex receives arterial supply from a subcapsular arteriolar plexus, rendering it vulnerable to infarction during systemic hypotension. An abrupt change in flow dynamics in the medullary sinusoids predisposes the gland to microvascular thrombosis and infarction. Necrotic areas are prone to hemorrhagic transformation during reperfusion. Anticoagulant use, thrombocytopaenia, and sepsis are the 3 most important risk factors associated with adrenal hemorrhage (27–28). Anticoagulants cause adrenal infarction/hemorrhage either directly or indirectly through induction of heparin-induced thromocytopaenia and thrombosis (HITT) *(29–30)*.

Adrenal infarction can arise from sepsis. Classically, the Waterhouse-Friderichsen syndrome is caused by meningococcemia *(31)*. However, hospital-acquired pathogens including *Pseudomonas aeruginosa, Escherichia coli* and *Staphylococcus aureus (32)* can cause a similar pathology. Occult malignancies cause adrenal insufficiency by infiltration or infarction. The latter may arise from thrombosis due to malignancy-induced prothrombotic state or anti-phospholipid syndrome *(33)*. Lymphoma can cause adrenal destruction through all 3 mechanisms.

Patients with HIV infection are at particularly high risk, as they are prone to opportunistic infections, exposure to drugs that interfere with glucocorticoid synthesis *(34–35)*, and malignancies. Adrenal destruction can result from opportunistic infections, such as cytomegalovirus and *Mycobacterium* avium-intravcellulare, or from an infiltrative malignancy such as Kaposi's sarcoma. Such patients are also vulnerable during critical illness from drugs treatment of opportunistic infection, such as ketoconazole, which reduces cortisol synthesis. Anti-retroviral medications especially protease inhibitors are potent cytochrome P450 inducer, which accelerate cortisol metabolism.

Secondary adrenal failure

Secondary adrenal failure can arise from organic hypothalamic pituitary diseases or from suppression of hypothalamic pituitary adrenal (HPA) axis from long term exogenous glucocorticoid use.

PITUITARY DISORDERS

Specific aetiologies of hypothalamic pituitary disease should be sought (Table 2). Symptoms of other pituitary hormonal deficits, such as infertility, cold intolerance, or hoarse voice may be present. A functional pituitary macroadenoma can cause hypopituitarism and secondary adrenal failure. Mass effects including visual field defects and cranial nerve palsies should be sought.

Isolated ACTH deficiency is a rare cause of secondary adrenal insufficiency. Diagnosis is often difficult and invariably delayed as the symptoms are non-specific and may include myalgia, arthralgia, fatigue, anorexia, weight loss, and depression *(36)*.

PATIENTS ON LONG TERM GLUCOCORTICOID THERAPY

Patients on long term glucocorticoid therapy are at a risk of acute adrenal crisis from underlying adrenal atrophy *(37–39)* secondary to ACTH suppression.

Table 2
**Symptoms and signs of acute adrenal crisis; distinction between primary
and secondary adrenal failure**

Symptoms	Fatigue, weakness, nausea, anorexia, vomiting, arthralgia, myalgia, poor concentration, depression
Signs	Dehydration (hypotension and tachycardia), mild fever, signs of other autoimmune conditions e.g., vitiligo

	Primary adrenal failure	Secondary adrenal failure
Mineralocorticoid deficiency	+	−
Glucocorticoid deficiency	+	+
Hyperpigmentation	+	−
Decreased libido	+	+/−
Pituitary hormone deficiencies	−	+/−
Hypoglycemia	−	+/−
Risk of acute adrenal crisis	+++	+

+ = present
− = absent

However, the risk of acute adrenal crisis is determined by the interplay between underlying glucocorticoid reserve and intercurrent stress (Fig. 2).

The extent of glucocorticoid suppression is determined by the potency of the steroid used, the duration of therapy, and the route of administration. While the risk appears to be the least when systemic administration is avoided, and both the dose and the duration are minimized, there is substantial individual variability. Adrenal crisis can occur following the use of a 'safe regime' such as single injection of intra-articular steroid (40), topical preparation (41), or inhaled steroid. Although systemic transfer is minimal, inappropriate inhalation technique and the use of more potent inhaled steroid (e.g., fluticasone) can lead to significant life-threatening suppression (42–44).

Despite clinicians' long experience with glucocorticoid therapy, the safest tapering regime for patients on long-term glucocorticoid therapy to prevent adrenal crisis has not been defined (45). Generally patients who are abruptly withdrawn from long-term supra-physiological doses of steroid (e.g., prednisolone 7.5 mg daily for more than 3 weeks) (46) are at the highest risk of adrenal crisis.

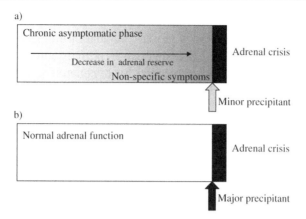

Fig. 2. Schematic diagram representing two scenario of adrenal crisis: (**a**) adrenal crisis precipitated by minor event in a patient with chronic progressive insufficiency (e.g., adrenalitis, adrenal infiltration) and (**b**) adrenal crisis caused by catastrophic adrenal destruction (e.g., adrenal hemorrhage or infarction).

DIAGNOSIS

Acute adrenal crisis is an endocrine emergency. The severity and onset of symptoms vary according to the level of defect in the HPA axis (primary vs secondary adrenal failure), and underlying aetiology (Table 2). A high index of clinical suspicion is the most important in establishing diagnosis. The approach to the diagnosis of adrenal insufficiency varies with different clinical settings (see section 2). Detailed history, examination, and investigations are indicated in the outpatient setting when patients present with subacute or chronic symptoms, while this may not be possible in the acutely unwell patient.

The acutely unwell patient

The clinical picture is dominated by profound shock in the most serious form of adrenal crisis and should be considered in any patient with unexplained circulatory collapse. It should be emphasized that the initial diagnosis of adrenal crisis is entirely based on clinical evaluation. Therapy must not be delayed by biochemical confirmation of adrenal insufficiency or by investigations to identify a cause.

Blood can be drawn prior to glucocorticoid replacement for measurement of full biochemical profile, including serum cortisol and ACTH. In the progressively unwell patient, a serum cortisol of <80 nmol/L is diagnostic and if accompanied by an elevated ACTH level of >10 pmol/L, indicates primary adrenal insufficiency. Although the mineralocorticoid axis is spared in patients with secondary adrenal failure, the picture of acute adrenal crisis is identical and may be as dramatic as patients with primary adrenal insufficiency.

Typical blood profile of acute adrenal crisis in primary adrenal failure reflects water and salt depletion, as characterised by hyponatraemia, hyperkalaemia, hyperchloraemic acidosis, and an elevated level of urea and creatinine. Anaemia and eosinophilia may be present, while hypercalcaemia is rare. In secondary adrenal insufficiency, hyponatraemia may result from lack of the inhibitory effect of glucocorticoids on ADH secretion. Hyperkalaemia is uncommon due to intact mineralocorticoid function.

Classic biochemical profile may not be evident in rapid onset adrenal failure (e.g., adrenal hemorrhage). Once basal bloods are drawn, treatment must not be withheld. Prompt glucocorticoid replacement with hydrocortisone is life-saving. If there is doubt after recovery, the diagnosis can be confirmed by further investigations as outlined below.

The patient in the subacute setting

In an outpatient setting, patients usually present with chronic progressive symptoms. The distinction between primary and secondary adrenal failure (Table 2) can usually be established from history and clinical examination (see section 2). The major symptoms of chronic insufficiency are chronic fatigue, anorexia, abdominal pain and weight loss, sometimes mimicking those of an occult malignancy.

Elective diagnosis

Confirmation of adrenal failure involves the demonstration of an inappropriately low serum cortisol concentration or inadequate response to stimulation.

CORTISOL MEASUREMENT

Interpretation of a serum cortisol concentration depends on several factors, including timing of blood collection, assay variability, medications affecting cortisol-binding globulin (CBG) and concurrent use of synthetic glucocorticoids.

Serum cortisol has a diurnal variation, with levels higher in the early morning, decreasing to a nadir as the day progresses. The diurnal rhythm, coupled with the variations between individuals, render it difficult to define a cut-off value for the diagnosis of adrenal insufficiency. A lower threshold improves specificity at the expense of sensitivity. In general, an early morning cortisol >450 nmol/L excludes adrenal insufficiency, while a level <100 nmol/L warrants further investigations for confirmation.

As cortisol circulates almost entirely bound to CBG, drugs which affect CBG will influence its level in the circulation. Oestrogens taken by the oral route enhance the levels of a number of hormone binding protein, including CBG *(47)*. Thus the concurrent use of oral oestrogen may mask biochemical evidence of adrenal insufficiency.

In contrast, total cortisol level may be affected in the opposite direction in critical illness. Sepsis and trauma reduce CBG synthesis *(48)* and its clearance is enhanced by neutrophil elastase *(49)*. Different serum cortisol concentration threshold levels (276–938 nmol/L) have been proposed to define glucocorticoid insufficiency in critical illness *(50–51)*. However, there is no consensus. A recent review by Cooper suggested a threshold of <414 nmol/L to be predictive of patients who would benefit from corticosteroid replacement in the setting of critical illness *(46)*.

Interpretation of serum cortisol measurement in patients taking synthetic glucocorticoids can be guided by a few caveats. In general, the degree and duration of suppression is dependent on the dose and duration of exogenous glucocorticoid use. Recovery of HPA axis begins to occur when glucocorticoid is tapered down to a physiological dose, usually <5 mg/day for prednisolone or 0.5 mg/day for dexamethasone. The interpretation of a serum cortisol measurement is dependent on the specificity of the assay. Most commercial assays demonstrate cross-reactivity to prednisolone but not dexamethasone. A cortisol measurement is most useful in evaluating recovery of the HPA axis when taken in the early morning at least 12 hours after the dose of exogenous glucocorticoid.

STIMULATION TESTS

Selection of stimulation tests depends on the clinical evaluation of the level of deficit.

The general principle is based on identifying an inadequate cortisol response to stimulation. For the patient suspected of primary adrenal failure, the short synacthen test (SST) is used; while those suspected of secondary adrenal failure, the insulin tolerance test (ITT) is the test of choice. The SST may still yield an apparently adequate response in secondary adrenal failure, especially early in the course of the disease.

In the outpatient setting, the SST should be performed in the morning when serum cortisol concentration is at its peak. Serum cortisol concentration is measured at 30 and 60 minutes in response to 250 mcg of Synacthen, a synthetic ACTH analogue. Generally a maximum response is observed at 30 minutes, with a normal level being >550 nmol/L (Table 3). Cortisol response may be blunted in patients on exogenous glucocorticoids. The interpretation of a suboptimal response is aided by the associated baseline ACTH measurement, which is high in primary adrenal failure, and normal or low with secondary adrenal

Table 3
Biochemical evaluation for acute adrenal crisis

1. Serum biochemistry (and screen for other autoimmune conditions such as hypothyroidism and diabetes if autoimmune adrenalitis is suspected)
2. Serum cortisol and ACTH concentration: serum cortisol level of >550 nmol/L excludes adrenal insufficiency and serum cortisol level <80 nmol/L is highly suggestive of adrenal insufficiency
3. Short synacthen test performed if serum cortisol equivocal
   - Measurement of serum cortisol 30 and 60 minutes following stimulation with 250 mcg of corticotropin (1-24)
   - Stimulated cortisol level at 60 minutes >550 nmol/L excluded primary deficiency
4. Insulin tolerance test for suspected secondary adrenal failure
   - Pituitary-adrenal sufficiency confirmed if peak cortisol level >550 nmol/L following adequate hypoglycaemia

Data adapted from Grinspoon SK, Biller BMK. Laboratory assessment of adrenal insufficiency. J Clin Endocriol Metab 1994;79:923-931

failure. The standard dose of 250 mcg of Synacthen is supra-physiological and may induce a falsely normal response in some patients with partial ACTH deficiency. For this reason, there has been interest in the use of a low dose 1 mcg Synacthen test, thereby reducing the likelihood of missing hypopituitarism (52–53).

The ITT evaluates the response of HPA axis to the potent stressor of hypoglycaemia, and it is generally the 'gold standard' in the confirmation of secondary adrenal failure. It has the advantage of also being a test of growth hormone reserve in patients with pituitary disease (54). Following injection of a standard dose of intravenous insulin (0.1 unit/kg) (55), plasma ACTH, and cortisol concentrations are serially measured. Upon achievement of adequate hypoglycaemia (<2.2 mmol/L), a peak cortisol response of between 500–600 nmol/L is generally accepted as adequate (56).

TREATMENT

Acute emergency treatment

Management of acute adrenal crisis includes restoration of intravascular volume and sodium and glucocorticoid replacement, and treating the underlying precipitant (Table 4).

Intensive fluid resuscitation is central to the initial treatment of acute adrenal crisis as hypovolemia is usually profound. At least 2–3L of normal saline should

Table 4
Management algorithm of acute adrenal crisis

1. Fluid resuscitation with normal saline (2-3L) depending on clin status.
2. Intravenous hydrocortisone 100 mg qid after blood sample for baseline investigations taken as detailed in Table 2.
3. Broad-spectrum antibiotics for febrile patients following full septic work-up.
4. Glucocorticoid (e.g., prednisolone 2.5-5 mg daily) and fludrocortisone (0.1-0.2 mg daily) once patient stabilised. Patients with secondary adrenal failure do not generally require fludrocortisone replacement.
5. Patient education regarding sick day management.

be instituted as quickly as possible to restore water balance, and importantly, reverse the severe sodium depletion. Glucocorticoid replacement is mandatory. Intravenous hydrocortisone with doses up to 300–400 mg daily is generally the initial regime because it possesses both mineralocorticoid and glucocorticoid activities. It is important to initiate treatment of concurrent illness, which precipitated the acute adrenal crisis whenever possible.

Long term hormone replacement

Upon clinical recovery, intravenous glucocorticoid dose is reduced and changed to an oral formulation. A number of preparations are available for treatment, including hydrocortisone, cortisone acetate, prednisone, prednisolone, and dexamethasone. Prednisolone has a longer half-life than hydrocortisone and may be administered once daily, and may enhance compliance. For patients with primary adrenal failure, mineralocorticoid replacement with fludrocortisone is usually given as soon as the patient has recovered. However, the sodium-retaining property of fludrocortisone takes several days to reach full effect.

Recent estimation of cortisol production rate using modern methods has led to a reappraisal of steroid replacement regime. A daily cortisol production rate of 9 mg/m2/day demonstrated by isotope dilution methodology is lower than previously shown and the traditional cortisol replacement dose of 30 mg/day is supra-physiological and may lead to adverse metabolic outcomes, such as diabetes, weight gain, and osteoporosis *(57–58)*. Generally the lowest replacement dose tolerated by the patient is preferred (10–20 mg/day). Doses can be divided to suit individual needs. Cortisol day-curves are advocated by some authors to fine tune dosage of steroid replacement *(59)*.

Table 5
Sick day management for patients on steroid replacement for adrenal insufficiency

1. Double dose of steroid replacement during acute febrile illness for 3 days.
2. Syrings with pre-drawn dexamethasone (4 mg/ml) should be kept at home for use when oral intake cannot be maintained or during major accidents.
3. Urgent presentation to the nearest hospital if vomiting continues or remaining unwell with increase steroid replacement

Patient education

It is most important to educate patients and their family the management of steroid replacement during acute illness, including a simple 'sick day' management plan (Table 5). Carrying a steroid card and wearing a medical bracelet highlighting the medical history of adrenal failure is essential.

It must be emphasized both to the patient and responsible family member that delayed or inappropriate steroid dose adjustment in patients with adrenal failure can be fatal during acute illness and may result in frequent hospital admission. In one study less than 50% of patients were carrying a steroid warning card and less than 60% of patients would take appropriate action during an intercurrent illness *(60)*. It is therefore most important for clinicians to educate their patients, with constant reinforcement at each follow-up consultation. Our service advocates the use of a written summary card detailing sick day management for each patient to reinforce verbal advice.

Patients with adrenal failure undergoing surgery

The HPA axis is strongly activated by any surgical procedures. Adrenal cortisol production increases from a usual rate of 10 mg/day to 50 mg/day during minor procedures, and up to 200 mg/day after major surgery *(4,61)*. While several studies demonstrated no adverse effects when patients were only given their usual dose of glucocorticoid peri-operatively *(62–63)*, we recommend increasing the dose to at least 200 mg/day (e.g., hydrocortisone 50 mg 4 times daily) to minimize any risk of peri-operative adrenal insufficiency. The risk of 1 to 2 days of high dose glucocorticoid is negligible, and the dose of glucocorticoid can be rapidly tapered after the stressful event.

SUMMARY

Acute adrenal crisis is an uncommon but important endocrine emergency. Severity of adrenal crisis depends on underlying aetiology, adrenal reserve, and intercurrent illness precipitating the acute crisis. Symptoms can be non-specific and signs may mimic other conditions (acute surgical abdomen), or be confounded by intercurrent precipitant. A high index of suspicion is paramount for diagnosis of an adrenal crisis, and should be considered especially in patients with profound unexplained shock or fever. Relative adrenal insufficiency in critical illness may be challenging to diagnose. Treatment of adrenal crisis should begin with treatment and should not be delayed by laboratory confirmation. Immediate fluid resuscitation with normal saline is crucial and should be promptly followed by glucocorticoid replacement. Intercurrent illness should be treated and patient education of sick day management is essential.

REFERENCES

1. Addison, T. On the Constitutional and Local Effects of Disease of the Supra-renal Capsules. Highley, London 1855.
2. Stachowiak MK, Rigual RJ, Lee. PHK Regulation of tyrosine hydroxylase and phenylethanolamine N-methyltransferse mRNA levels in the sympathoadrenal system by the pituitary-adrenocortical axis. *Brain Res* 1998; 427:275–286.
3. Rasmussen H. The calcium messenger system. *N Engl J Med* 1986; 314:1164
4. Lamberts, SW, Bruining, HA, deJong, FH. Corticosteroid therapy in severe illness. *N Engl J Med* 1997; 337:1285–92
5. Kalsner S. Mechanism of hydrocortisone potentiation of responses to epinephrine and nore-pinephrine in rabbit aorta. *Circ Res* 1969 Mar; 24(3):383–95.
6. Besse JC, Bass AD. Potentiation by hydrocortisone of responses to catecholamines in vascular smooth muscle. *J Pharmacol Exp Ther* 1966 Nov; 154(2):224–38
7. Yard AC, Kadowitz PJ. Studies on the mechanism of hydrocortisone potentiation of vasoconstrictor responses to epinephrine in the anesthetized animal. *Eur J Pharmacol* 1972 Oct; 20(1):1–9.
8. Yang S, Zhang L. Glucocorticoids and vascular reactivity. *Curr Vasc Pharmacol* 2004 Jan; 2(1):1 12
9. Xu R, Sowers JR, Skafar DF, Ram JL. Hydrocortisone modulates the effect of estradiol on endothelial nitric oxide synthase expression in human endothelial cells. *Life Sci* 2001 Oct 26; 69(23):2811–7.
10. Lewis GD, Campbell WB, Johnson AR. Inhibition of prostaglandin synthesis by glucocorticoids in human endothelial cells. *Endocrinology* 1986 Jul; 119(1):62–9.
11. Stith RD, Bhaskar M, Reddy YS, Brackett DJ, Lerner MR, Wilson MF. Cardiovascular changes in chronically adrenalectomized conscious rats. *Circ Shock* 1989 Aug; 28(4): 395–403.
12. Bouachour G, Tirot P, Varache N, Gouello JP, Harry P, Alquier P. Hemodynamic changes in acute adrenal insufficiency. *Intensive Care Med* 1994; 20(2):138–41.
13. Nehama Zuckerman-Levin, Dov Tiosano, Graeme Eisenhofer, Stefan Bornstein and Ze'ev Hochberg. The Importance of Adrenocortical Glucocorticoids for Adrenomedullary and Physiological Response to Stress: A Study in Isolated Glucocorticoid Deficiency. *J Clin Endocrinol Metab* 2001; 86:5920–5924.

14. Dallman MF, Fleur SE, Pecoraro NC, Gomez F, Houshyar H, Akana SF. Minireview: Glucocorticoids – food intake, abdominal obesity and wealth nations in 2004. *Endocrinology* 2004; 145:2633–38.

15. Di S, Malcher-Lopex R, Halmos KC, Tasker JG. Nongenomic glucocorticoid inhibition via endocannabinoid release in the hypothalamus: fast feedback mechanism. *J Neurosci* 2003; 23:4850–4857.

16. Houssay BA, Biasotti A. The hypophysis, carbohydrate metabolism and diabetes. *Endocrinology* 1931; 15:511–523.

17. Epel E, Lapidus R, McEwen B, Brownell K. Stress may add bite to appetite in women: a laboratory study of stress-induced cortisol and eating behavior. *Psychoneuroendocrinology* 2001; 26:37–49.

18. Chrousos, GP. The hypothalamic-pituitary-adrenal axis and immune-mediated inflammation. Seminars in Medicine of the Beth Israel Hospital 1995; 332:1351–1362.

19. Gallin JI, Goldstein IM, Snyderman R. Overview. In: Gallin JL, Goldstein IM, Snyderman R. eds. Inflammation: basic principles and clinical correlates. New York: Raven Press, 1988: 1–3.

20. Chrousos GP, Gold PW. The concepts of stress and stress disorders: overview of physical and behavioral homeostasis. *JAMA* 1992; 267:1244–52

21. Chrousos GP. Regulation and dysregulation of the hypothalamic-pituitary-adrenal axis: the corticotropin-releasing hormone perspective. *Endocrinol Metab Clin North Am* 1992; 21:833–858

22. Cronstein BN, Kimmel SC, Levin RI, Martiniuk F, Weissmann G. A mechanism for the autoinflammatory effects of corticosteroids: the glucocorticoid receptor regulates leukocyte adhesion to endothelial cells and expression of endothelial-leukocyte adhesion molecule 1 and intracellular adhesion molecule 1. *Proc Natl Acad Sci USA* 1992; 89:9991–5.

23. Laureti S; Aubourg P; Calcinaro F; Rocchiccioli F; Casucci G; Angeletti G; Brunetti P; Lernmark A; Santeusanio F; Falorni A. Etiological diagnosis of primary adrenal insufficiency using an original flowchart of immune and biochemical markers. *J Clin Endocrinol Metab* 1998; 83:3163–68.

24. Myhre, AG, Undlien, DE, Løvås, K, et al. Autoimmune adrenocortical failure in Norway. Autoantibodies and human leukocyte antigen class II associations related to clinical features. *J Clin Endocrinol Metab* 2002; 87:618.

25. Zelissen, PM, Bast, EJ, Croughs, RJ. Associated autoimmunity in Addison's disease. *J Autoimmun* 1995; 8:121.

26. Erturk, E, Jaffe, CA, Barkan, AL. Evaluation of the integrity of the hypothalamic-pituitary-adrenal axis by insulin hypoglycemia test. *J Clin Endocrinol Metab* 1998; 83:2350–54.

27. Kovacs, KA, Lam, YM, Pater, JL. Bilateral massive adrenal hemorrhage. Assessment of putative risk factors by the case-control method. *Medicine* (Baltimore) 2001; 80:45–53.

28. Greenfield JR, Chisholm DJ. Adrenal apoplexy: an inconspicuous cause of hypotension in the intensive care patient. *Med J Aust* 2001; 175:384–5

29. Rowland CH, Woodford PA, De Lisle-Hammond J, Nair B. Heparin-induced thrombocytopenia-thrombosis syndrome and bilateral adrenal haemorrhage after prophylactic heparin use. *Aust N Z J Med* 1999; 29:741–2

30. Delhumeau A, Moreau X, Chapotte C, Houi N, Bigorgne JC. Heparin-associated thrombocytopenia syndrome: an underestimated etiology of adrenal hemorrhage. *Intensive Care Med* 1993; 19:475–7.

31. Migeon, CJ, Kenny, FM, Hung, W, Voorhess, ML. Study of adrenal function in children with meningitis. Pediatrics 1967; 40:163.

32. Margaretten, W, Nakai, H, Landing, BH. Septicemic adrenal hemorrhage. *Am J Dis Child* 1963; 105:346.
33. Fujishima N, Komatsuda A, Ohyagi H, Fujishima M, Tada M, Ohtani H, Wakui H, Hirokawa M, Sawada K. Adrenal insufficiency complicated with antiphospholipid syndrome (APS). *Intern Med* 2006; 45:963–6
34. Samaras K, Pett S, Gowers A, McMurchie M, Cooper DA. Iatrogenic Cushing's syndrome with osteoporosis and secondary adrenal failure in human immunodeficiency virus-infected patients receiving inhaled corticosteroids and ritonavir-boosted protease inhibitors: six cases. *J Clin Endocrinol Metab* 2005; 90:4394–8.
35. Razzaq F, Dunbar EM, Bonington A. The development of cytomegalovirus-induced adrenal failure in a patient with AIDS while receiving corticosteroid therapy. *HIV Med* 2002; 3: 212–4.
36. Greenfield JR, Samaras K. Evaluation of pituitary function in the fatigued patient: a review of 59 cases. *Eur J Endocrinol* 2006; 154:147–57.
37. Simpson, ER, Waterman, MR. Regulation of the synthesis of steroidogenic enzymes in adrenal cortical cells by ACTH. *Annu Rev Physiol* 1988; 50:427–40.
38. Cronin, CC, Callaghan, N, Kearney, PJ, et al. Addison disease in patients treated with glucocorticoid therapy. *Arch Intern Med* 1997; 157:456–458.
39. Jacobs, TP, Whitlock, RT, Edsall, J, Holub, DA. Addisonian crisis while taking high-dose glucocorticoids. An unusual presentation of primary adrenal failure in two patients with underlying inflammatory diseases. *JAMA* 1988; 260:2082–2084.
40. Duclos M, Guinot M, Colsy M, Merle F, Baudot C, Corcuff JB, Lebouc Y. High risk of adrenal insufficiency after a single articular steroid injection in athletes. *Med Sci Sports Exerc* 2007 Jul; 39(7):1036–43.
41. Gilbertson EO, Spellman MC, Piacquadio DJ, Mulford MI. Super potent topical corticosteroid use associated with adrenal suppression: clinical considerations. *J Am Acad Dermatol* 1998 Feb; 38(2 Pt 2):318–21
42. Brown PH, Greening AP, Crompton GK. Hypothalamo-pituitary-adrenal axis suppression in asthmatic adults taking high dose beclomethasone dipropionate. *Br J Clin Pract* 1992; 46:102–4.
43. Greenfield JR, Samaras K. Suppression of HPA axis in adults taking inhaled corticosteroids. *Thorax* 2006; 61:272–3
44. Todd GR. Adrenal crisis due to inhaled steroids is underestimated. *Arch Dis Child* 2003; 88:554–5.
45. Richter B, Neises G, Clar C. Glucocorticoid withdrawal schemes in chronic medical disorders. A systematic review. *Endocrinol Metab Clin North Am* 2002 Sep; 31(3):751–78
46. Cooper, MS, Stewart, PM. Corticosteroid insufficiency in acutely ill patients. *N Engl J Med* 2003; 348:727–734
47. Klose, M, Lange, M, Rasmussen, AK, Skakkebaek NE, Hilsted L, Haug E, Andersen M, Feldt-Rasmussen U. Factors Influencing the Adrenocorticotropin Test: Role of Contemporary Cortisol Assays, Body Composition, and Oral Contraceptive Agents. *J Clin Endocrinol Metab* 2007; 92:1326–1333.
48. Beishuizen A, Thijs LG, Vermes I. Patterns of corticosteroid-binding globulin and the free cortisol index during septic shock and multitrauma. *Intensive Care Med* 2001; 27: 1584–91.
49. Hammond GL, Smith CL, Paterson NA, Sibbald WJ. A role for corticosteroid-binding globulin in delivery of cortisol to activated neutrophils. *J Clin Endocrinol Metab* 1990; 71: 34–9.

50. Bouachour G, Tirot P, Varache N, Govello JP, Harry P, Alquier P. Hemodynamic changes in acute adrenal insufficiency. *Intensive Care Med* 1994; 20:138–141.
51. Barquist E, Kirton O. Adrenal insufficiency in the surgical intensive care unit patient. *J Trauma* 1997; 42:27–31.
52. Park YJ, Park KS, Kim JH, Shin CS, Kim SY, Lee HK. Reproducibility of the cortisol response to stimulation with the low dose (1 microg) of ACTH. *Clin Endocrinol* (Oxf) 1999; 51:153–158.
53. Rasmuson, S, Olsson, T, Hagg, E. A low dose ACTH test to assess the function of the hypothalamic-pituitary-adrenal axis. *Clin Endocrinol* 1996; 44:151–156.
54. Hoffman DM, O'Sullivan AJ, Baxter RC, Ho KK. The diagnosis of growth hormone deficiency in adults. *Lancet* 1994; 343:1064–1068.
55. Trainer PJ, Besser M. 1995 The Bart's Endocrine Protocols. Churchchill Livingstone; 4–6.
56. Nieman, LK. Dynamic evaluation of adrenal hypofunction. *J Endocrinol Invest* 2003; 26: 74–82
57. Filipsson H, Monson JP, Koltowska-Haggstrom M, Mattsson A, Johannsson G. The impact of glucocorticoid replacement regimens on metabolic outcome and comorbidity in hypopituitary patients. *J Clin Endocrinol Metab* 2006; 91:3954–61.
58. Lukert BP. Editorial: glucocorticoid replacement – how much is enough? *J Clin Endocrinol Metab* 2006; 91:793–4.
59. Crown A, Lightman S. Why is the management of glucocorticoid deficiency still controversial: a review of the literature. *Clin Endocrinol* (Oxf). 2005; 63:483–92.
60. Peacey SR, Pope RM, Naik KS, Hardern RD, Page MD, Belchetz PE. Corticosteroid therapy and intercurrent illness: the need for continuing patient education. *Postgrad Med J* 1993; 69:282–4.
61. Salem M; Tainsh RE Jr; Bromberg J; Loriaux DL; Chernow B. Perioperative glucocorticoid coverage: a reassessment 42 years after the emergence of a problem. *Ann Surg* 1994; 219:416–25
62. Glowniak, JV, Loriaux, DL. A double-blind study of perioperative steroid requirements in secondary adrenal insufficiency. *Surgery* 1997; 121:123–9
63. Kehlet, H, Binder, C. Adrenocortical function and clinical course during and after surgery in unsupplemented glucocorticoid-treated patients. *Br J Anaesth* 1973; 45:1043.

4 Acute Calcium Disorders

Sophie J. Van Cromphaut, MD, PhD
and Roger Bouillon, MD, PhD

CALCIUM CONCENTRATION IN EXTRACELLULAR FLUIDS

Extracellular calcium homeostasis is kept within tight limits despite the large bidirectional fluxes of calcium across the intestine, bone, and especially the kidney in comparison with the total extracellular calcium content, which is about 1 to 2 grams. Many ions (phosphate, magnesium and H^+) and humoral factors (such as interleukins) influence calcium homeostasis. However, parathyroid hormone (PTH) and the active vitamin D hormone, 1,25-dihydroxyvitamin D_3 [$1,25(OH)_2D_3$], represent the two critical factors cooperating in a short and a long feedback loop (Fig. 1).

The concentration of total extracellular calcium varies normally between 8.5 and 10.5 mg/dl (or 2.12 and 2.63 mM, but usually even within more narrow limits). Calcium circulates in the extracellular fluid (ECF) in three distinct fractions: about 50% is ionized [the free calcium ion (Ca^{2+})]. 40% of extracellular

From: *Contemporary Endocrinology: Acute Cause to Consequence*
Edited by: G. Van den Berghe, DOI: 10.1007/978-1-60327-177-6_4,
© Humana Press, New York, NY

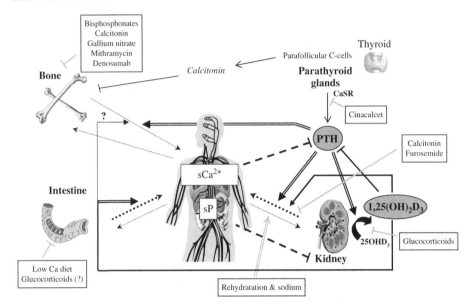

Fig. 1. Extracellular calcium homeostasis: feed back regulatory mechanisms and mode of action of anti-hypercalcemic strategies or drugs.

calcium is protein-bound (to albumin or complexed to globulins) and not filterable by the kidney. A small proportion, 10%, is complexed to anions such as bicarbonate, citrate, sulphate, phosphate and lactate *(1)*. Only the ionized fraction is feedback regulated and biologically important. Hence only Ca^{2+} is subject to transport into cells and capable of activating cellular processes, including cell division, cell adhesion, plasma membrane integrity, protein secretion, muscle contraction, neuronal excitability, glycogen metabolism and coagulation.

Marked changes in serum protein concentration affect total calcium concentration, whereas Ca^{2+} may remain relatively stable: a change of total serum albumin of 1 g/dl is associated with a 0.8 mg/dl change in total calcium. In contrast, changes in blood pH can alter the equilibrium constant of the albumin – Ca^{2+} complex, since acidosis decreases and alkalosis increases protein binding of Ca^{2+}. Accordingly, in the presence of major shifts in serum protein or pH, it is most prudent to directly measure the Ca^{2+} level in order to determine the presence of hypo- or hypercalcemia *(2)*.

The constancy of the serum Ca^{2+} concentration results from the balance between calcium influx and outflux from the three major calcium handling tissues (gut, bone, and kidney). Noteworthy, disruption of serum calcium homeostasis by major calcium fluxes across the placenta (during pregnancy) or breast (during lactation) is usually prevented by a variety of adaptations. Finally, calcium shifts across the skin or between the intra- and extracellular compartment rarely disturb extracellular calcium homeostasis.

PATHOGENESIS AND ETIOLOGY OF HYPER- AND HYPOCALCEMIA

Hypercalcemia

Hypercalcemia develops when the rate of influx of calcium from bone and/or intestine to the blood and extracellular fluid compartment exceeds the renal capacity to eliminate it *(3,4,5)*. More exceptionally, the kidney fails to excrete a normal calcium load. Figure 4 lists different causes of hypercalcemia, including some infrequent or less well understood mechanisms.

ROLE OF INTESTINAL CALCIUM ABSORPTION

Calcium is absorbed from the intestinal lumen to the circulatory system either through passive, mostly paracellular, diffusion (by a poorly understood mechanism, predominant in distal parts of the small intestine) or by an active cellular uptake and transport mechanism. The latter transcellular calcium absorption is energy dependent and predominant in duodenum. The pathway involves the movement of luminal calcium across the microvillar membrane into the enterocyte, which is regulated by the highly calcium selective epithelial channels, Transient Receptor Potential Vanilloid 6 (TRPV6) and to a lesser extent, TRPV5. This process is highly vitamin D dependent and may be the genuine rate limiting step in intestinal calcium absorption *(6,7)*. Subsequently, calcium is transferred through the cytosol via the intracellular calcium binding protein calbindin-$D_{9 K}$. Finally, at the basolateral site of the enterocyte, the plasma membrane calcium ATPase (PMCA1b) controls calcium extrusion from the enterocyte into the lamina propria and eventually into the blood stream. Passive calcium absorption will rarely cause hypercalcemia because of its relative low absorption efficacy. Increased intestinal calcium absorption will occur in the presence of exogenous (in the context of vitamin D intoxication or excess intake of 1α-hydroxylated vitamin D metabolites) or endogenous $1,25(OH)_2D_3$ as a result of ectopic production in monocytes in patients affected with sarcoidosis or related granulomatous diseases *(8)*.

ROLE OF BONE RESORPTION

Excessive bone resorption is the major cause of hypercalcemia (Figs. 2 and 4). Osteoclasts are primarily responsible for the degradation of mineralized bone matrix (calcium and protein combined) during bone development, homeostasis,

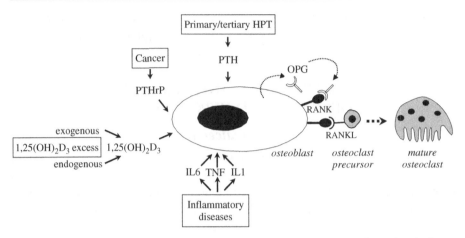

Fig. 2. The common essential mechanism in osteoclastogenesis involves the molecular interaction of RANK with RANK-L. OPG inhibits RANKL binding to its receptor.

and repair *(5)*. These highly specialized, multinucleated cells are recruited from hematopoietic precursors and have a relatively short life span. Numerous cellular, hormonal, and humoral mechanisms are required for osteoclastogenesis, but recent studies have been unveiling the central pathways for the regulation of bone formation/resorption coupling. The common essential mechanism involves the molecular interaction of receptor activator of nuclear factor-κB (RANK), its ligand (RANK-L), and osteoprotegerin (OPG), a decoy receptor of RANK-L. The differentiation and maturation of osteoclasts are highly dependent on the interaction of RANK expressed on the precursor cells and RANK-L expressed on osteoblasts and bone stromal cells (reviewed in *(9)*). This explains why different signals and signaling systems such as PTH, PTH related protein (PTHrP), vitamin D, and cytokines substitute each other in osteoclast differentiation and activation (Fig. 2). Severe and potentially life threatening acute hypercalcemia is mainly caused by either malignancy-associated hypercalcemia (MAH) or, less frequently by primary or tertiary hyperparathyroidism (PHPT or THPT).

Malignancy-Associated Hypercalcemia. MAH classically occurs in 10–15% of the patients with advanced cancer. The incidence is now decreasing because of an earlier and prolonged use of bisphosphonates in cancer patients *(10)*. MAH may be induced by any type of tumor, but most commonly by breast and lung carcinomas *(11)*. MAH is generally a complication of advanced cancer and a marker of a high bone resorption status, indicative for a high risk of skeletal complications and mortality *(12)*.

Cancer may affect bone by two distinct mechanisms: either (1) indirectly through elaboration of factors that act systemically on target organs of bone and kidney to disrupt normal calcium homeostasis, termed humoral hypercalcemia of malignancy (HHM); or (2) locally and directly via secondary spread of tumor to bone *(11)*.

PTHrP was discovered in 1980 as the major mediator of HHM *(13)*. Eight of the first 13 amino acid residues of the NH_2 terminus of PTH and PTHrP are identical, resulting in the same interaction with a common receptor (PTH1R) and have similar effects on calcium and phosphate homeostasis *(14)*. PTHrP basically modulates cell growth and differentiation and is widely expressed in many fetal and adult tissues *(14)*. Several groups have confirmed that 50–90% of patients with solid tumors and hypercalcemia and 20–60% of patients with hematological malignancies and hypercalcemia have elevated circulating PTHrP levels. Constitutively, PTHrP hypersecretion by these neoplasms, essentially in the absence of skeletal metastases, mimics the effects of PTH on bone and kidney.

As in PHPT, hypercalcemia is accompanied by hypophosphatemia, reduced tubular reabsorption of phosphorus, enhanced tubular reabsorption of calcium, and increased excretion of nephrogenous cyclic AMP, reflecting the PTH-like actions of PTHrP on the kidney. By contrast, serum $1,25(OH)_2D_3$ concentrations are frequently low or low normal in HHM, probably reflecting higher levels of ambient Ca^{2+}, while $1,25(OH)_2D_3$ levels are generally high or high normal in PHPT.

As far as the effects on bone are concerned, secretion of humoral and paracrine factors by tumor cells stimulates osteoclast proliferation and activity, resulting in a marked increase in collagen crosslinks excretion *(12)*. In addition, inhibition of osteoblast activity often leads to a characteristic uncoupling of bone resorption and formation *(11)*. Decreased osteoblast activity in MAH contributes to the rapid rise in serum calcium but the underlying mechanism remains poorly understood: cytokines such as IL-6 and TGF-β probably play a role *(11)* and relative immobilization often exacerbates the phenomenon.

The acute rise in serum calcium of MAH contrasts with the relatively stable levels of serum calcium observed in PHPT where coupling of bone resorption and formation is usually preserved leading to a more 'chronic' condition. As a consequence, the ratio between deoxypyridinoline – a marker of bone resorption – and osteocalcin – a marker of bone formation – is normal in primary hyperparathyroidism but markedly increased in MAH. The latter observation holds true for both types of MAH, whether of humoral (paraneoplastic) or of local osteolytic origin *(11)*.

Primary and Tertiary Hyperparathyroidism. PHPT is a common endocrine disorder. Currently the prevalence rates are about 1 to 4 per

1000, with a female/male ratio of 3/1 *(15)*. The disease is characterized by hypercalcemia in the face of increased levels of PTH, or by PTH levels in the normal range, but inappropriately high relative to the hypercalcemia. PHPT, formerly a disease of 'bones, stones, and psychic groans' has evolved into a mainly asymptomatic disorder in Western countries *(16)*. These patients present now with serum modest hypercalcemia (often within 1 mg/dl above the upper limits) and PTH concentrations of 1.5 to 2.0 times normal. Serum phosphorus levels are in the lower normal range and urinary calcium levels are at the upper normal limits. 25OHD$_3$ concentrations tend to be in the low normal, whereas 1,25(OH)$_2$D$_3$ levels are elevated in 40% of patients. A benign, solitary adenoma is found in 80% of patients with PHPT. In most of the remaining patients, a pathologic process characterized by hyperplasia of several or all four parathyroid glands is involved: sporadically or in association with multiple endocrine neoplasia (MEN) type I, MEN type IIa or Hyperparathyroidism-Jaw Tumor (HPT-JT) Syndrome. Mutations in the respective menin ret and HRPT2 genes are implicated in these rare inherited syndromes *(17)*.

THPT represents the autonomous function of parathyroid tissue that develops in the face of long-standing secondary HPT. The most common circumstance in which this occurs is in chronic renal failure where hypocalcaemia, hyperphosphatemia, and impaired renal 1,25(OH)$_2$D$_3$ synthesis with attendant reductions in serum 1,25(OH)$_2$D$_3$ concentration contribute to excess PTH synthesis, secretion, and ultimately parathyroid gland hyperplasia *(18)*. Furthermore, chronic phosphate treatment may in some cases of hypophosphatemic osteomalacia induce intermittent slight hypocalcemia and also stimulate PTH secretion *(19)*.

Disuse. Immobilization with or without bone fractures also enhances net calcium release from bone especially when bone turnover is already stimulated such as in critically ill patients *(20,21)*.

ROLE OF RENAL CALCIUM RE-ABSORPTION

Net urinary calcium excretion results from the balance between the filtered load (determined by serum Ca^{2+} concentration, renal perfusion, and glomerular filtration rate) and tubular calcium reabsorption *(22)*. The normal filtered load ($\pm$ 10 g per day) exceeds by far the plasma pool of Ca^{2+} but is nearly quantitatively reabsorbed by several consecutive mechanisms in the proximal tubule and cortical thick ascending limb by paracellular mechanisms linking calcium and sodium reuptake. Active, transcellular reabsorption is restricted to the distal convoluted tubule (DCT) and connecting segments (CNT) and accounts only for 5–10% of total calcium reabsorption along the nephron. However, it is responsive to PTH (with lesser contributions by calcitonin and 1,25(OH)$_2$D$_3$), and plays a role in the fine tuning of whole body calcium homeostasis *(22)*. At the cellular

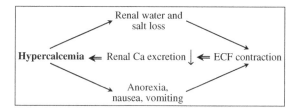

Fig. 3. The vicious circle of hypercalcemia and hypovolemia.

level, calcium enters the renal epithelial cell via TRPV5 because of a steep inward electrochemical gradient across the apical membrane. In the cell, calcium is bound to calbindin-D_{28K} that ferries calcium from the apical side to the basolateral side where the Na^+/Ca^{2+}-exchanger (NCX1) and PMCA1b extrude calcium into the blood compartment *(22)*. Decreased urinary calcium excretion may be observed during therapy with thiazide diuretics *(23)* or during extracellular fluid retraction. In various acute disorders hypercalcemia lowers renal perfusion, causing a reduction in renal calcium excretion mainly due to the coupling of renal sodium and calcium reabsorption. Hypercalcemia by itself may induce antidiuretic hormone insensitivity and as a consequence polyuria and/or gastrointestinal discomfort or vomiting thereby reducing fluid intake and increasing fluid loss *(24)*. The resulting extracellular fluid retraction further aggravates the hypercalcemia and a vicious circle ensues (Fig. 3).

ROLE OF CALCIUM SETPOINT AND PTH DYNAMICS

In 1993 the calcium-sensing receptor (CaSR) was discovered as a G protein–coupled receptor. Serum Ca^{2+} binds to the extracellular portion of the CaSR and relays intracellular signals (intracellular calcium, protein kinase C, and phosphoinositides) that, in turn, suppress the secretion of PTH, with a resultant decrease in the serum Ca^{2+} *(25)*.

Familial Hypocalciuric hypercalcemia (FHH) is a rare autosomal dominant trait characterized by moderate hypercalcemia and relative hypocalciuria: urine calcium is low in relationship to the prevailing hypercalcemia. The molecular basis is mostly an inactivating mutation in the CaSR gene *(26)*. The diminished ability of the renal CaSR to detect ECF calcium leads in heterozygotes to enhanced renal tubular reabsorption of calcium. In addition, increased ECF calcium is inadequately sensed by the altered parathyroid gland CaSR with mild parathyroid hyperplasia and 'normal' PTH levels despite mild hypercalcemia. Patients are generally asymptomatic. Sporadically, Neonatal Severe Primary hyperparathyroidism (NSHPT) presents within a week of birth of homozygous or compound heterozygotes individuals with life-threatening hypercalcemia, high PTH levels, massive parathyroid gland hyperplasia, relative hypocalciuria, and skeletal abnormalities (demineralization, widening of the metaphyses, osteitis fibrosa, and fractures) *(26)*.

Lithium carbonate, at 900 to 1500 mg/day, has occasionally been reported to cause hypercalcemia. Lithium may reduce renal calcium clearance and alter the set-point for PTH secretion such that higher ECF calcium levels than normal are required to suppress PTH *(27)*. The hypercalcemia is generally reversible with discontinuation of therapy.

Hypocalcemia

Protein-corrected hypocalcemia is far less frequent than hypercalcemia owing to the normal setpoint of calcium. Actually, PTH constitutes a better defense mechanism against hypocalcemia than hypercalcemia (Fig. 1). Indeed, a fall in serum Ca^{2+} evokes a prompt rise in PTH release, which raises Ca^{2+} by increasing renal tubular calcium reabsorption and renal phosphate clearance, activating new bone resorption loci, and augmenting osteoclast work at existing resorption loci and increasing renal 1α-hydroxylase activity producing increased $1,25(OH)_2D_3$ serum levels.

Hypoparathyroidism (or PTH resistance) of variable etiology and lack of $1,25(OH)_2D_3$ or its action are the most common etiologies of hypocalcemia *(28,6,14)*. Renal insufficiency is associated with hypocalcemia due to impaired vitamin D metabolism and low intestinal Ca absorption, phosphate retention, serum protein abnormalities, PTH resistance, and/or aluminum toxicity *(29)*. Severe magnesium deficiency also causes impaired PTH secretion and consequently functional hypoparathyroidism *(30)*. Of course, too zealous treatment of hypercalcemia may lead to hypocalcemia, especially by use of bisphosphonates *(31)*. Recalcification that occurs in bone postoperatively, after abrupt correction of thyrotoxicosis or hyperparathyroidism is referred to as 'hungry bone syndrome', due to a rapid increase in bone remodeling: hypocalcemia occurs if the rate of skeletal mineralization exceeds the rate of osteoclast mediated bone resorption.

Critical Illness

Acute, non-calcium-related diseases may also be associated with changes in serum ionized calcium levels: hypocalcemia, hypercalcemia, or even both in different phases of the same condition have been described (Figs. 4 and 5).

Hypocalcemia due to calcium sequestration by free fatty acids is a typical complication of severe, acute pancreatitis *(32)*. Important hypercalcemia may be found in acute Addison's disease *(33)*.

Twelve to 88% of critically ill patients would present with hypocalcemia depending on the definition of hypocalcemia and the patient population *(34)*.

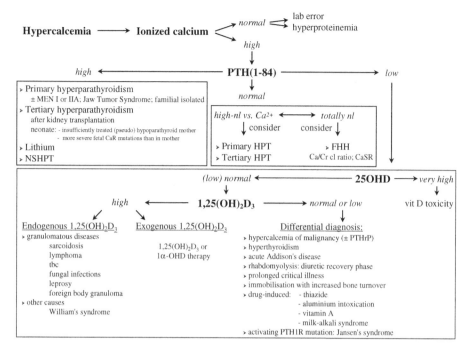

Fig. 4. Classification of hypercalcemia: a diagnostic algorithm.

Underlying mechanisms are complex: depressed PTH function possibly related to the up-regulation of the CaSR, failure of Ca^{2+} mobilization from bone secondary to abnormal blood flow, intracellular movement of Ca^{2+}, hypomagnesemia, altered renal excretion of phosphate, and/or citrate binding of calcium following blood transfusion have all been proposed as a part of the pathogenesis (35,34). Treatment should be considered if clinically relevant (36). Interestingly, patient with prolonged critical illness may develop hypercalcemia (37). Further investigation is needed to unravel the mechanisms involved in this phenomenon, but excessive bone resorption is undoubtedly linked to prolonged critical illness (20). It is presently not clear whether a special form of hyperparathyroidism may intervene (37). Circulating $1,25(OH)_2D_3$ levels are generally found to be low in prolonged critical illness (20). Still, $1,25(OH)_2D_3$ levels may occasionally be increased during sepsis through (lipopolysacchararides induced) toll-like receptor stimulation of 1α-hydroxylase in macrophages or monocytes (38,39).

Abnormal calcium metabolism is common in rhabdomyolysis-induced acute renal failure. During the oliguric phase, patients are frequently hypocalcemic,

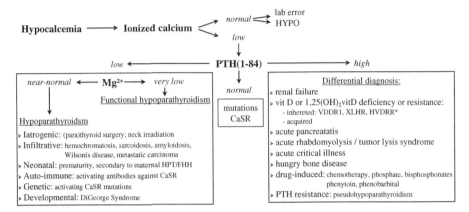

Fig. 5. Classification of hypocalcemia: a diagnostic algorithm. ∗ VDDR1: vitamin D dependent rickets type 1; HVDDR: human vitamin D resistant rickets; XLHR: X-linked hypophosphatemic rickets.

which may be explained by the release of intracellular phosphate and PTH resistance *(40)*. Hypocalcemia may even occur without renal failure. However, the diuretic recovery phase of induced acute renal failure may be complicated by hypercalcemia: several mechanisms have been proposed, including mobilization of calcium from muscle deposits, secondary HPT, and elevated levels of $1,25(OH)_2D_3$ *(41,42)*.

DIAGNOSTIC PROCEDURES

A simple algorithm using ionized calcium, PTH, 25OHD$_3$, and occasionally $1,25(OH)_2D_3$ is usually sufficient for a correct classification of hypercalcemia and hypocalcemia (Figs. 4 and 5). This approach could then further direct the procedures allowing detailed diagnosis and in some cases genetic/familial screening. For instance, in non-PTH related hypercalcemia, PTHrP measurement and other diagnostic procedures are needed for final diagnostic fine tuning.

Mild hyper- or hypocalcemia will seldom present as a medical or surgical emergency: as these disturbances in calcium homeostasis develop gradually in a wide variety of diseases, they usually cause only mild complaints or clinical symptoms. However patients in need of acute medical or surgical care because of non-calcemic related disorders may exhibit mild abnormalities in calcium homeostasis which can provide additional early clues regarding the etiology of the disease.

SYMPTOMS AND CLINICAL SPECTRUM
OF HYPER- AND HYPOCALCEMIA (TABLE 1)

Extreme hypercalcemia or hypocalcemia are exceptional, but may comprise a life-threatening medical emergency.

As a matter of fact, severe hypercalcemia can impair mental functions leading to confusion or even coma. It can cause marked polyuria with dehydration and may induce cardiac arrhythmias (especially bradycardia or atrioventricular block). Hypercalcemia in digitalis-treated patients may exacerbate digitalis toxicity *(43)*. Furthermore, hypercalcemia may trigger acute pancreatitis *(32)*. Most patients will remain asymptomatic as long as serum calcium does not exceed 12 mg/dl, whereas values above 14 mg/dl become problematic.

Hypocalcemia boosts neuromuscular excitability. Hence, severe hypocalcemia may produce muscle cramps (e.g., carpopedal spasms, tetany) or seizures of all types. Cardiac abnormalities (prolonged Q-T interval) are

Table 1
Clinical manifestations of acute hypercalcemia and hypocalcemia

	Hypercalcemia	*Hypocalcemia*
Neuro-muscular:	weakness	irritability: - paresthesias, muscle cramps, tetany - Chvostek's and Trousseau's sign - laryngeal spasms, bronchial spasms
Neurological:	confusion, depression	irritability, confusion, psychosis
	stupor, coma	seizures (focal, petit mal, grand mal)
Gastro-intestinal:	anorexia	dysphagia
	nausea, vomitting	abdominal pain, biliary colic
Renal:	polyuria polydipsia	
ECG:	shortened QT interval	prolonged QT interval
Cardiac:	bradycardia, first degree AV block	cardiomyopathy
	increased digitalis sensitivity	congestive heart failure

rarely life threatening. Blood coagulation may be impaired due to extreme hypocalcemia, but also in polytransfused patients.

TREATMENT OF ACUTE HYPERCALCEMIA

If the patient's serum calcium concentration is less than 12 mg/dL, treatment should focus at the underlying disorder. Patients with clinical manifestations of acute hypercalcemia and a calcemia greater than 12 mg/dL require urgent measures. The four basic goals in the management of acute hypercalcemia, regardless of its origin, are: (1) to restore hydratation; (2) to stimulate renal calcium excretion; (3) to inhibit osteoclastic bone resorption, and (4) if achievable, to treat the underlying disorder. General treatment options and strategies of hypercalcemia are also illustrated in Fig. 1.

Rehydration

Rehydration with intravenous saline at a rate of 2.5 to 4 L daily is imperative in the initial approach of severe hypercalcemia *(33,44)*. Expansion of the intravascular volume with sodium interrupts the vicious cycle of hypercalcemia by increasing the glomerular filtration of calcium and decreasing tubular reabsorption of sodium and calcium (Fig. 3). Rehydration improves the clinical status, even though it generally results in only a mild, transient reduction of calcemia (by approximately 1.6–2.4 mg/dL) *(33,44)*. This therapy should be used cautiously in patients with compromised cardiovascular or renal function.

Bone Resorption

Because accelerated bone resorption is a key factor in the majority of patients with acute hypercalcemia, it should be addressed promptly after sufficient hydratation. Bisphosphonates have supplanted most other drugs inhibiting bone resorption.

BISPHOSPHONATES

Bisphosphonates are effective osteoclast inhibitors. These pyrophosphate analogs have a high affinity for hydroxyapatite and bind directly to mineralized bone. On osteoclast stimulation of bone resorption, they are released and internalized by the osteoclasts, interfering with osteoclast formation, function, and survival.

Clodronate was one of the first bisphosphonates applied in the management of hypercalcemia. Bisphosphonates are preferentially administered intravenously when acute hypercalcemia is concerned. Currently, pamidronate (90 mg for the most severe hypercalcemic states, otherwise 30–60 mg intravenously in 500 ml of 0.9% saline or 5% dextrose over 4 hours *(45)*) and zoledronate (4 mg intravenously in 5 ml over 15 minutes *(46)*) are the agents of choice because of their potency, efficacy and wide experience. The doses of bisphosphonates used to stabilize primary hyperparathyroidism patients before surgery, are often lower than those used in cancer patients *(47)*. Potential nephrotoxicity is avoided by respecting adequate infusion periods of at least 2 hours and 15 minutes for palmidronate or zoledronate respectively *(48)*. Serum calcium will gradually decline, beginning 24–48 hours after the initial dose and will only normalize after 4 days. However, this effect may last from days to weeks. Repeating of the treatment is not recommended for at least 8 days. From experience with repeated infusions in patients with cancer-related bone disease, the dose of 8 mg zoledronate is not recommended for long-term treatment because of nephrotoxicity. Bisphosphonates may induce transient hypocalcemia, hypophosphatemia and fever, flu-like symptoms, or myalgia in approximately one fourth of patients.

Two pooled, randomized, double blind, double dummy trials in 275 evaluable patients with moderate or severe MAH (corrected calcemia = 12 mg/dl) compared zoledronate (4 mg or 8 mg) to pamidronate (90 mg). At day 10, success rates (corrected calcemia ≤ 10.8 mg/dl) of 88%, 87%, and 70% respectively demonstrated the higher efficiency of zoledronate compared with pamidronate. The difference was not impressive in patients with bone metastases, but quite marked in patients with hypercalcemia of humoral origin *(49)*. Another randomized, double blind, double dummy trial compared the long-term (25-month) safety and efficacy of zoledronate (4 mg or 8 mg (reduced to 4 mg) every 3–4 weeks) with pamidronate (90 mg every 3–4 weeks) in patients with bone lesions secondary to advanced breast carcinoma or multiple myeloma. Compared with pamidronate, zoledronate (4 mg) reduced the overall risk of developing skeletal complications (including MAH) by an additional 16% *(P=0.030)* *(50)*.

Since 2003, the observation and reporting of the adverse effect profile of bisphosphonates, including the development of osteonecrosis of the jaw (ONJ), has boosted, coinciding with the prolonged exposure to potent bisphosphonates in symptomatic malignant bony disease *(51,48)*. In 2004, the International Myeloma Foundation conducted a web-based survey to assess the risk factors for ONJ. Respondents were myeloma and breast cancer patients. At 36 months censure of data, ONJ development was higher in patients receiving zoledronate (10%) compared with pamidronate (4%), and the mean time to the onset of ONJ was 18 months for zoledronate and 6 years for pamidronate (P=0.002) *(51)*. Underlying dental problems, such as infection or dental extraction were much more frequent in the ONJ group *(51)*. In light of these reports Novartis convened an international advisory board of experts to provide updated recommendations on the clinical diagnosis, prevention, and management of ONJ in oncology *(52)*.

Patients should receive dental examinations prior to and during bisphosphonate therapy. Any necessary dental procedure should, if possible, be completed prior to initiating bisphosphonate therapy. Several prospective studies are presently investigating optimal dosing regimens and treatment duration of bisphosphonate cancer therapy, both in terms of efficacy and safety. Additionally, a comprehensive research plan was launched to provide more definitive guidance with regard to the pathogenesis, risk factors, effective preventive measures and treatments for ONJ (52).

CALCITONIN

Calcitonin is a natural anti-osteoclastic peptide hormone with a negligible toxicity. It has a beneficial rapid onset of action, causing serum calcium to fall generally by 2 mg/dL within 2 to 6 hours of administration. Its calciuretic effect intensifies its hypocalcemic activity (53). Compared to the therapeutic effect of bisphosphonates, the efficacy of calcitonin is inconsistent, partial and transient though. Hypercalcemia usually recurs after a few days and is refractory to an increase of the dose. Salmon calcitonin (4–8 IU/kg/day, intravenously, intramuscularly or subcutaneously) could be used concurrently with bisphosphonates during the first 2 to 3 days of treatment in cases of severe hypercalcemia since the calcium-lowering effects of bisphosphonates are generally only evident 1 or 2 days after administration (54).

GLUCOCORTICOIDS

Glucocorticoids remain indispensable in the management of hypercalcemia caused by steroid-responsive disorders such as hematological malignancies (myeloma or lymphoma (55)) and granulomatous diseases (sarcoidosis (56) and others). Corticosteroids inhibit the (extra)-renal $1,25(OH)_2D_3$ production and are presumed to counteract the effects of endo- or exogenous $1,25(OH)_2D_3$ excess. The reduction of elevated $1,25(OH)_2D_3$ levels actually precedes the fall in serum calcium levels in corticosteroid-treated sarcoidosis (56). Glucocorticoid-induced intestinal malabsorption of calcium is a fairly consistent 'textbook' finding. However recent animal studies exploring the molecular substrate for this malabsorption yielded conflicting data regarding the influence of short term, highly dosed glucocorticoid treatment (57,58). Hydrocortisone (200 to 300 mg intravenously over 24 hours), or its equivalent, is given intravenously for 3 to 5 days.

Interestingly, corticosteroids have a more delayed effect on exogenous vitamin D-induced hypercalcemia, compared with pamidronate treatment, suggesting that increased bone resorption is the major determinant of hypercalcemia in this setting (59).

Glucocorticoid treatment is mandatory in acute primary and secondary adrenal insufficiency, regardless of the severity of the associated hypercalcemia.

PLICAMYCIN (MITHRAMYCIN)

Plicamycin is a cytotoxic antibiotic that inhibits RNA synthesis in osteoclasts *(60)*. Serum calcium invariably falls, as early as 6–12 hours after administration and reaches a nadir by 2 to 3 days, with persisting normocalcemia from days to weeks depending on the extent of ongoing bone resorption. The dose may be repeated at 24 to 48 hour intervals. Its use is limited by major potential toxicity (bone marrow, liver, kidney), particularly with repetitive administration even at the recommended dose (15 to 25 mg/kg intravenously over 4 to 6 hours *(60,33)*). The drug is presently held in reserve for particularly difficult and unusual situations.

GALLIUM NITRATE

Gallium nitrate was originally developed as a chemotherapy agent but was found to markedly reduce hypercalcemia in patients with osteolytic bone metastases. Its mechanism of action is elusive, but it is thought to inhibit osteoclast activity *(61)*. Nonetheless, the risk of nephrotoxicity dampened the enthusiasm for this drug. A recent report suggests a potential benefit of gallium nitrate (200 mg/m^2 per kg intravenously for 5 consecutive days) in the treatment of serious flare hypercalcemia following the initiation of tamoxifen therapy in hypercalcemic patients with metastatic advanced breast cancer *(62)*.

OTHER COMPOUNDS

Several groups are investigating new inhibitors of bone resorption. Targeting the RANK-RANKL-OPG system was first successfully explored *(in vitro*, in animal models and in a phase 1 clinical trial with a recombinant OPG construct (AMGN-0007) in patients with multiple myeloma or breast carcinoma who exhibited lytic bone lesions *(63,64)*. Subsequently denosumab (AMG 162) a fully human mAb directed against RANKL, showed a safe and more efficient anti-resorptive profile than Fc-OPG. Denosumab is currently under investigation in several phase 3 clinical trials for pre-metastatic (prostate cancer) and metastatic cancer (prostate and breast cancer, solid tumors, myeloma), with skeletal-related events as primary endpoints *(64)*. Restraining cancer-related bone disease has potential implications for the prevention or therapy of MAH.

Renal Calcium Excretion

FUROSEMIDE

Loop diuretics, such as furosemide, inhibit both sodium and calcium reabsorption at the cortical thick ascending limbs (CTAL) of the kidney. However, forced saline diuresis with 6 liters or more per 24 hours combined with large doses of furosemide is a risky, outdated procedure. On the other hand, if high levels of PTHrP (or PTH) mediate the presenting hypercalcemia, inhibition of bone resorption alone may be inadequate to control serum calcium *(65)*. Accordingly, the association of furosemide (10 tot 20 mg intravenously) may be considered to overcome the possible contributory role of circulating PTHrP on the kidney, but only *after* rehydration.

DIALYSIS

Dialysis is effective, but should be reserved for severely hypercalcemic patients refractory to other therapies or who have renal insufficiency *(66)*. Hypercalcemia emergent during prolonged critical illness with acute renal failure requiring continuous venovenous hemofiltration or dialysis is a sign of severe bone hyperresorption *(20)*. In this setting, bone protective measures outweigh the necessity of omitting calcium in substitution fluid or dialysate *(67)*.

Etiology

Ideally, long-term control of serum calcium is achieved by effective treatment of the underlying disorder.

HYPERCALCEMIA OF MALIGNANCY

Hypercalcemia generally complicates advanced and refractory cancer. Consequently, marked reduction of tumor burden is often not attainable. Several studies have reported that PTHrP contributes to the local growth of the tumor *(68)*. Consequently, reduction of PTHrP levels may contribute not only to the long-term amelioration of skeletal and calcium homeostasis but also to a reduction in tumor burden. Approaches to reduce PTHrP production remain experimental though *(68)*.

HYPERPARATHYROIDISM

Surgery. Surgery (removal of the culprit parathyroid adenoma) often brings cure in patients with symptomatic or complicated PHPT *(47)*. For asymptomatic patients with no serious renal or bone mineral density risk, long-term surveillance may represent acceptable management *(16)*. In view of the fact that the renal lesion and therefore hypercalcemia persists after parathyroidectomy, it is important to identify FHH patients to ensure that they are not subjected to parathyroidectomy. In symptomatic THPT patients, surgical treatment, either removal of about 5/8 of the parathyroid mass or total parathyroidectomy with autografting of parathyroid tissue fragments into the muscle of the forearm, is often indicated *(69)*.

Calcimimetics. Calcimimetic agents, such as cinacalcet, represent the latest exciting pharmacological approach to target PTH secretion in hyperparathyroidism. These drugs suppress PTH secretion by sensitizing the CaSRs to extracellular Ca^{2+}. Cinacalcet has been approved for treatment of dialysis patients with uncontrolled secondary HPT. Of course these patients do not present with hypercalcemia, but still calcemia is moderately reduced *(70)*. However, increasing data support the use of calcimimetics (schedules varying between 30 mg/d and 90 mg/6 hour, orally) in the management of hypercalcemic THPT in kidney graft recipients *(71)* , PHPT *(72)* and FHH *(73)* patients and patients with inoperable parathyroid carcinoma *(74)*.

TREATMENT OF ACUTE HYPOCALCEMIA

Severe, rapidly emergent hypocalcemia will induce tetany, seizures, or laryngeal spasms, warranting parenteral calcium administration *(75)*. Quite the opposite, chronic hypocalcemia will mostly be asymptomatic even with extremely low calcium levels and hence will not require aggressive treatment.

The goal of intravenous calcium therapy is to relieve the acute manifestations of hypocalcemia and not to acutely normalize serum calcium *(75)*. Calcium gluconate contains about 90 mg of elemental calcium per 10 mL and usually 10 to 20 ml is infused over 10 minutes. This procedure can be repeated until the symptoms of hypocalcemia have cleared. With persistent hypercalcemia, for instance caused by the hungry bone syndrome following parathyroidectomy or by acute pancreatitis, continuous intravenous administration may be necessary. Recommended protocols diverge. One could aim at raising serum Ca^{2+} up to a low normal range by infusing 15 mg/kg bw of elemental calcium over 4 to 8 hours, under close monitoring of serum Ca^{2+}.

If possible, oral calcium supplementation (1 to 2 grams of elemental calcium) and, if indicated, vitamin D derivatives should be initiated concurrently as a more chronic approach to restore calcium homeostasis *(75)*. It is essential to exclude hypomagnesia in any hypocalcemic patient and to administer magnesium intravenously in any case of doubt. Calcemia will only normalize if correction of magnesium levels restores PTH secretion.

Intravenous calcium administration may be hazardous and should be carefully monitored. Severe arrhythmias may occur if calcium is injected too rapidly.

Especially patients taking digitalis may have increased sensitivity to intravenous calcium *(43)*. Solutions containing over 200 mg/100 mL of elemental calcium will cause venous irritation: calcium gluconate is less caustic and thus preferred over calcium chloride. Extravasation into soft tissues may lead to skin necrosis as a result of calcium phosphate crystal precipitation *(76)*. Actually, metastatic calcifications (in the lungs, kidney, or other soft tissues) are most likely if the calcium-phosphate ratio exceeds the solubility product. Hence, patients receiving intravenous calcium in the presence of high serum phosphate levels such as in the tumor lysis syndrome are at risk and should only be treated with intravenous calcium if symptomatic *(77)*.

REFERENCES

1. Walser M. Ion association. VI. Interactions between calcium, magnesium, inorganic phosphate, citrate and protein in normal human plasma. *J Clin Invest* 1961; 40:723–30.
2. Slomp J, van der Voort PH, Gerritsen RT et al. Albumin-adjusted calcium is not suitable for diagnosis of hyper- and hypocalcemia in the critically ill. *Crit Care Med* 2003; 31: 1389–93.
3. Moyses-Neto M, Guimaraes FM, Ayoub FH et al. Acute renal failure and hypercalcemia. *Ren Fail* 2006; 28:153–9.
4. Newman EM, Bouvet M, Borgehi S et al. Causes of hypercalcemia in a population of military veterans in the United States. *Endocr Pract* 2006; 12:535–41.
5. Bruzzaniti A, Baron R Molecular regulation of osteoclast activity. *Rev Endocr Metab Disord* 2006; 7:123–39.
6. Van Cromphaut SJ, Dewerchin M, Hoenderop JG et al. Duodenal calcium absorption in vitamin D receptor-knockout mice: functional and molecular aspects. *Proc Natl Acad Sci U S A* 2001; 98:13324–9.
7. Bianco SD, Peng JB, Takanaga H et al. Marked disturbance of calcium homeostasis in mice with targeted disruption of the Trpv6 calcium channel gene. *J Bone Miner Res* 2007; 22: 274–85.
8. Sharma OP. Hypercalcemia in granulomatous disorders: a clinical review. *Curr Opin Pulm Med* 2000; 6:442–7.
9. Suda T, Takahashi N, Udagawa N et al. Modulation of osteoclast differentiation and function by the new members of the tumor necrosis factor receptor and ligand families. *Endocr Rev* 1999; 20:345–57.
10. Pavlakis N, Schmidt R, Stockler M. Bisphosphonates for breast cancer. *Cochrane Database Syst Rev* 2005; CD003474.
11. Guise TA, Mundy GR. Cancer and bone. *Endocr Rev* 1998; 19:18–54.
12. Coleman RE. Clinical features of metastatic bone disease and risk of skeletal morbidity. *Clin Cancer Res* 2006; 12:6243s-9s.
13. Stewart AF, Horst R, Deftos LJ et al. Biochemical evaluation of patients with cancer-associated hypercalcemia: evidence for humoral and nonhumoral groups. *N Engl J Med* 1980; 303:1377–83.
14. Gensure RC, Gardella TJ, Juppner H. Parathyroid hormone and parathyroid hormone-related peptide, and their receptors. *Biochem Biophys Res Commun* 2005; 328:666–78.

15. Heath DA. Primary hyperparathyroidism. Clinical presentation and factors influencing clinical management. *Endocrinol Metab Clin North Am* 1989; 18:631–46.

16. Silverberg SJ, Bilezikian JP. The diagnosis and management of asymptomatic primary hyperparathyroidism. *Nat Clin Pract Endocrinol Metab* 2006; 2:494–503.

17. Zikusoka MN, Kidd M, Eick G et al. The molecular genetics of gastroenteropancreatic neuroendocrine tumors. *Cancer* 2005; 104:2292–309.

18. Goodman WG. Medical management of secondary hyperparathyroidism in chronic renal failure. *Nephrol Dial Transplant* 2003; 18 Suppl 3:iii2–iii8.

19. Davies M. Hyperparathyroidism in X-linked hypophosphataemic osteomalacia. *Clin Endocrinol (Oxf)* 1995; 42:205–6.

20. Van den Berghe G, Van Roosbroeck D, Vanhove P et al. Bone turnover in prolonged critical illness: effect of vitamin D. *J Clin Endocrinol Metab* 2003; 88:4623–32.

21. Stewart AF, Adler M, Byers CM et al. Calcium homeostasis in immobilization: an example of resorptive hypercalciuria. *N Engl J Med* 1982; 306:1136–40.

22. Lambers TT, Bindels RJ, Hoenderop JG. Coordinated control of renal Ca2+ handling. *Kidney Int* 2006; 69:650–4.

23. Suki WN. Effects of diuretics on calcium metabolism. *Adv Exp Med Biol* 1982; 151: 493–500.

24. Schrier RW. Body water homeostasis: clinical disorders of urinary dilution and concentration. *J Am Soc Nephrol* 2006; 17:1820–32.

25. Brown EM, Pollak M, Seidman CE et al. Calcium-ion-sensing cell-surface receptors. *N Engl J Med* 1995; 333:234–40.

26. Pollak MR, Chou YH, Marx SJ et al. Familial hypocalciuric hypercalcemia and neonatal severe hyperparathyroidism. Effects of mutant gene dosage on phenotype. *J Clin Invest* 1994; 93:1108–12.

27. Haden ST, Stoll AL, McCormick S et al. Alterations in parathyroid dynamics in lithium-treated subjects. *J Clin Endocrinol Metab* 1997; 82:2844–8.

28. Bringhurst FR, Demay MB, Kronenberg HM et al. Hormones and Disorders of Mineral Metabolism. In: Larsen PR, Kronenberg HM, Melmed S, Polonsky KS, eds. Williams Textbook of Endocrinology, 10th ed., vol. 1. Philadelphia: Saunders, 2003:1303–74.

29. Locatelli F, Cannata-Andia JB, Drueke TB et al. Management of disturbances of calcium and phosphate metabolism in chronic renal insufficiency, with emphasis on the control of hyperphosphataemia. *Nephrol Dial Transplant* 2002; 17:723–31.

30. Lim P, Dong S, Khoo OT. Intracellular magnesium depletion in chronic renal failure. *N Engl J Med* 1969; 280:981–4.

31. Tanvetyanon T, Stiff PJ. Management of the adverse effects associated with intravenous bisphosphonates. *Ann Oncol* 2006; 17:897–907.

32. Dettelbach MA, Deftos LJ, Stewart AF. Intraperitoneal free fatty acids induce severe hypocalcemia in rats: a model for the hypocalcemia of pancreatitis. *J Bone Miner Res* 1990; 5:1249–55.

33. Bilezikian JP. Clinical review 51: Management of hypercalcemia. *J Clin Endocrinol Metab* 1993; 77:1445–9.

34. Dickerson RN. Treatment of hypocalcemia in critical illness – part 1. *Nutrition* 2007; 23:358–61.

35. Drop LJ, Laver MB. Low plasma ionized calcium and response to calcium therapy in critically ill man. *Anesthesiology* 1975; 43:300–6.

36. Dickerson RN. Treatment of hypocalcemia in critical illness – part 2. *Nutrition* 2007; 23:436–7.

37. Forster J, Querusio L, Burchard KW et al. Hypercalcemia in critically ill surgical patients. *Ann Surg* 1985; 202:512–8.

38. Stoffels K, Overbergh L, Giulietti A et al. Immune regulation of 25-hydroxyvitamin-D3-1alpha-hydroxylase in human monocytes. *J Bone Miner Res* 2006; 21:37–47.

39. Lin WJ, Yeh WC. Implication of Toll-like receptor and tumor necrosis factor alpha signaling in septic shock. *Shock* 2005; 24:206–9.

40. Warren JD, Blumbergs PC, Thompson PD. Rhabdomyolysis: a review. *Muscle Nerve* 2002; 25:332–47.

41. Shrestha SM, Berry JL, Davies M et al. Biphasic hypercalcemia in severe rhabdomyolysis: serial analysis of PTH and vitamin D metabolites. A case report and literature review. *Am J Kidney Dis* 2004; 43:e31–5.

42. Akmal M, Bishop JE, Telfer N et al. Hypocalcemia and hypercalcemia in patients with rhabdomyolysis with and without acute renal failure. *J Clin Endocrinol Metab* 1986; 63: 137–42.

43. Vella A, Gerber TC, Hayes DL et al. Digoxin, hypercalcaemia, and cardiac conduction. *Postgrad Med J* 1999; 75:554–6.

44. Hosking DJ, Cowley A, Bucknall CA. Rehydration in the treatment of severe hypercalcaemia. *Q J Med* 1981; 50:473–81.

45. Nussbaum SR, Younger J, Vandepol CJ et al. Single-dose intravenous therapy with pamidronate for the treatment of hypercalcemia of malignancy: comparison of 30-, 60-, and 90-mg dosages. *Am J Med* 1993; 95:297–304.

46. Body JJ, Lortholary A, Romieu G et al. A dose-finding study of zoledronate in hypercalcemic cancer patients. *J Bone Miner Res* 1999; 14:1557–61.

47. Marcus R. Diagnosis and treatment of hyperparathyroidism. *Rev Endocr Metab Disord* 2000; 1:247–52.

48. Mehrotra B, Ruggiero S. Bisphosphonate complications including osteonecrosis of the jaw. *Hematology Am Soc Hematol Educ Program* 2006; 356–60, 515.

49. Major P, Lortholary A, Hon J et al. Zoledronic acid is superior to pamidronate in the treatment of hypercalcemia of malignancy: a pooled analysis of two randomized, controlled clinical trials. *J Clin Oncol* 2001; 19:558–67.

50. Rosen LS, Gordon D, Kaminski M et al. Long-term efficacy and safety of zoledronic acid compared with pamidronate disodium in the treatment of skeletal complications in patients with advanced multiple myeloma or breast carcinoma: a randomized, double-blind, multicenter, comparative trial. *Cancer* 2003; 98:1735–44.

51. Durie BG, Katz M, Crowley J. Osteonecrosis of the jaw and bisphosphonates. *N Engl J Med* 2005; 353:99–102.

52. Weitzman R, Sauter N, Eriksen EF et al. Critical review: updated recommendations for the prevention, diagnosis, and treatment of osteonecrosis of the jaw in cancer patients–May 2006. *Crit Rev Oncol Hematol* 2007; 62:148–52.

53. Hosking DJ, Gilson D. Comparison of the renal and skeletal actions of calcitonin in the treatment of severe hypercalcaemia of malignancy. *Q J Med* 1984; 53:359–68.

54. Fatemi S, Singer FR, Rude RK. Effect of salmon calcitonin and etidronate on hypercalcemia of malignancy. *Calcif Tissue Int* 1992; 50:107–9.

55. Percival RC, Yates AJ, Gray RE et al. Role of glucocorticoids in management of malignant hypercalcaemia. *Br Med J (Clin Res Ed)* 1984; 289:287.

56. Sandler LM, Winearls CG, Fraher LJ et al. Studies of the hypercalcaemia of sarcoidosis: effect of steroids and exogenous vitamin D3 on the circulating concentrations of 1,25-dihydroxy vitamin D3. *Q J Med* 1984; 53:165–80.

57. Van Cromphaut SJ, Stockmans I, Torrekens S et al. Duodenal calcium absorption in dexamethasone-treated mice: functional and molecular aspects. *Arch Biochem Biophys* 2007; 460:300–5.

58. Huybers S, Naber TH, Bindels RJ et al. Prednisolone-induced Ca2+ malabsorption is caused by diminished expression of the epithelial Ca2+ channel TRPV6. *Am J Physiol Gastrointest Liver Physiol* 2007; 292:G92–7.

59. Selby PL, Davies M, Marks JS et al. Vitamin D intoxication causes hypercalcaemia by increased bone resorption which responds to pamidronate. *Clin Endocrinol (Oxf)* 1995; 43:531–6.

60. Perlia CP, Gubisch NJ, Wolter J et al. Mithramycin treatment of hypercalcemia. *Cancer* 1970; 25:389–94.

61. Leyland-Jones B. Treatment of cancer-related hypercalcemia: the role of gallium nitrate. *Semin Oncol* 2003; 30:13–9.

62. Arumugam GP, Sundravel S, Shanthi P et al. Tamoxifen flare hypercalcemia: an additional support for gallium nitrate usage. *J Bone Miner Metab* 2006; 24:243–7.

63. Dougall WC, Chaisson M. The RANK/RANKL/OPG triad in cancer-induced bone diseases. *Cancer Metastasis Rev* 2006; 25:541–9.

64. Schwarz EM, Ritchlin CT. Clinical development of anti-RANKL therapy. *Arthritis Res Ther* 2007; 9 Suppl 1:S7

65. Gurney H, Grill V, Martin TJ. Parathyroid hormone-related protein and response to pamidronate in tumour-induced hypercalcaemia. *Lancet* 1993; 341:1611–13.

66. Cardella CJ, Birkin BL, Rapoport A. Role of dialysis in the treatment of severe hypercalcemia: report of two cases successfully treated with hemodialysis and review of the literature. *Clin Nephrol* 1979; 12:285–90.

67. Koo WS, Jeon DS, Ahn SJ et al. Calcium-free hemodialysis for the management of hypercalcemia. *Nephron* 1996; 72:424–8.

68. Goltzman D, Karaplis AC, Kremer R et al. Molecular basis of the spectrum of skeletal complications of neoplasia. *Cancer* 2000; 88:2903–8.

69. Kebebew E, Duh QY, Clark OH. Tertiary hyperparathyroidism: histologic patterns of disease and results of parathyroidectomy. *Arch Surg* 2004; 139:974–7.

70. Block GA, Martin KJ, de Francisco AL et al. Cinacalcet for secondary hyperparathyroidism in patients receiving hemodialysis. *N Engl J Med* 2004; 350:1516–25.

71. Srinivas TR, Schold JD, Womer KL et al. Improvement in hypercalcemia with cinacalcet after kidney transplantation. *Clin J Am Soc Nephrol* 2006; 1:323–6.

72. Shoback DM, Bilezikian JP, Turner SA et al. The calcimimetic cinacalcet normalizes serum calcium in subjects with primary hyperparathyroidism. *J Clin Endocrinol Metab* 2003; 88:5644–9.

73. Festen-Spanjer B, Haring CM, Koster JB et al. Correction of hypercalcaemia by cinacalcet in familial hypocalciuric hypercalcaemia. *Clin Endocrinol (Oxf)* 2007; 68(2):324–5. Epub 2007 Sep 4.

74. Silverberg SJ, Rubin MR, Faiman C et al. Cinacalcet Hydrochloride Reduces the Serum Calcium Concentration in Inoperable Parathyroid Carcinoma. *J Clin Endocrinol Metab* 2007; 92(10):3803–8. Epub 2007 Jul 31.

75. Tohme JF, Bilezikian JP. Hypocalcemic emergencies. *Endocrinol Metab Clin North Am* 1993; 22:363–75.

76. Lin CY, Hsieh KC, Yeh MC et al. Skin necrosis after intravenous calcium chloride administration as a complication of parathyroidectomy for secondary hyperparathyroidism: report of four cases. *Surg Today* 2007; 37:778–81.

77. Rampello E, Fricia T, Malaguarnera M. The management of tumor lysis syndrome. *Nat Clin Pract Oncol* 2006; 3:438–47.

5

Phaeochromocytoma and Other Diseases of the Sympathetic Nervous System

Dr. Umasuthan Srirangalingam, BSc (Hons.), MB ChB, MRCP and Professor Shern L. Chew, BSc (Hons.), MB BChir, MD, FRCP.

BASIC PRINCIPLES

Development of the Sympathoadrenal System

The origins of the sympathoadrenal system begin with the development of the neural plate from the ectodermal germ layer in the 3rd week of gestation (1). By week 5, primitive sympathetic ganglia have formed and by week 8, afferent and efferent connections have been made with the spinal nerves.

Initially, during the process of neural tube closure, cells detach from the basal plate of the neural tube and neural crest and migrate along the ventromedial path to become the cells of the future sympathoadrenal system (2) These neural crest cells migrate to the rostral part of the adjacent somite and then coalesce in the rudimentary ganglia forming in the region the dorsal aorta. Growth,

From: *Contemporary Endocrinology: Acute Cause to Consequence*
Edited by: G. Van den Berghe, DOI: 10.1007/978-1-60327-177-6_5,
© Humana Press, New York, NY

migration, and differentiation of neural crest cells are guided by the intrinsic cellular properties, the interplay of local attractive and repulsive environmental cues, and cell-cell interactions *(3)*. Neural crest precursors begin to differentiate into sympathetic neurones under the influence of members of the bone morphogenetic protein (BMP) family *(4)*. Developing sympathetic axons grow along the path of blood vessels to target organs driven by the chemoattractive neurotrophin, artemin, which is expressed in the vascular smooth muscle cells *(5)*. Once close to target organs, neurotrophic factors can influence the entry of sympathetic axons with the relevant receptors *(2)* for example, sympathetic neurones expressing α4-integrins bind vascular cell adhesion molecule-1 in developing heart myocytes *(6)*. Fibroblast growth factor causes neurite differentiation while glucocorticoids cause chromaffin cell differentiation *(7)*.

Pre-ganglionic sympathetic neurons originate from the intermediolateral nucleus in the lateral horn of the spinal cord (T1-L3). These neurones exit the cord and synapse in several ways. Some synapse with post-ganglionic neurones in the paravertebral sympathetic chain at the same level, rostrally or caudally of the exit segment. The post-ganglionic neurones then join the spinal nerves and synapse in the effector organs (viscera, skin, vasculature, mucous membranes, and glands). Some travel through the paravertebral sympathetic chain ganglia (without synapsing) to eventually synapse with post-ganglionic neurones in prevertebral ganglion, for example, ceoliac, superior mesenteric, and inferior mesenteric ganglia. Other pre-ganglionic sympathetic neurons synapse with chromaffin cells in the adrenal medulla; a modified sympathetic ganglion. Sympathetic innervations from the superior cervical ganglia to the pelvic-hypogastric plexus provide an infrastructure to maintain ongoing homeostatic control of the viscera and to also coordinated the response of viscera during stress.

Catecholamine Synthesis and Metabolism

The amino acid tyrosine is the starting point for the synthesis of catecholamines (Fig. 1). The rate-limiting enzyme, tyrosine hydroxylase catalyzes the conversion of tyrosine to dopa (3,4-dihydroxyphenylalanine). Catecholamines form a feed-back loop controlling the levels of tyrosine hydroxylase. Aromatic L-amino acid decarboxylase (AADC) causes the decarboxylation of dopa to dopamine *(8)*. Dopamine is then transported to the granulated vesicles in chromaffin cells or the synaptic vesicles of sympathetic nerves where the enzyme β-hydroxylase catalyzes its hydroxylation to noradrenaline. Noradrenaline is converted to adrenaline by phenylethanolamine N-methyltransferase (PNMT) in the adrenal medulla. Adrenaline is then taken up by vesicles in the chromaffin cells, ready for exocytosis in response to cholinergic sympathetic stimulation.

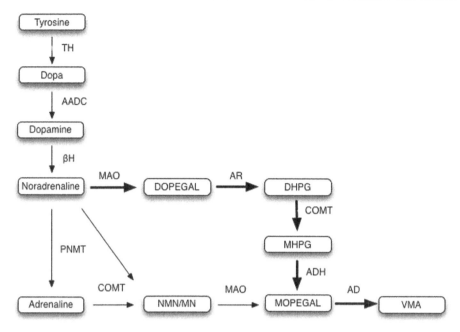

Fig. 1. Synthesis and degradation of catecholamines. Boxes denote catecholamine intermediates, unboxed words denote enzymes. TH – tyrosine hydroxylase; AADC – Aromatic L-amino acid decarboxylase; βH – β-hydroxylase; PMNT – phenylethanolamine N-methyltransferase; MAO – monoamine oxidase; COMT - catechol-O-methyltransferase; AR – aldehyde reductase; ADH – alcohol dehydrogenase; AD – aldehyde dehydrogenase; DOPEGAL – 3,4-dihydroxyphenylglycolaldehyde; NMN – normetanephrine; MN – metanephrines; DHPG – 3,4-dihydroxyphenylglycol; MHPG – 3-methoxy-4-hydroxyphenylglycol; MOPEGAL – 3-methoxy-4-hydroxyphenylglycolaldehyde; VMA – vanillylmandelic acid. Thick arrows indicate predominant mechanism of degradation.

The major end product in catecholamine synthesis is vanillylmandelic acid (VMA) *(9)*. The principal sites of catecholamine degradation include the sympathetic neurones, the adrenal medulla and the liver *(10)*. Enzymes involved in the degradation of catecholamines include catechol-O-methyltransferase (COMT), monoamine oxidase (MAO), aldose, and aldehyde reductase. Catechol-O-methyltransferase is only present extra-neuronally while monoamine oxidase is present both intra and extra-neuronally and this distribution of enzymes determines the process of degradation *(11)*. The major proportion of initial catecholamine metabolism occurs in the sympathetic neurones *(12)* and subsequently in the liver where 3-methoxy-4-hydroxyphenylglycol (MHPG) is converted to VMA *(13, 14)*. Figure 1 illustrates the principal steps in the synthesis and metabolism of catecholamines. Dopamine is converted to the end product homovanilic acid (HVA) via monoamine oxidase, aldehyde dehydrogenase, and catechol-O-methyltransferase. Unlike VMA production which is predominantly from the liver, most homovanilic acid is produced peripherally *(15)*.

Adrenoceptors

The receptors in the sympathetic ganglion and the adrenal medulla are nicotinic acetylcholine receptors. The other post-ganglionic neurones synapse with the adrenoceptors. Adrenoceptors are divided into α-adrenoceptors (α_1 and α_2) and the β-adrenoceptors (β_1, β_2, and β_3). Further subdivisions have identified a total of 9 adrenoceptors to date *(16)*. The broad distribution of adrenoceptor subtypes in the viscera lead to the protean variation in response to stimulation. Table 1 shows the distribution of the predominant adrenoceptors in the key viscera.

Alpha1-adrenoceptor effects are mediate by phospholipase C via Gq/11 (eventually leading to calcium release), α_2-adrenoceptor cause adenylate cyclase inhibition via G_i (leading to reduced generation of cAMP and reduced calcium

Table 1
Adrenoceptor distribution and predominant sympathetic visceral effects

Organ	Receptors	Effect
Arteries		
skin/mucosa	α_1 α_2	Constriction
skeletal muscle	α_1 α_2	Constriction
	β_2	Vasodilatation
Coronary arteries	α_1 α_2	Constriction
	β_2	Vasodilatation
Pulmonary arteries	α_1	Constriction
	β_2	Vasodilatation
Heart- conducting system	β_1 β_2	↑ chronicity, ↑ ionotropic force
Skeletal muscle	β_2	↑ ionotropic force, ↑ glycogenolysis
Lungs – trachea/bronchi	β_2	Dilatation
Eyes		
Radial muscles/iris	α_1	mydriasis (pupil dilatation)
Ciliary muscle	β_2	relaxation → distant focus
GI tract		
Motility/tone	α_1 α_2 β_1 β_2	Relaxation
Sphincters	α_1	Constriction
Sweat Glands	α_1	Sweating

release), and β-adrenoceptor cause adenylate cyclase stimulation via G_s (calcium release via increase generation in cAMP) *(17)*.

Both noradrenaline and adrenaline have equal affinity for α and $β_1$-adrenoceptors but the $β_2$-adrenoceptors have a higher affinity for adrenaline and the $β_3$ -adrenoceptors a higher affinity for noradrenaline *(16)*.

Catecholamine effects are determined by the adrenoceptor subtype; the coupled G-protein; the affinity of the agonist for the receptor; concentration of catecholamine; dissipation of catecholamine; number of receptors, and degree of receptor desensitisation *(18)*.

The actions of dopamine are mediated mainly by the dopamine receptors (D1-D5), however at higher circulating levels dopamine can activate both α and β-adrenoceptors. Peripheral dopamine effects include changes in blood flow, glomerular filtration rate, sodium excretion, catecholamine release, and ionotropic effects on the heart. Dopamine can act on pre-synaptic D2 receptors to inhibit noradrenaline release.

Fight or Flight

The sympathoadrenal system can be said to play two main roles; firstly to counterbalance the parasympathetic system in normal functioning and secondly to provide the 'extra gear' required during the 'fight or flight' response *(19)*. This requires optimal fuel delivery to the vital organs, that is, skeletal muscle, heart, brain, and lungs. To perform these functions, an intricate system of counterweighted controls has been developed, causing organ specific alterations in physiology and metabolism. Catecholamines are delivered to the effector organs via synapses with the post-ganglionic sympathetic neurone or via the circulation. Each pre-ganglionic sympathetic nerve can synapse with many post-ganglionic neurones and therefore sympathetic stimulation causes a co-ordinated wave of responses *(20)*. The advantages of a dual delivery of catecholamines include; prolonged duration of action of catecholamines via the circulation (half life in the circulation is 1–2 minutes, compared with milliseconds at the synaptic cleft); differential effect of adrenaline from the adrenal medulla on effector organs; stimulation of additional viscera without direct sympathetic innervations, for example, bronchioles, hepatocytes, and adipose tissue; 'back-up' system ensuring catecholamine delivery during stress confers a significant survival advantage.

Noradrenaline mediated vasoconstriction via $α_1$-receptors of the vasculature to 'non-essential' organs including the gastro-intestinal tract, kidney, and skin allows blood to be diverted to essential organs.

In the heart both $β_1$ and $β_2$-adrenoceptors are present with the $β_1$-adrenoreceptor being predominant. Both noradrenaline and adrenaline act on the β_1 receptors resulting in increased contractility, chronicity and rate of conduction. Adrenaline effects on β_2-adrenoreceptors maximise this response.

In the lungs, bronchiole dilatation allows increased oxygen uptake and carbon dioxide clearance for muscular respiration. There is no direct sympathetic nervous innervation to the bronchioles, therefore activation occurs via the circulation of adrenaline to the β_2-adrenoceptors.

The liver increases its production of glucose for skeletal muscle and the brain, initially by glycogenolysis and then predominantly by gluconeogenesis. These processes occur via adrenaline effects on the β_2-adrenoceptors.

The release of insulin is inhibited by the α_2-adrenoceptors in the pancreas to maximise the availability of glucose.

In adipose tissue, adrenaline, via its effects on the β_3-adrenoceptors (also α_2, β_1, β_2) causes increased lipolysis resulting in the release of free fatty acids for use as energy by skeletal muscle and an increase in thermogenesis.

The eye adapts with sympathetic stimulation resulting in pupil dilatation by contraction of the radial muscle of the iris (via α_1-adrenoceptors) and lens adjustment for distant vision by the ciliary muscles (β_2-adrenoceptors).

Sweating occurs over the skin as a result of sweat gland stimulation by cholinergic and $\alpha 1$-adrenergic stimulation. This allows thermoregulation, dissipation of heat and reduces friction between moving limbs.

The effects of dopamine are dependent on the circulating levels and can range from peripheral vasodilatation, natriuresis and diuresis at low circulating levels, mediated by D1 receptors, to peripheral vasoconstriction and increased chronotropic and ionotropic stimulation to the heart at higher circulating levels via the α and β_1-adrenoceptors respectively.

PHAEOCHROMOCYTOMA AND PARAGANGLIOMA

Definitions

The WHO 2004 definition of a phaeochromocytoma is a tumour arising from catecholamine-producing chromaffin cells in the adrenal medulla – an intra-adrenal paraganglioma. Paragangliomas are extra-adrenal chromaffin tumours of either sympathetic (secretory) or parasympathetic (mainly non-secretory) origin *(21)*, located between the base of skull and the pelvis. Both occur in sporadic and familial forms.

Aetiology

The old rule that only 10% of such tumours are familial is an underestimate. Registries of subjects with apparently sporadic phaeochromocytomas and paragangliomas, that is, no family history of similar disease, reveal that up to 30% of subjects have germ-line mutations in known familial genes *(22–24)*. These syndromes include Von Hippel-Lindau disease, Multiple Endocrine Neoplasia type 2, Familial Paraganglioma Syndromes type 1,3,4, and Neurofibromatosis type 1 caused by the VHL, RET, SDH-D, SDH-C, SDH-B, NF-1 genes respectively. Paragangliomas are also associated with the sporadic Carney's Triad syndrome of paragangliomas with gastric stromal tumours (GISTs) and pulmonary chondromas *(25)* and the recently described familial Carney-Stratakis syndrome (paraganglioma and gastric stromal tumours alone) associated with SDH mutations *(26)*.

Somatic mutations of the Rearranged during tranfection (RET), VHL, and SDH genes have been identified in phaeochromocytomas and paragangliomas in subjects without identifiable germline mutations *(27–31)*. Though in the large majority of cases genetic information will not be available in the acute setting, such information can allow a prediction of tumour behaviour (including future risk of malignancy) and the possibility of identifying disease at an early stage in the affected subject and other family members.

Epidemiology

The annual incidence of phaeochromocytoma is estimated at 1 to 8 per million *(32–35)*. Amongst hypertensive subjects the prevalence is between 0.1 to 0.6% *(36)*. However, up to 75% of phaeochromocytomas are only discovered at autopsy *(37)* suggesting higher overall rates of disease *(38)*.

Sex distribution is equal and the highest incidence is in the 4th to 5th decade *(39)*; however, tumours associated with syndromal disease tend to occur at a younger age *(22)*. Phaeochromocytoma account for between 4 to 8% of incidentally diagnosed adrenal tumours *(40, 41)* and between 80 to 90% of chromaffin tissue tumours, whilst paragangliomas make up the remainder (10 to 20%) *(32, 42)*. Most paragangliomas are intra-abdominal (75%) whilst the remaining 25% are extra-abdominal (10% thoracic, 10% pelvic, and 4% in head and neck region) *(42)*. Malignancy rates run at approximately 10% for phaeochromocytomas and up to 40% for paragangliomas *(39, 42)*.

Pathogenesis

The association of phaeochromocytoma and paraganglioma with several familial syndromes provides an insight into the pathogenesis of disease. These include Von Hippel-Lindau (VHL) disease, Multiple endocrine neoplasia type 2 (MEN 2), Familial Paraganglioma Syndromes type 1, 3, 4 (PGL-1, PGL- 3, PGL-4), and Neurofibromatosis type 1 (NF1). The associated features and genetic defects are described in Table 2. As per Knudson's two hit hypothesis, a second hit is needed to accompany the abnormal germline allelic mutation to cause disease *(43)*.

Table 2
Disease syndromes associated with phaeochromocytoma and paraganglioma.
Associated genetic defects and associated features. MEN – multiple endocrine
neoplasia; VHL – Von Hippel Lindau. PGL-Familial Paraganglioma Syndrome.
Modified from Lenders et al. *(36)*

Disease	Gene	Associated features
MEN 2A	RET	Medullary thyroid carcinoma Hyperparathyroidism Phaeochromocytoma Hirschsprung's disease
MEN 2B	RET	Medullary thyroid carcinoma Hyperparathyroid Phaeochromocytoma Ganglioneuromatosis of GI tract Marfanoid habitus Hyperflexible joints
VHL Disease	VHL	Retinal haemangiomas CNS haemangioblastoma Phaeochromocytoma Renal cell carcinoma Pancreatic cysts and neoplasms Endolymphatic sac tumours Epididymal cystadenomas
PGL-1	SDH-D	Phaeochromocytoma Paraganglioma Gastrointestinal stromal tumours
PGL-3	SDH-C	Paraganglioma Gastrointestinal stromal tumours
PGL-4	SDH-B	Phaeochromocytoma Paraganglioma Gastrointestinal stromal tumours Renal cell carcinoma
Neurofibromatosis	NF1	Café-au-lait spots Lisch nodules Axillary freckling Optic glioma

Table 2
(Continued)

Disease	Gene	Associated features
		Neurofibromas
		Phaeochromocytoma
		Tibial bowing
Carney's Triad	Sporadic	Gastrointestinal stromal tumours
		Extra-adrenal paragangliomas
		Pulmonary chondromas
		Oesophageal leiomyomas

Recent studies using global expression profiling have demonstrated 2 clusters of transcription associations *(44)*. The most extensively studied cluster is that of the genetic defects in the VHL, SDH-D, and SDH-B genes. This cluster has transcription signatures suggestive of hypoxia, angiogenesis, and oxidoreductase imbalance (Fig. 2). Other mechanism may involve the high levels of reactive oxygen species (ROS) generated and mitochondrial resistance to apoptosis *(49, 50)*.

The second transcription signature was noted with Multiple Endocrine Neoplasia type 2 and Neurofibromatosis and the associated genes RET and NF1 respectively *(44)*. Though mutations in these genes have been linked to tumourigenesis, a direct link to phaeochromocytoma has not been established. The RET proto-oncogene encodes a transmembrane receptor with an extracellular cysteine-rich domain and an intracellular tyrosine kinase domain *(51)*. Mutations in this gene lead to constitutive activation of the receptors and increased catalytic activity of the intracellular kinase domain predisposing to tumour formation *(52, 53)*. NF1 acts as a tumour suppressor gene, encodes the protein neurofibromin and is found in tissue of neuroectodermal origin *(54)*. This protein acts as a Ras GTPase activating protein (Ras GAP) which inactivates Ras (GTPase) by hydrolysis *(55)*. Ras signal transduction is important in the regulation of apoptosis and therefore mutations on NF1 can be linked to tumourigenesis *(56)*.

Catecholamine in Disease

Between 80–93% of phaeochromocytomas and approximately 20% of paragangliomas secrete catecholamines or their metabolites *(57–59)*. The majority of abdominal tumours (80 to 100%) secrete catecholamines in comparison to less than 5% of head and neck paragangliomas *(59)*. Several factors determine the characteristics of catecholamine secretion. These include associated genetic

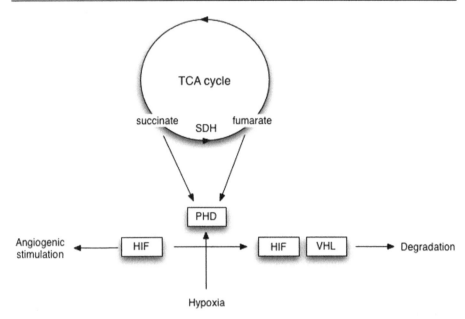

Fig. 2. Proposed mechanism for pathogenesis of phaeochromocytomas and paragangliomas via VEGF-HIF pathway. The VHL protein, under normoxic conditions, restricts hypoxic signalling by binding to hydroxylated hypoxic inducible factor 1α (HIF 1α) resulting in ubiquitinated degradation *(45)*. Lack of the VHL protein in disease leads to unsuppressed angiogenic stimulation of hypoxic inducible genes, for example, vascular endothelial growth factor (VEGF), hexokinase, lactate dehydrogenase, thrombospondin via HIF-1α which accelerates tumourigenesis *(46, 47)*. Several mechanisms are suggested for the role of SDH in the pathogenesis of disease. Prolyl hydroxylases are enzymes which hydroxylates HIF-1α prior to its degradation. SDH dysfunction leads to a build up of succinate which inhibits the prolyl hydroxylase resulting in non-degradation of HIF-1α and unsuppressed angiogenic stimulation *(48)*.

abnormality; site of tumour and the balance between catecholamine metabolism and secretion.

High levels of adrenaline secretion are associated with adrenal lesions *(58)* due to the presence of the enzyme phenylethanolamine N-methyltransferase, causing the conversion of noradrenaline to adrenaline *(60)*. Indeed a proportion of phaeochromocytomas secrete adrenaline only *(61)*. Extra-adrenal paragangliomas are synonymous with predominant noradrenaline secretion *(59, 62)*. Different syndromes produce characteristic catecholamines secretion patterns. Hence tumours associated with MEN2 and NF1 result in the secretion of both adrenaline and noradrenaline whilst those associated SDH and VHL, noradrenaline predominates *(60, 63, 64)*. Malignant disease has been associated with higher levels of noradrenaline and dopamine secretion and a lower ratio of adrenaline to adrenaline and noradrenaline *(58, 65, 66)*.

Other Active Products

Phaeochromocytomas have been shown to also secrete other vasoactive peptides and hormones including; neuropeptide Y; adrenomedullin; atrial natriuretic peptide; met-enkephalin; dopa; calcitonin gene-relate peptide; vasoactive intestinal peptide(VIP); parathormone (PTH); PTH related peptide (PTHrP) and adrenocorticotrophic hormone (ACTH) *(67)*. Ectopic ACTH has been shown to cause bilateral adrenal hyperplasia and Cushing's syndrome in both phaeochromocytomas and paragangliomas *(68, 69)*. These tumours also secrete pro-inflammatory cytokines such as IL-1 and IL-6 *(70, 71)*. Both cytokines can influence steroidogenesis by inducing production of corticotrophin-releasing hormone (CRH) and ACTH in tumour cells *(72, 73)* and initiating a systematic inflammatory response *(71, 74)*. Adrenomedullin can act as a potent vasodilator and may provide a compensatory mechanism to catecholamine induced vasoconstriction; however, it is a biologically ubiquitous peptide not specific to phaeochromocytoma with a plethora of other functions from cellular growth and differentiation to modulation of hormone secretion *(75)*.

Presentation

The majority of subjects present with symptoms as a result of catecholamine excess or mass effect *(65)*. However, there is a lack of correlation between catecholamine levels, severity of hypertension, and symptoms *(76)*. Increasing levels of abdominal imaging have resulted in the identification of phaeochromocytoma 'incidentalomas'. As screening of families with germline mutations becomes comprehensive, more subjects with pre-symptomatic disease are being identified. Table 3 provides a list of features which may point to a diagnosis of a catecholamine secreting tumour.

Catecholamine secreting tumours are 'the great mimic' of many medical conditions and the presentation can be hugely varied. Table 4 provides a list of differentials and highlights conditions where the possibility of catecholamine secreting tumours should be considered. Clinical features fall into 2 categories; those during a paroxysm and sustained effects as a result of hypertension. Paroxysms may occur on a daily basis to every few months. Paroxysms on average last between 15 and 60 minutes but can last a few minutes to several hours *(77)*. They may occur spontaneously or secondary to a precipitant (Table 5). Sustained features included cardiomyopathy, hypertensive nephropathy in the form of nephrosclerosis and hypertensive retinopathy.

The classical triad of headaches, palpitations and diaphoresis are the most common symptoms. Presence of these 3 symptoms has been reported to have a sensitivity and specificity of over 90% in hypertensive subjects *(78)*. Other symptoms are listed in Table 6. Hypertension may be sustained in a half or paroxysmal in a third of subjects. Up to a sixth of subjects have normal blood

Table 3

**Features suggestive of a diagnosis of phaeochromocytoma
or secreting paraganglioma**

Clues to diagnosis

Hypertension + triad symptoms
Poorly controlled hypertension
Paroxysmal symptoms
Relevant precipitants
Associated hypotension
Hypotension refractory to fluid/ionotropes
Relevant syndromal features
Family history – hypertension, abdominal
    tumours, or sudden death in young subjects

pressure (Bravo EL 1994). Indeed hypotension or clinic shock can result from predominantly adrenaline or dopamine secretion *(80, 81)*. Noradrenaline secretion has also been associated with hypotension though the mechanism remains unclear *(82)*. Such blood pressure liability has been attributed to episodic catecholamine release, impaired sympathetic reflexes, and chronic volume depletion *(83)*.

Catecholamine secreting tumours may present acutely as cardiovascular, neurological, gastroenterological, renal, and psychiatric disease.

Cardiovascular disease presents either acutely, during paroxysms, for example, myocardial infarction, aortic dissection, arrhythmia, acute pulmonary oedema, or as a result of hypertension over a longer period, for example, reversible cardiomyopathy (dilating or hypertrophic). Rhythm disturbances are predominantly tachyarrhymthias but may also paradoxically be bradyarrhymthmias (including asystole) mediated by the baroreceptors response to hypertensive surges. Pulmonary oedema can occur as a consequence of cardiogenic shock or a non-cardiogenic form, secondary to altered pulmonary circulation dynamics *(82)*.

Neurological presentations as a result of hypertension include cerebral haemorrhage and infarction (Fig. 3C), subarachnoid haemorrhage, seizures, and visual deterioration secondary to hypertensive retinopathy. Posterior reversible encephalopathy syndrome (PRES) which includes the association of headache, confusion, seizure, visual loss in association with a predominant posterior leukoencephalopathy secondary to oedema *(84)* has been associated with phaeochromocytoma *(85)*. Spinal metastasis may cause cord compression presenting as a paraparesis *(86)*.

Table 4
Differential diagnosis for symptoms associated with phaeochromocytoma and paraganglioma. MAO – monoamine oxidase; POTS – postural orthostatic tachycardia syndrome. Modified from Lenders et al. (36)

Cardiovascular	Neurological	Endocrine
Heart failure	Migraine	Hyperthyroidism
Arrhythmias	Stroke	Carcinoid
Ischaemic heart disease	Seizure	Hypoglycaemia
Baroreflex failure	Visual loss	Medullary thyroid carcinoma
	Diencephalic epilepsia	Menopausal syndrome
	Meningioma	
	POTS	
	Serotonin syndrome	
Drugs	**Psychiatric**	**Miscellaneous**
Sympathomimetic drugs	Panic disorder	Pre-eclampsia
MAO inhibitors	Anxiety	Mastocytosis
Clonidine withdrawal	Psychosis	Porphyria
Cocaine		Neuroleptic malignant syndrome
		Malignant hyperpyrexia

A gastrointestinal presentation as an acute abdomen may be due to tumour haemorrhage, bowel ischaemia or infarction secondary to vasoconstriction, paralytic ileus, bowel obstruction and perforation. Occult phaeochromocytoma can be mistaken for other acute abdominal presentations and only become apparent with hypertensive surges during abdominal surgery.

Acute renal failure due to accelerated hypertension, renal ischaemia, and rhabdomyolysis secondary to muscle ischaemia have all be described (87).

Accelerated hypertension may cause multi-organ failure in association with hypertension/hypotension, elevated temperature and encephalopathy (88).

Anxiety symptoms may be mistaken for neurotic disorders and psychotic symptoms have been an initial presenting feature of catecholamine secreting tumours (89, 90).

Fever, symptoms related to anaemia and thrombo-embolic disease may all result from the pro-inflammatory response mediated by IL-1 and IL-6 (74).

Subjects with dopamine-only secreting tumours may be asymptomatic, present with symptoms of mass effect or an inflammatory-type syndrome as a result of malignant disease (91, 92). Normotension or hypotension as a result of dopamine receptor stimulation may be noted. Classical adrenergic symptoms

Table 5
Precipitants of catecholamine release

Precipitants

Spontaneous
Exercise
Medication e.g., metoclopromide
                 sympathomimetics
                 tricyclic antidepressants
Anaesthesia
Micturition
Surgical manipulation
Defaecation
Trauma
Pregnancy
Lifting
Straining
Bending

Table 6
Symptoms and clinical signs of disease in catecholamine secreting tumours.
SVT – supra-ventricular tachycardia; LVH - left ventricular hypertrophy
Modified from Lenders et al. *(36)* and Manelli et al. *(79)*

Symptoms	*Clinical findings*
Headache	Hypertension- episodic, sustained
Palpitations	Postural hypotension
Sweating	Tachycardia
Pallor	Perspiration
Nausea	Pallor
Flushing	Tachypnoea
Weight loss	Weight loss
Tiredness	Hypergylcaemia
Anxiety	Hypertensive retinopathy/papilloedema
Chest pain	ECG findings
Shortness of breath	– arrhythmia (sinus tachycardia, SVT, ectopics)
Constipation	– cardiomegaly (LVH, T wave inversion)
	– infarction/ischemia (ST elevation/depression,
	T wave inversion)

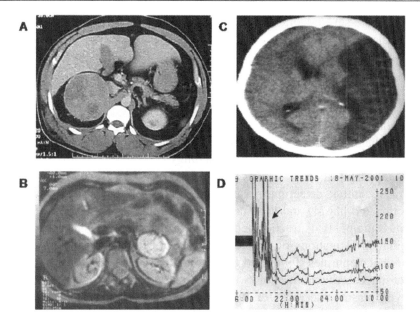

Fig. 3. A. CT scan (pre-contrast) of a large right side adrenal phaeochromocytoma. Note inhomogeneous appearance. **B**. MRI scan (T2-weighted image) of a left-sided adrenal phaeochromocytoma showing high signal intensity due to hypervascularity. **C**. CT head scan showing a large left cerebral infarct due to hypertension. **D**. Blood pressure trace in subject during hypertensive crisis and subsequent control following administration of phenoxybenzamine intravenously (*arrow*).

have been reported with dopamine-only secreting tumours *(91)* and may result from α and β-adrenoceptor stimulation at higher circulating levels.

Identification of syndromal features during clinic examination will improve surveillance for subsequent disease. Multifocal or metastatic disease may be more prevalent, there may be associated extraparaganglial disease and disease in other affected family members can be identified. Table 2 lists the associated syndrome and clinical features.

Differential Diagnosis

A number of conditions may mimic the clinical presentation of phaeochromocytoma (Table 4). These include cocaine use (via block of uptake 1), amphetamine use, malignant neuroleptic syndrome, and even thyrotoxicosis. The difficulty is that such patients may also have elevations of catecholamines and metabolites but will have normal imaging. A medication and illicit drug history and examination of the thyroid are mandatory. Patients with renal failure may also have severe labile hypertension and elevated plasma catecholamines, causing diagnostic concern.

INVESTIGATIONS

Biochemical and other Parameters

Once a catecholamine secreting lesion is suspected it is essential to initially make the diagnosis biochemically, given the high incidence of incidental adrenal lesions *(93)*. Once established, these findings can then be radiologically and functionally confirmed.

In most centres, detection of catecholamine excess is via the measurement of fractionated plasma and/or urinary catecholamines or metanephrines. However, measurements of fractionated plasma or urinary metanephrines are now the initial investigations of choice *(94)*. The sensitivity for measurement of plasma metanephrines (99%) and urinary metanephrines (97%) is higher than for plasma catecholamines (86%), and urinary catecholamines (84%) *(94)*. However, plasma measures of metanephrines using the radioimmuno-assay method appear slightly less robust than the studies using the highly purified liquid chromatography (HPLC) method *(95)*. The high levels of catechol-O-methyltransferase (COMT) in phaeochromocytomas results in metabolism of catecholamines into metanephrines *(96)*. The often paroxysmal nature of catecholamine release and the short half-life of catecholamine in the circulation (1–2 minutes) compared to metanephrines, mean the latter are more amenable to detection *(96, 97)*. Indeed measures of total urinary metanephrines appear to correlate with overall tumour burden whilst catecholamines do not *(96, 98)*. These measures have superseded the use of other intermediates and final products in catecholamine metabolism (e.g., VMA, HVA) both in terms of sensitivity and specificity. A clear limitation in the measurement of metanephrines, however, is the ability to detect dopamine-only secreting tumours especially given that these tumours can be difficult to detect due to lack of symptoms. In these cases, a measurement of plasma dopamine or methoxytyramine (O-methylated metabolite) provides higher diagnostic accuracy than urinary dopamine *(99)*.

Catecholamine levels in subjects with acute or chronic stress are appropriately elevated *(100)* and therefore delineating high levels due to a phaeochromocytoma or paraganglioma can be difficult in the acute setting. This is compounded by the use of catecholamine ionotropes in the critical care setting. Studies show that plasma adrenaline can increase up to 300 times normal levels during acute stress *(100)*.

Suppression testing with clonidine and pentolinium and provocation tests with glucagon to detect catecholamine secreting tumours are less frequently used due to the improved sensitivity and specificity of metanephrines measurements. The clonidine suppression test has been shown to have a high specificity but a low sensitivity and therefore its use is in identifying subjects with false positive biochemical screening *(101)*.

Other metabolic associations can include hyperglycaemia (reduced insulin release, inhibition hepatic/muscle uptake), hypercalcaemia (ecoptic PTH or PTHrP), hypokalaemic alkalosis (ecoptic ACTH or CRH leading to excess cortisol secretion) *(67)*. Serum calcitonin and calcium may also be elevated in association with MEN 2.

Phaeochromocytomas have been associated with paraneoplastic erythrocytosis due to erythropoeitin overproduction *(102)*. Another study notes the higher measures of leukocytes, neutrophils, and platelets in hypertensives with phaeochromocytomas compared with other forms of hypertension *(103)*. As noted earlier, the inflammatory response mediate by cytokines such as IL-6 can result in raised inflammatory markers, thrombocytosis, hyperfibrinogenaemia, and anaemia *(71, 104)* The anaemia may be masked, however, by haemoconcentration secondary to volume depletion.

Plasma chromogranin A, a protein co-secreted with catecholamines in phaeochromocytoma is present both in benign and malignant, functional and non-functional disease *(105, 106)*. It has been used to identify disease, monitor disease relapse, and progression *(107)*. Other markers that may differentiate between benign and malignant disease include chromogranin B, chromogranin C (secretogranin II), prohormone convertases 1 and 2, neuron-specific enolase, ACTH, and aromatic L-amino acid decarboxylase (ALAAD) *(58, 107)*.

Radiological Imaging

Both CT and MR scanning provide equally sensitive and specific imaging modalities to detect phaeochromocytomas and paragangliomas, however, choices regarding imaging may be based on local availability and expertise. Figure 3 (3A and 3B) shows tumour images with both modalities. Several of the germline mutations predispose to extra-abdominal disease and therefore it is important to have complete imaging from the base of the skull to the pelvis, though in the acute setting this may not be appropriate. A stepwise approach may be more suitable, that is, abdomen and pelvis followed by neck and then thorax, should disease not be found initially.

CT scanning will allow the differentiation of benign adrenal adenomas from phaeochromocytoma. On non-contrast scans most benign adenomas have an attenuation of <10 Hounsfield (Hu) units based on their high lipid content. Lesions with attenuation between 40–50 Hu without evidence of haemorrhage or calcifications may be compatible with a diagnosis of a chromaffin tumour *(108)*. On a delayed, contrast-enhanced CT, an absolute percentage washout of less than 60% is in keeping with non-adenomatous lesions *(108)*. Haemorrhage and necrosis can give an inhomogeneous appearance. Overall sensitivity for CT varies between 77 and 98% while specificity is lower at 29–92% *(109)*. Importantly, ionic contrast agents can precipitate a hypertensive crisis and therefore subjects should be fully α and β-blocked prior to imaging or alternatively a preference given to non-ionic contrast agents *(110)*.

MR imaging of phaeochromocytomas demonstrate variable signal intensity on T1 weighted imaging but high signal intensity on T2 weighted imaging (high fluid content due to hypervascularity) *(108)*. Haemorrhage and necrosis in the tumours can result in reduced signal on the T2 weighted image *(109)*. Importantly, phaeochromocytomas do not lose signal on out of phase images in contrast to adrenal adenomas. MR provides a useful tool for the identification of extra-adrenal paraganglioma *(111)*. It has a sensitivity of 90–100% and a specificity of 50–100% *(109)*.

Ultrasound may be useful in localising paragangliomas of the neck *(109)*.

Functional Imaging

Functional imaging allows confirmation of radiological and biochemical findings but is of particular benefit in the identification of multiple tumours, metastatic disease, and lesions not identified with radiological imaging *(112)*. Specific imaging relies on the uptake of compounds by chromaffin tissue via the human norepinephrine transporter (hNET) at the plasma membrane and vesicular monoamine transporters (VMAT) on storage vesicles *(113)*. Compounds used include meta-iodobenzylguanidine (MIBG) and various positron emission tomography (PET) ligands, while non-specific imaging includes the use of somatostatin analogues (e.g., ^{111}In–pentetreotide) and [^{18}F]fluorodeoxyglucose (FDG) PET *(109)*. MIBG and somatostatin receptor scintigraphy have the additional benefit of determining future treatment options in the case of metastatic disease.

Functional imaging using ^{123}I MIBG, a guanethidine analogue, has a sensitivity of 83–100% and a specificity of 95–100% *(114, 115)*. As MIBG is mostly excreted via the kidney, localising bladder and pelvic paragangliomas can be problematic. Figure 4 demonstrates at positive ^{123}I MIBG scan of an adrenal phaeochromocytoma.

Radiolabelled somatostatin analogues, for example ^{111}In–pentetreotide, exploit the presence of somatostatin receptors in chromaffin tumours, particularly the type 2 and 4 receptors *(116)*. Though the sensitivity of somatostatin scintigraphy is significantly less than with MIBG in chromaffin tumour

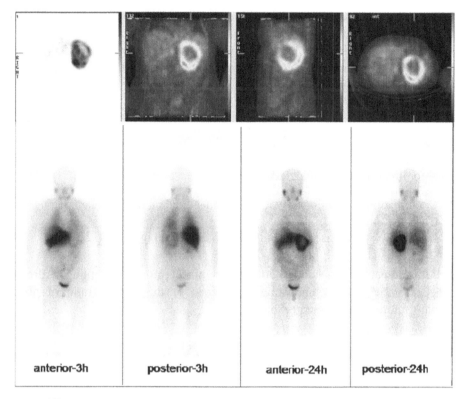

| anterior-3h | posterior-3h | anterior-24h | posterior-24h |

Fig. 4. [123]I MIBG images of a left-sided adrenal phaeochromocytoma. Upper panel – single photon emission computed tomography (SPECT) image. Note central paucity of enhancement consistent with central tumour necrosis. Lower panel, 2 images to the left taken at 3 hours and 2 images to right, lower panel taken at 24 hours. Tumour enhancement with radionucleotide more prominent at 24 hours.

identification *(117, 118)*, the detection of metastatic lesions not seen with MIBG imaging suggests a complementary role for it *(114, 117)*.

PET provides another form of functional imaging which is of use where other functional imaging is negative and in particular with dopamine-only secreting lesions *(91)*. Both specific ligands including, [^{11}C]hydroxyephedrine; [11C]epinephrine; [^{18}F] Dihydroxyphenylalanine (DOPA) and [^{18}F] fluorodopamine (DA) and non-specific ligands, which utilise increased glucose uptake by tumours, such as [^{18}F]fluoro-2-deoxy-D-glucose (FDG) are in use *(109)*. Clearly specific functional imaging is preferential. In a recent study of SDH-B subjects with malignant chromaffin tumours [^{18}F] FDG PET appeared more sensitive (100%) compared to other ligands including ^{123}I MIBG (80%) and [^{18}F] DA (88%) in detecting disease *(119)*. [^{18}F] FDG PET has a role in detecting tumours which have de-differentiated or are rapidly growing which specific ligands would not detect *(109)*.

Future advances in the field will include the use of new more specific radioligands *(67)* and the integration of radiological and functional imaging modalities to allow improved disease identification and localisation such as ^{131}I MIBG/MR and PET/CT *(120, 121)*.

Venous Sampling

This can be a useful adjuvant investigation if expertise is available. Indications for this investigation include:

1. Confirmation of functionality of a lesion identified on radiological imaging
2. Confirmation of bilateral disease
3. Localisation of disease not identified with functional imaging *(122)*.

Full adrenergic blockade should be in place prior to sampling. Adrenal phaeochromocytomas demonstrate a reversal of the normal ratio of noradrenaline:adrenaline to greater than 1.

MANAGEMENT

BP Control/ Adrenergic Blockade

The cornerstone of management of catecholamine secreting lesions is blood pressure control. No evidence-based trials are available to guide management but recommendations have been made on the basis of international consensus *(123)*. Alpha and β-blockade are the mainstay of treatment though other anti-hypertensives including calcium antagonists and angiotensin converting enzyme (ACE) inhibitors are used. Table 7 provides a summary of commonly used medication and doses. Dosages for all anti-hypertensives should be titrated according to blood pressure and side-effects. Parasympathetic head and neck paragangliomas and dopamine only secreting lesions are exceptions where blockade may not be required *(125)*. It was noted however, that hypertensive surges with tumour manipulation are seen in tumours associated with no catecholamine secretion and normotension pre-operatively *(125)*.

Alpha-blockers used include phenoxybenzamine, doxazocin, prazocin, and tetrazocin. Phenoxybenzamine is the only irreversible α_1/α_2-adrenergic blocker. This can be given orally and intravenously. In the acute setting, phenoxybenzamine can be given intravenously at a dose of 1 mg/kg in 250 ml of 5% dextrose over 2–4 hours. Figure 3D demonstrates its rapid onset of action. Orally, doses are started at 5–10 mg twice a day and can be titrated up to 1 mg/kg in divided

Table 7

Drug and dosages used in the management of catecholamine secreting tumours. Modified from Chew et al. (124)

Type	Drug	Dose range	Comments
Alpha-adrenoceptor blocker	Phenoxybenzamine	5 – 10 mg oral qds	non-competitive, non-selective
Beta-adrenoceptor blocker	Propranolol	0.5 – 1 mg/kg infusion daily 20 – 80 mg oral tds	non-selective
Alpha-adrenoceptor blocker	Phentolamine	1 mg intravenous bolus 1 mg intravenous bolus	non-selective, 50 min half-life
Beta-adrenoceptor blocker	Esmolol	400 mcg/kg/min infusion	short-acting, 9 min half-life
Alpha-adrenoceptor blocker	Prazosin	5 mg oral od	selective alpha-1
Beta-adrenoceptor blocker	Bisoprolol	10 – 20 mg oral od	cardioselective
Alpha-adrenoceptor blocker	Urapidil	10 – 15 mg infusion per hour	selective alpha-1, 3-h half-life
Calcium channel blocker	Nicardipine	60 – 120 mg oral daily	
Calcium channel blocker	Nifedipine	2.5 – 7.5 mcg/kg/min infusion 30 – 90 mg oral daily	
Vasodilator	Sodium nitroprusside	0.5 – 1.5 mcg/Kg/min	

doses (maximum daily dose of 2 mg/kg). Common side effects include postural hypotension, lethargy, and nasal stuffiness. Pre-synaptic α_2-adrenergic blockade on sympathetic neurones inhibits negative feedback resulting in increased release of noradrenaline at cardiac sympathetic nerve terminals leading to reflex tachycardia (126). The advantage of phenoxybenzamine is the longer duration of irreversible blockade, however, this can result in a higher risk of post-operative hypotension (127) and intra-operative bleeding. Excess somnolence in the first 48 hours as a result of central α_2-adrenergic blockade can hamper post-operative recovery (126).

Doxazocin, prazocin, and tetrazocin are competitive specific α_1-adrenoceptor antagonists. Though first dose hypotension is an issue, less associated post-operative hypotension and the absence of reflex tachycardia (no pre-synaptic α_2-adrenergic blockade) mean β-blockade may not be required (126).

Beta-blockade can improve blood pressure control and the associated tachyarrhythmia. They should only be initiated after α-blockade due to the risk of a hypertensive crisis from unopposed α_1-mediated vasoconstriction. Commonly used β-blockers include the β_1-selective agents, atenolol, and metoprolol and the non-selective β_1/β_2 blocker propranolol. Labetolol, a dual α and β-blocker is not a recommended initial agent for adrenergic blockade because of its predominant β over α action which can paradoxically induce a hypertensive crisis. It can, however, be used in addition to established α/β blockade.

Calcium antagonists used for blood pressure control include amlodipine, nicardipine, nifedipine and verapamil. Though there is no direct adrenergic blockade, these agents block catecholamine induced calcium influx into the vascular smooth muscle resulting in muscular relaxation and vasodilatation (128). Advantages of calcium antagonist use include their use as adjuvant agents in those not controlled by α and β-blockade and that they are not associated with significant hypotension.

Metyrosine is an analogue of tyrosine that blocks catecholamine production by inhibiting tyrosine hydroxylase. It is used as an adjuvant to adrenergic blockade. Drug availability and potential side effects including depression, sedation, anxiety, extra-pyramidal signs, diarrhoea, crystalluria and galactorrhoea can limit its use. Dosages start at 250 mg three times a day up to 4 g/day in divided doses. In combination with α-blockade it has been shown to reduce the intra-operative hypertensive surges and the requirement for treatment (129).

The somatostatin analogue octreotide has been used in cases with poor blood pressure control with adrenergic blockade. In the acute setting, it can be given via a subcutaneous 24 h infusion. The suggested mechanism is via inhibition of cell depolarisation and calcium influx in tumour cells resulting in reduced catecholamine release (130).

The aim of adrenergic blockade is haemodynamic stability, volume expansion, and full α and β-adrenergic blockade in anticipation of surgery. Though there is no consensus as to how long before surgery blockade should be initiated, in most centres it is commenced at least 1–2 weeks prior. Blood pressure should be brought down to at least 140/90 mm/Hg with reduced labile episodes and associated tachycardia. Postural hypotension should begin to improve as the circulating volume expands. Intravenous fluid administration may be required and occasionally a blood transfusion is necessary if haemodilution is marked. Patients may have additional α-blockade for 3 days with intravenous phenoxybenzamine before surgery *(124)*.

Prior to surgery a complete work-up should identify and optimise any medical conditions which may influence surgical outcome, particularly cardiovascular status *(125)*. Adrenergic blockade is withheld on the day of surgery to reduce the risk of post-operative hypotension.

In cases of clear syndromal disease where subjects have other disease in association with phaeochromocytomas and paragangliomas, the emphasis is always on the initial management of the catecholamine secreting tumour to remove the risk of life-threatening complications when other disease is managed.

In the subject with a catecholamine secreting tumour who is critically ill or awaiting surgery, important considerations included the use of intra-arterial catheter for assessment of blood pressure, central intravenous catheter for rapid administration of anti-hypertensive agents, and assessment of intra-vascular volume *(131)*. Prior to surgery anxiolytic therapy is important for patient comfort as well as reducing the risk of haemodynamic instability *(131)*.

Surgery

Surgery is the mainstay of treatment and the laparoscopic approach to adrenalectomy is preferred to the open approach when possible *(132–134)*. Despite adequate preparation, hypertensive episodes still occur with tumour manipulation. The risk of uncontrolled bleeding without compensatory sympathetic vasoconstriction is significant. Operative success is dependent on the use of surgical and anaesthetic teams experienced in the management of catecholamine secreting tumours.

Intraoperatively, hypertensive surges are traditionally controlled with sodium nitroprusside and the non-specific α-blocker phentolamine. Sodium nitroprusside action results from the release of nitric oxide, a potent vasodilator. Its usefulness stems from its rapid onset of action within seconds of administration. It can be used inter-operatively and during hypertensive crisis not responding to α-blockade acutely. It can be given intravenously at a dose of 0.5–10 μg/kg/min. Degradation of sodium nitroprusside liberates cyanide ions which are converted to thiocyanate in the liver. Its use is limited to 72 hours and thiocyanate levels need to be monitored. Phentolamine is a non-selective α-blocker which causes marked vasodilatation which can result in precipitous fall in blood pressure. Other agents used intraoperatively include nitroglycerine, MgSO4, and urapidil (α_1-adrenergic antagonist). Magnesium inhibits the release of catecholamines from the adrenal medulla *(135)* and adrenergic nerve terminals *(136)*.

Tachyarrhythmia may be managed with lidocaine, labetalol, or the short-acting cardioselective β-blocker esmolol once α-blockade is in place *(126, 137)*.

During surgery, meticulous care is required monitoring blood pressure and fluid status. Post-operative hypotension can be significant for several reasons; intra-operative blood loss in the context of a contracted vascular volume; the source of the catecholamine excess has been removed; the blocked adrenoceptors cannot mediate vasoconstriction and the prior excess of catecholamines would desensitise the remaining receptors. Blood pressure should be monitored closely up to 48 hours after surgery and hypotension is managed with appropriate fluid replacement and vasopressor agents if necessary. After tumour removal, the risk of hypoglycaemia is increased as the result of hyperinsulinaemia (loss of α_2 mediate inhibition of insulin release from the pancreas) *(131)* along with the reduction in glycogenolysis and gluconeogenesis. Importantly prior β-blockade may mask hypoglycaemic symptoms *(138)*.

Other Treatment

Surgery, if amenable, is the mainstay of treatment for initial disease and indeed for metastatic disease. This can reduce catecholamine excretion, remove metastasis from anatomically compromising sites and possibly improve response to chemotherapy and ^{131}I-MIBG therapy *(139)*. Other methods such as radiofrequency ablation, cryoablation, and arterial embolisation can provide short-term, symptomatic benefit *(139–141)*.

To date the only other treatment modalities to show consistent benefit include chemotherapy and ^{131}I-MIBG therapy. Chemotherapy with cyclophosphamide, vincristine, and dacarbazine (CVD) appears the most effective regime with over half of subjects having at least a partial response to therapy *(142)*. However, disease appears to relapse after 2 years *(143, 144)*. Other regimes with some evidence of response include cisplatin and etoposide *(145)*, lomustine (CCNU) and cepacitabine (pro-drug of 5 Florouracil) *(146)*, and more recently the combination of temozolomide and thalidomide *(147)*.

^{131}I-MIBG therapy for metastatic disease results in a response (mainly partial) in approximately a third of subjects, stable disease in half and disease progression in a fifth of subjects *(107, 148)*. Treatment is well tolerated with the main side effects relating to bone marrow toxicity *(149)*. However, disease progression after an initial response was commonly seen within 2 years *(149)*.

Dosing and treatment interval regimes are variable and continue to be an area of ongoing study including the use of high dose[131]I-MIBG therapy *(150, 151)*. Determination of VMAT expression and therefore MIBG uptake may identify those most likely to respond to this therapy *(152)*.

Somatostatin analogue therapy in the form of octreotide and lanreotide has not shown a benefit *(153)* but radiolabelled analogues, commonly with yttrium 90 or indium 111 have shown some limited benefits. The distribution of somato-statin receptors in catecholamine producing tumours (predominantly sst3) *(154)* may limit the benefit of these analogues (high affinity sst2) but suggest newer analogues, for example, SOM230/pasireotide (high affinity sst3) may be of more benefit *(155)*.

Other possible strategies for therapy include the use of multi-targeted kinase inhibitor, for example, sorafenib and sunitinib to target the angiogenic HIF-VEGF pathway implicated in VHL and SDH disease. The chaperone pro-tein HSP 90, is important in the folding and delivery of proteins (e.g., telom-erase hTERT and HIF-1α in key pathways in tumourigenesis *(156)*. Specific inhibitors, for example, geldanamycin may provide a means to inhibit tumour growth *(157)*.

Prognosis

The risk of malignancy is increased in association with SDH-B muta-tions *(158)*, extra-adrenal paraganglioma *(39,42,79)*, tumours >5 cm *(39)* and tumours greater than 80 g *(42, 66)*. There are no histological features which can predict the risk of malignancy. Dopamine-only secreting tumours have been associated with higher rates of malignancy. Reasons cited for this asso-ciation include poor tumour differentiation (indicated by reduced levels of β-hydroxylase, the enzyme responsible for the conversion to noradrenaline), the lack of typical symptoms resulting in later presentation, larger tumours, and higher rates of malignancy *(91)*. Malignancy rates in sporadic phaeochromocy-toma are approximately 9% *(159)*.

In sporadic catecholamine secreting tumours, the 5 year survival is quoted as 96% *(160)*. In those with metastatic disease, the 5 year survival is 50% *(66, 139)*. Patients with bony metastasis may have long survival times, in some cases up to 20 years *(161)*.

SUMMARY

The rarity of phaeochromocytoma and paraganglioma, the frequency of the associated symptoms and the potential devastating consequences of such dis-ease mean that making a diagnosis is both difficult and yet crucial. It will allow a potential cure and the avoidance of significant associated mortality and morbidity. Several factors are essential for the successful management of these tumours. Most important is to consider the diagnosis with a suggestive history at the outset. It is essential to keep an open mind with potentially atypical presentations. Secondly, careful pre-operative preparation is the key to a positive surgical outcome. Finally the involvement of the multidisciplinary team in centres with relevant experience is a necessity. Understanding the basic pathophysiology and the genetic basis of disease enables us to predict disease patterns and tailor surveillance and may eventually point to new therapeutic interventions. In the event of metastatic disease, it should be borne in mind that survival can be prolonged in some instances and therefore any treatment should be carefully considered so as not to compromise the patient more than the disease itself.

Acknowledgments We would like to acknowledge the assistance of Dr Norbert Avril in providing the [123] I-MIBG imaging used in Fig. 4.

REFERENCES

1. Le Douarin NM. The Neural Crest: Cambridge University Press, Cambridge.; 1982.
2. Young HM, Anderson RB, Anderson CR. Guidance cues involved in the development of the peripheral autonomic nervous system. Auton Neurosci 2004; 112:1–14.
3. Ayer-Le Lievre CS, Le Douarin NM. The early development of cranial sensory ganglia and the potentialities of their component cells studied in quail-chick chimeras. Dev Biol 1982; 94:291–310.
4. Schneider C, Wicht H, Enderich J, Wegner M, Rohrer H. Bone morphogenetic proteins are required in vivo for the generation of sympathetic neurons. Neuron 1999; 24:861–70.
5. Honma Y, Araki T, Gianino S, et al. Artemin is a vascular-derived neurotropic factor for developing sympathetic neurons. Neuron 2002; 35:267–82.
6. Wingerd KL, Goodman NL, Tresser JW, et al. Alpha 4 integrins and vascular cell adhesion molecule-1 play a role in sympathetic innervation of the heart. J Neurosci 2002; 22: 10772–80.
7. Carnahan JF, Patterson PH. Isolation of the progenitor cells of the sympathoadrenal lineage from embryonic sympathetic ganglia with the SA monoclonal antibodies. J Neurosci 1991; 11:3520–30.
8. Blaschko H. The activity of l(–)-dopa decarboxylase. J Physiol 1942; 101:337–49.
9. Armstrong MD, Mc MA, Shaw KN. 3-Methoxy-4-hydroxy-D-mandelic acid, a urinary metabolite of norepinephrine. Biochim Biophys Acta 1957; 25:422–3.
10. Eisenhofer G, Kopin IJ, Goldstein DS. Catecholamine metabolism: a contemporary view with implications for physiology and medicine. Pharmacol Rev 2004; 56:331–49.
11. Graefe KH, Henseling M. Neuronal and extraneuronal uptake and metabolism of catecholamines. Gen Pharmacol 1983; 14:27–33.
12. Eisenhofer G. Plasma normetanephrine for examination of extraneuronal uptake and metabolism of noradrenaline in rats. Naunyn Schmiedebergs Arch Pharmacol 1994; 349:259–69.

13. Mardh G, Luehr CA, Vallee BL. Human class I alcohol dehydrogenases catalyze the oxidation of glycols in the metabolism of norepinephrine. Proc Natl Acad Sci U S A 1985; 82:4979–82.

14. Eisenhofer G, Rundquist B, Aneman A, et al. Regional release and removal of catecholamines and extraneuronal metabolism to metanephrines. J Clin Endocrinol Metab 1995; 80:3009–17.

15. Lambert GW, Eisenhofer G, Jennings GL, Esler MD. Regional homovanillic acid production in humans. Life Sci 1993; 53:63–75.

16. Bylund DB, Eikenberg DC, Hieble JP, et al. International Union of Pharmacology nomenclature of adrenoceptors. Pharmacol Rev 1994; 46:121–36.

17. Zhong H, Minneman KP. Alpha1-adrenoceptor subtypes. Eur J Pharmacol 1999; 375: 261–76.

18. Tsujimoto G, Manger WM, Hoffman BB. Desensitization of beta-adrenergic receptors by pheochromocytoma. Endocrinology 1984; 114:1272–8.

19. McCorry LK. Physiology of the autonomic nervous system. Am J Pharm Educ 2007; 71:78.

20. Wang FB, Holst MC, Powley TL. The ratio of pre- to postganglionic neurons and related issues in the autonomic nervous system. Brain Res Brain Res Rev 1995; 21:93–115.

21. DeLellis RA LR, Heitz PU, Eng C (eds). Tumours of Endocrine Organs. Pathology and Genetics. World Health Organization. IARC Press Lyon 2004.

22. Neumann HP, Bausch B, McWhinney SR, et al. Germ-line mutations in nonsyndromic pheochromocytoma. N Engl J Med 2002; 346:1459–66.

23. Bauters C, Vantyghem MC, Leteurtre E, et al. Hereditary phaeochromocytomas and paragangliomas: a study of five susceptibility genes. J Med Genet 2003;40:e75.

24. Amar L, Bertherat J, Baudin E, et al. Genetic testing in pheochromocytoma or functional paraganglioma. J Clin Oncol 2005; 23:8812–8.

25. Carney JA, Sheps SG, Go VL, Gordon H. The triad of gastric leiomyosarcoma, functioning extra-adrenal paraganglioma and pulmonary chondroma. N Engl J Med 1977; 296:1517–8.

26. McWhinney SR, Pasini B, Stratakis CA. Familial gastrointestinal stromal tumors and germline mutations. N Engl J Med 2007; 357:1054–6.

27. Eng C, Crossey PA, Mulligan LM, et al. Mutations in the RET proto-oncogene and the von Hippel-Lindau disease tumour suppressor gene in sporadic and syndromic phaeochromocytomas. J Med Genet 1995;32:934–7.

28. van der Harst E, de Krijger RR, Bruining HA, et al. Prognostic value of RET proto-oncogene point mutations in malignant and benign, sporadic phaeochromocytomas. Int J Cancer 1998;79:537–40.

29. Gimm O, Armanios M, Dziema H, Neumann HP, Eng C. Somatic and occult germ-line mutations in SDHD, a mitochondrial complex II gene, in nonfamilial pheochromocytoma. Cancer Res 2000;60:6822–5.

30. Dannenberg H, De Krijger RR, van der Harst E, et al. Von Hippel-Lindau gene alterations in sporadic benign and malignant pheochromocytomas. Int J Cancer 2003; 105:190–5.

31. van Nederveen FH, Korpershoek E, Lenders JW, de Krijger RR, Dinjens WN. Somatic SDHB mutation in an extraadrenal pheochromocytoma. N Engl J Med 2007; 357:306–8.

32. Beard CM, Sheps SG, Kurland LT, Carney JA, Lie JT. Occurrence of pheochromocytoma in Rochester, Minnesota, 1950 through 1979. Mayo Clin Proc 1983; 58:802–4.

33. Hartley L, Perry-Keene D. Phaeochromocytoma in Queensland–1970–83. Aust N Z J Surg 1985; 55:471–5.

34. Stenstrom G, Svardsudd K. Pheochromocytoma in Sweden 1958–1981. An analysis of the National Cancer Registry Data. Acta Med Scand 1986; 220:225–32.

35. Andersen GS, Toftdahl DB, Lund JO, Strandgaard S, Nielsen PE. The incidence rate of phaeochromocytoma and Conn's syndrome in Denmark, 1977–1981. J Hum Hypertens 1988; 2:187–9.

36. Lenders JW, Eisenhofer G, Mannelli M, Pacak K. Phaeochromocytoma. Lancet 2005; 366:665–75.

37. Sutton MG, Sheps SG, Lie JT. Prevalence of clinically unsuspected pheochromocytoma. Review of a 50-year autopsy series. Mayo Clin Proc 1981; 56:354–60.

38. McNeil AR, Blok BH, Koelmeyer TD, Burke MP, Hilton JM. Phaeochromocytomas discovered during coronial autopsies in Sydney, Melbourne and Auckland. Aust N Z J Med 2000; 30:648–52.

39. O'Riordain DS, Young WF, Jr., Grant CS, Carney JA, van Heerden JA. Clinical spectrum and outcome of functional extraadrenal paraganglioma. World J Surg 1996; 20:916–21; discussion 22.

40. Mantero F, Terzolo M, Arnaldi G, et al. A survey on adrenal incidentaloma in Italy. Study Group on Adrenal Tumors of the Italian Society of Endocrinology. J Clin Endocrinol Metab 2000; 85:637–44.

41. Mansmann G, Lau J, Balk E, Rothberg M, Miyachi Y, Bornstein SR. The clinically inapparent adrenal mass: update in diagnosis and management. Endocr Rev 2004; 25: 309–40.

42. Whalen RK, Althausen AF, Daniels GH. Extra-adrenal pheochromocytoma. J Urol 1992; 147:1–10.

43. Knudson AG, Jr., Strong LC, Anderson DE. Heredity and cancer in man. Prog Med Genet 1973; 9:113–58.

44. Dahia PL, Ross KN, Wright ME, et al. A HIF1alpha regulatory loop links hypoxia and mitochondrial signals in pheochromocytomas. PLoS Genet 2005; 1:72–80.

45. Kamura T, Sato S, Iwai K, Czyzyk-Krzeska M, Conaway RC, Conaway JW. Activation of HIF1alpha ubiquitination by a reconstituted von Hippel-Lindau (VHL) tumor suppressor complex. Proc Natl Acad Sci U S A 2000; 97:10430–5.

46. Kim WY, Kaelin WG. Role of VHL gene mutation in human cancer. J Clin Oncol 2004; 22:4991–5004.

47. Stratmann R, Krieg M, Haas R, Plate KH. Putative control of angiogenesis in hemangioblastomas by the von Hippel-Lindau tumor suppressor gene. J Neuropathol Exp Neurol 1997; 56:1242–52.

48. Selak MA, Armour SM, MacKenzie ED, et al. Succinate links TCA cycle dysfunction to oncogenesis by inhibiting HIF-alpha prolyl hydroxylase. Cancer Cell 2005; 7:77–85.

49. Yankovskaya V, Horsefield R, Tornroth S, et al. Architecture of succinate dehydrogenase and reactive oxygen species generation. Science 2003;299:700–4.

50. Gottlieb E, Tomlinson IP. Mitochondrial tumour suppressors: a genetic and biochemical update. Nat Rev Cancer 2005;5:857–66.

51. Takahashi M, Buma Y, Iwamoto T, Inaguma Y, Ikeda H, Hiai H. Cloning and expression of the ret proto-oncogene encoding a tyrosine kinase with two potential transmembrane domains. Oncogene 1988;3:571–8.

52. Santoro M, Carlomagno F, Romano A, et al. Activation of RET as a dominant transforming gene by germline mutations of MEN2A and MEN2B. Science 1995;267:381–3.

53. Ichihara M, Murakumo Y, Takahashi M. RET and neuroendocrine tumors. Cancer Lett 2004;204:197–211.

54. Cichowski K, Jacks T. NF1 tumor suppressor gene function: narrowing the GAP. Cell 2001; 104:593–604.

55. Martin GA, Viskochil D, Bollag G, et al. The GAP-related domain of the neurofibromatosis type 1 gene product interacts with ras p21. Cell 1990; 63:843–9.

56. Bollag G, Clapp DW, Shih S, et al. Loss of NF1 results in activation of the Ras signaling pathway and leads to aberrant growth in haematopoietic cells. Nat Genet 1996; 12:144–8.

57. Peaston RT, Weinkove C. Measurement of catecholamines and their metabolites. Ann Clin Biochem 2004; 41:17–38.

58. van der Harst E, de Herder WW, de Krijger RR, et al. The value of plasma markers for the clinical behaviour of phaeochromocytomas. Eur J Endocrinol 2002; 147:85–94.

59. Erickson D, Kudva YC, Ebersold MJ, et al. Benign paragangliomas: clinical presentation and treatment outcomes in 236 patients. J Clin Endocrinol Metab 2001; 86:5210–6.

60. Eisenhofer G, Walther MM, Huynh TT, et al. Pheochromocytomas in von Hippel-Lindau syndrome and multiple endocrine neoplasia type 2 display distinct biochemical and clinical phenotypes. J Clin Endocrinol Metab 2001; 86:1999–2008.

61. Smythe GA, Edwards G, Graham P, Lazarus L. Biochemical diagnosis of pheochromocytoma by simultaneous measurement of urinary excretion of epinephrine and norepinephrine. Clin Chem 1992; 38:486–92.

62. Crout JR, Sjoerdsma A. Catecholamines in the localization of pheochromocytoma. Circulation 1960; 22:516–25.

63. Kalff V, Shapiro B, Lloyd R, et al. The spectrum of pheochromocytoma in hypertensive patients with neurofibromatosis. Arch Intern Med 1982; 142:2092–8.

64. Benn DE, Gimenez-Roqueplo AP, Reilly JR, et al. Clinical presentation and penetrance of pheochromocytoma/paraganglioma syndromes. J Clin Endocrinol Metab 2006; 91: 827–36.

65. Timmers HJ, Kozupa A, Eisenhofer G, et al. Clinical Presentations, Biochemical Phenotypes, and Genotype-Phenotype Correlations in Patients with Succinate Dehydrogenase Subunit B-Associated Pheochromocytomas and Paragangliomas. J Clin Endocrinol Metab 2007; 92:779–86.

66. John H, Ziegler WH, Hauri D, Jaeger P. Pheochromocytomas: can malignant potential be predicted? Urology 1999; 53:679–83.

67. Zapanti E, Ilias I. Pheochromocytoma: physiopathologic implications and diagnostic evaluation. Ann N Y Acad Sci 2006; 1088:346–60.

68. Aniszewski JP, Young WF, Jr., Thompson GB, Grant CS, van Heerden JA. Cushing syndrome due to ectopic adrenocorticotropic hormone secretion. World J Surg 2001; 25: 934–40.

69. Otsuka F, Miyoshi T, Murakami K, et al. An extra-adrenal abdominal pheochromocytoma causing ectopic ACTH syndrome. Am J Hypertens 2005; 18:1364–8.

70. Bornstein SR, Ehrhart-Bornstein M, Gonzalez-Hernandez J, Schroder S, Scherbaum WA. Expression of interleukin-1 in human pheochromocytoma. J Endocrinol Invest 1996; 19:693–8.

71. Minetto M, Dovio A, Ventura M, et al. Interleukin-6 producing pheochromocytoma presenting with acute inflammatory syndrome. J Endocrinol Invest 2003; 26:453–7.

72. Omura M, Sato T, Cho R, et al. A patient with malignant paraganglioma that simultaneously produces adrenocorticotropic hormone and interleukin-6. Cancer 1994; 74:1634–9.

73. Venihaki M, Ain K, Dermitzaki E, Gravanis A, Margioris AN. KAT45, a noradrenergic human pheochromocytoma cell line producing corticotropin-releasing hormone. Endocrinology 1998; 139:713–22.

74. Takagi M, Egawa T, Motomura T, et al. Interleukin-6 secreting phaeochromocytoma associated with clinical markers of inflammation. Clin Endocrinol (Oxf) 1997; 46:507–9.

75. Hinson JP, Kapas S, Smith DM. Adrenomedullin, a multifunctional regulatory peptide. Endocr Rev 2000; 21:138–67.
76. Bravo EL, Tarazi RC, Gifford RW, Stewart BH. Circulating and urinary catecholamines in pheochromocytoma. Diagnostic and pathophysiologic implications. N Engl J Med 1979; 301:682–6.
77. Sheps SG, Jiang NS, Klee GG. Diagnostic evaluation of pheochromocytoma. Endocrinol Metab Clin North Am 1988; 17:397–414.
78. Plouin PF, Degoulet P, Tugaye A, Ducrocq MB, Menard J. [Screening for phaeochromocytoma : in which hypertensive patients? A semiological study of 2585 patients, including 11 with phaeochromocytoma (author's transl)]. Nouv Presse Med 1981; 10: 869–72.
79. Mannelli M, Ianni L, Cilotti A, Conti A. Pheochromocytoma in Italy: a multicentric retrospective study. Eur J Endocrinol 1999; 141:619–24.
80. Baxter MA, Hunter P, Thompson GR, London DR. Phaeochromocytomas as a cause of hypotension. Clin Endocrinol (Oxf) 1992; 37:304–6.
81. Bergland BE. Pheochromocytoma presenting as shock. Am J Emerg Med 1989; 7:44–8.
82. de Leeuw PW, Waltman FL, Birkenhager WH. Noncardiogenic pulmonary edema as the sole manifestation of pheochromocytoma. Hypertension 1986; 8:810–2.
83. Gifford RW, Jr., Manger WM, Bravo EL. Pheochromocytoma. Endocrinol Metab Clin North Am 1994; 23:387–404.
84. Hinchey J, Chaves C, Appignani B, et al. A reversible posterior leukoencephalopathy syndrome. N Engl J Med 1996; 334:494–500.
85. Moorthy S ST, Prabhu NK, Sree KK, Nair RG. Posterior reversible encephalopathy syndrome in a child with pheochromocytoma. Indian J Radiol Imaging 2002; 12:321–4.
86. Brouwers FM, Lenders JW, Eisenhofer G, Pacak K. Pheochromocytoma as an endocrine emergency. Rev Endocr Metab Disord 2003; 4:121–8.
87. Shemin D, Cohn PS, Zipin SB. Pheochromocytoma presenting as rhabdomyolysis and acute myoglobinuric renal failure. Arch Intern Med 1990; 150:2384–5.
88. Newell KA, Prinz RA, Pickleman J, et al. Pheochromocytoma multisystem crisis. A surgical emergency. Arch Surg 1988; 123:956–9.
89. Bahemuka M. Phaeochromocytoma with schizophreniform psychosis. Br J Psychiatry 1983;142:422–3.
90. Benabarre A, Bosch X, Plana MT, et al. Relapsing paranoid psychosis as the first manifestation of pheochromocytoma. J Clin Psychiatry 2005;66:949–50.
91. Dubois LA, Gray DK. Dopamine-secreting pheochromocytomas: in search of a syndrome. World J Surg 2005; 29:909–13.
92. Proye C, Fossati P, Fontaine P, et al. Dopamine-secreting pheochromocytoma: an unrecognized entity? Classification of pheochromocytomas according to their type of secretion. Surgery 1986; 100:1154–62.
93. Cook DM, Loriaux DL. The incidental adrenal mass. Am J Med 1996; 101:88–94.
94. Lenders JW, Pacak K, Walther MM, et al. Biochemical diagnosis of pheochromocytoma: which test is best? JAMA 2002;287:1427–34.
95. Unger N, Pitt C, Schmidt IL, et al. Diagnostic value of various biochemical parameters for the diagnosis of pheochromocytoma in patients with adrenal mass. Eur J Endocrinol 2006;154:409–17.
96. Eisenhofer G, Keiser H, Friberg P, et al. Plasma metanephrines are markers of pheochromocytoma produced by catechol-O-methyltransferase within tumors. J Clin Endocrinol Metab 1998;83:2175–85.

97. Sinclair D, Shenkin A, Lorimer AR. Normal catecholamine production in a patient with a paroxysmally secreting phaeochromocytoma. Ann Clin Biochem 1991; 28 (Pt 4): 417–9.

98. Amar L, Peyrard S, Rossignol P, Zinzindohoue F, Gimenez-Roqueplo AP, Plouin PF. Changes in urinary total metanephrine excretion in recurrent and malignant pheochromocytomas and secreting paragangliomas. Ann N Y Acad Sci 2006; 1073:383–91.

99. Eisenhofer G, Goldstein DS, Sullivan P, et al. Biochemical and clinical manifestations of dopamine-producing paragangliomas: utility of plasma methoxytyramine. J Clin Endocrinol Metab 2005; 90:2068–75.

100. Wortsman J, Frank S, Cryer PE. Adrenomedullary response to maximal stress in humans. Am J Med 1984; 77:779–84.

101. Eisenhofer G, Goldstein DS, Walther MM, et al. Biochemical diagnosis of pheochromocytoma: how to distinguish true- from false-positive test results. J Clin Endocrinol Metab 2003; 88:2656–66.

102. Wiesener MS, Seyfarth M, Warnecke C, et al. Paraneoplastic erythrocytosis associated with an inactivating point mutation of the von Hippel-Lindau gene in a renal cell carcinoma. Blood 2002; 99:3562–5.

103. Zelinka T, Petrak O, Strauch B, et al. Elevated inflammation markers in pheochromocytoma compared to other forms of hypertension. Neuroimmunomodulation 2007; 14:57–64.

104. Fukumoto S, Matsumoto T, Harada S, Fujisaki J, Kawano M, Ogata E. Pheochromocytoma with pyrexia and marked inflammatory signs: a paraneoplastic syndrome with possible relation to interleukin-6 production. J Clin Endocrinol Metab 1991; 73:877–81.

105. Portel-Gomes GM, Grimelius L, Johansson H, Wilander E, Stridsberg M. Chromogranin A in human neuroendocrine tumors: an immunohistochemical study with region-specific antibodies. Am J Surg Pathol 2001; 25:1261–7.

106. Guignat L, Bidart JM, Nocera M, Comoy E, Schlumberger M, Baudin E. Chromogranin A and the alpha-subunit of glycoprotein hormones in medullary thyroid carcinoma and phaeochromocytoma. Br J Cancer 2001; 84:808–12.

107. Chrisoulidou A, Kaltsas G, Ilias I, Grossman AB. The diagnosis and management of malignant phaeochromocytoma and paraganglioma. Endocr Relat Cancer 2007; 14: 569–85.

108. Sahdev A, Reznek RH. Imaging evaluation of the non-functioning indeterminate adrenal mass. Trends Endocrinol Metab 2004; 15:271–6.

109. Ilias I, Pacak K. Current approaches and recommended algorithm for the diagnostic localization of pheochromocytoma. J Clin Endocrinol Metab 2004; 89:479–91.

110. Mukherjee JJ, Peppercorn PD, Reznek RH, et al. Pheochromocytoma: effect of nonionic contrast medium in CT on circulating catecholamine levels. Radiology 1997; 202:227–31.

111. Sahdev A, Sohaib A, Monson JP, Grossman AB, Chew SL, Reznek RH. CT and MR imaging of unusual locations of extra-adrenal paragangliomas (pheochromocytomas). Eur Radiol 2005; 15:85–92.

112. Shulkin BL, Ilias I, Sisson JC, Pacak K. Current trends in functional imaging of pheochromocytomas and paragangliomas. Ann N Y Acad Sci 2006; 1073:374–82.

113. Kolby L, Bernhardt P, Levin-Jakobsen AM, et al. Uptake of meta-iodobenzylguanidine in neuroendocrine tumours is mediated by vesicular monoamine transporters. Br J Cancer 2003; 89:1383–8.

114. van der Harst E, de Herder WW, Bruining HA, et al. [(123)I]metaiodobenzylguanidine and [(111)In]octreotide uptake in begnign and malignant pheochromocytomas. J Clin Endocrinol Metab 2001; 86:685–93.

115. Nielsen JT, Nielsen BV, Rehling M. Location of adrenal medullary pheochromocytoma by I-123 metaiodobenzylguanidine SPECT. Clin Nucl Med 1996; 21:695–9.

116. Epelbaum J, Bertherat J, Prevost G, et al. Molecular and pharmacological characterization of somatostatin receptor subtypes in adrenal, extraadrenal, and malignant pheochromocytomas. J Clin Endocrinol Metab 1995; 80:1837–44.

117. Tenenbaum F, Lumbroso J, Schlumberger M, et al. Comparison of radiolabeled octreotide and meta-iodobenzylguanidine (MIBG) scintigraphy in malignant pheochromocytoma. J Nucl Med 1995; 36:1–6.

118. Kaltsas G, Korbonits M, Heintz E, et al. Comparison of somatostatin analog and meta-iodobenzylguanidine radionuclides in the diagnosis and localization of advanced neuroendocrine tumors. J Clin Endocrinol Metab 2001; 86:895–902.

119. Timmers HJ, Kozupa A, Chen CC, et al. Superiority of fluorodeoxyglucose positron emission tomography to other functional imaging techniques in the evaluation of metastatic SDHB-associated pheochromocytoma and paraganglioma. J Clin Oncol 2007; 25:2262–9.

120. Fujita A, Hyodoh H, Kawamura Y, Kanegae K, Furuse M, Kanazawa K. Use of fusion images of I-131 metaiodobenzylguanidine, SPECT, and magnetic resonance studies to identify a malignant pheochromocytoma. Clin Nucl Med 2000; 25:440–2.

121. Blodgett TM, Meltzer CC, Townsend DW. PET/CT: form and function. Radiology 2007; 242:360–85.

122. Chew SL, Dacie JE, Reznek RH, et al. Bilateral phaeochromocytomas in von Hippel-Lindau disease: diagnosis by adrenal vein sampling and catecholamine assay. Q J Med 1994; 87:49–54.

123. Pacak K, Eisenhofer G, Ahlman H, et al. Pheochromocytoma: recommendations for clinical practice from the First International Symposium. October 2005. Nat Clin Pract Endocrinol Metab 2007; 3:92–102.

124. Chew SL. Recent developments in the therapy of phaeochromocytoma. Expert Opin Investig Drugs 2004; 13:1579–83.

125. Mannelli M. Management and treatment of pheochromocytomas and paragangliomas. Ann N Y Acad Sci 2006; 1073:405–16.

126. Prys-Roberts C. Phaeochromocytoma–recent progress in its management. Br J Anaesth 2000; 85:44–57.

127. Bergman SM, Sears HF, Javadpour N, Keiser HR. Postoperative management of patients with pheochromocytoma. J Urol 1978; 120:109–12.

128. Lehmann HU, Hochrein H, Witt E, Mies HW. Hemodynamic effects of calcium antagonists. Review. Hypertension 1983;5:II66–73.

129. Steinsapir J, Carr AA, Prisant LM, Bransome ED, Jr. Metyrosine and pheochromocytoma. Arch Intern Med 1997; 157:901–6.

130. Koriyama N, Kakei M, Yaekura K, et al. Control of catecholamine release and blood pressure with octreotide in a patient with pheochromocytoma: a case report with in vitro studies. Horm Res 2000; 53:46–50.

131. Kinney MA, Narr BJ, Warner MA. Perioperative management of pheochromocytoma. J Cardiothorac Vasc Anesth 2002; 16:359–69.

132. Janetschek G, Finkenstedt G, Gasser R, et al. Laparoscopic surgery for pheochromocytoma: adrenalectomy, partial resection, excision of paragangliomas. J Urol 1998; 160: 330–4.

133. Walz MK, Peitgen K, Neumann HP, Janssen OE, Philipp T, Mann K. Endoscopic treatment of solitary, bilateral, multiple, and recurrent pheochromocytomas and paragangliomas. World J Surg 2002; 26:1005–12.

134. Hwang J, Shoaf G, Uchio EM, et al. Laparoscopic management of extra-adrenal pheochromocytoma. J Urol 2004; 171:72–6.

135. Douglas WW, Rubin RP. The mechanism of catecholamine release from the adrenal medulla and the role of calcium in stimulus-secretion coupling. J Physiol 1963; 167: 288–310.

136. von Euler US, Lishajko F. Effects of Mg2+ and Ca2+ on noradrenaline release and uptake in adrenergic nerve granules in differential media. Acta Physiol Scand 1973; 89: 415–22.

137. Nicholas E, Deutschman CS, Allo M, Rock P. Use of esmolol in the intraoperative management of pheochromocytoma. Anesth Analg 1988; 67:1114–7.

138. Bravo EL. Pheochromocytoma. Curr Ther Endocrinol Metab 1997; 6:195–7.

139. Eisenhofer G, Bornstein SR, Brouwers FM, et al. Malignant pheochromocytoma: current status and initiatives for future progress. Endocr Relat Cancer 2004; 11:423–36.

140. Kebebew E, Duh QY. Benign and malignant pheochromocytoma: diagnosis, treatment, and follow-Up. Surg Oncol Clin N Am 1998; 7:765–89.

141. Pacak K, Fojo T, Goldstein DS, et al. Radiofrequency ablation: a novel approach for treatment of metastatic pheochromocytoma. J Natl Cancer Inst 2001; 93:648–9.

142. Averbuch SD, Steakley CS, Young RC, et al. Malignant pheochromocytoma: effective treatment with a combination of cyclophosphamide, vincristine, and dacarbazine. Ann Intern Med 1988; 109:267–73.

143. Tada K, Okuda Y, Yamashita K. Three cases of malignant pheochromocytoma treated with cyclophosphamide, vincristine, and dacarbazine combination chemotherapy and alpha-methyl-p-tyrosine to control hypercatecholaminemia. Horm Res 1998; 49:295–7.

144. Noshiro T, Honma H, Shimizu K, et al. Two cases of malignant pheochromocytoma treated with cyclophosphamide, vincristine and dacarbazine in a combined chemotherapy. Endocr J 1996; 43:279–84.

145. Schlumberger M, Gicquel C, Lumbroso J, et al. Malignant pheochromocytoma: clinical, biological, histologic and therapeutic data in a series of 20 patients with distant metastases. J Endocrinol Invest 1992; 15:631–42.

146. Kaltsas GA, Mukherjee JJ, Isidori A, et al. Treatment of advanced neuroendocrine tumours using combination chemotherapy with lomustine and 5-fluorouracil. Clin Endocrinol (Oxf) 2002; 57:169–83.

147. Kulke MH, Stuart K, Enzinger PC, et al. Phase II study of temozolomide and thalidomide in patients with metastatic neuroendocrine tumors. J Clin Oncol 2006; 24:401–6.

148. Scholz T, Eisenhofer G, Pacak K, Dralle H, Lehnert H. Clinical review: Current treatment of malignant pheochromocytoma. J Clin Endocrinol Metab 2007;92:1217–25.

149. Sisson JC. Radiopharmaceutical treatment of pheochromocytomas. Ann N Y Acad Sci 2002;970:54–60.

150. Rose B, Matthay KK, Price D, et al. High-dose 131I-metaiodobenzylguanidine therapy for 12 patients with malignant pheochromocytoma. Cancer 2003;98:239–48.

151. Fitzgerald PA, Goldsby RE, Huberty JP, et al. Malignant pheochromocytomas and paragangliomas: a phase II study of therapy with high-dose 131I-metaiodobenzylguanidine (131I-MIBG). Ann N Y Acad Sci 2006;1073:465–90.

152. Kolby L, Bernhardt P, Johanson V, et al. Can quantification of VMAT and SSTR expression be helpful for planning radionuclide therapy of malignant pheochromocytomas? Ann N Y Acad Sci 2006; 1073:491–7.

153. Lamarre-Cliche M, Gimenez-Roqueplo AP, Billaud E, Baudin E, Luton JP, Plouin PF. Effects of slow-release octreotide on urinary metanephrine excretion and plasma

chromogranin A and catecholamine levels in patients with malignant or recurrent phaeochromocytoma. Clin Endocrinol (Oxf) 2002; 57:629–34.

154. Mundschenk J, Unger N, Schulz S, Hollt V, Steinke R, Lehnert H. Somatostatin receptor subtypes in human pheochromocytoma: subcellular expression pattern and functional relevance for octreotide scintigraphy. J Clin Endocrinol Metab 2003; 88:5150–7.

155. Bruns C, Lewis I, Briner U, Meno-Tetang G, Weckbecker G. SOM230: a novel somatostatin peptidomimetic with broad somatotropin release inhibiting factor (SRIF) receptor binding and a unique antisecretory profile. Eur J Endocrinol 2002; 146:707–16.

156. Powers MV, Workman P. Targeting of multiple signalling pathways by heat shock protein 90 molecular chaperone inhibitors. Endocr Relat Cancer 2006; 13 Suppl 1:S125–35.

157. Sausville EA, Tomaszewski JE, Ivy P. Clinical development of 17-allylamino, 17-demethoxygeldanamycin. Curr Cancer Drug Targets 2003; 3:377–83.

158. Amar L, Baudin E, Burnichon N, et al. Succinate dehydrogenase B gene mutations predict survival in patients with malignant pheochromocytomas or paragangliomas. J Clin Endocrinol Metab 2007.

159. Bravo EL, Tagle R. Pheochromocytoma: state-of-the-art and future prospects. Endocr Rev 2003; 24:539–53.

160. Manger WM, Gifford RW, Jr. Hypertension secondary to pheochromocytoma. Bull N Y Acad Med 1982; 58:139–58.

161. Yoshida S, Hatori M, Noshiro T, Kimura N, Kokubun S. Twenty-six-years' survival with multiple bone metastasis of malignant pheochromocytoma. Arch Orthop Trauma Surg 2001; 121:598–600.

6

Hyperglycemic Crises: Diabetic Ketoacidosis (DKA) and Hyperglycemic Hyperosmolar State (HHS)

Abbas E. Kitabchi, PhD, MD
and Joseph N. Fisher, MD

CONTENTS

Diabetic ketoacidosis (DKA) and the hyperglycemic hyperosmolar state (HHS) are acute metabolic complications of diabetes that are potentially fatal and require prompt, informed medical attention for successful treatment. DKA is the most common acute hyperglycemic complication of diabetes, the annual incidence estimated from 4 to 8 episodes per 1000 patient admissions with diabetes *(1)*. A recent report by the Centers for Disease Control *(2)* indicated that there had been more than a 45% increase in the incidence of hospitalizations in the United States for DKA between 1980 and 2003, (Fig. 1a) but with a 22% age-adjusted decline in the mortality rate of DKA in the same interval. (Fig. 1b)

From: *Contemporary Endocrinology: Acute Cause to Consequence*
Edited by: G. Van den Berghe, DOI: 10.1007/978-1-60327-177-6_6,
© Humana Press, New York, NY

(a)

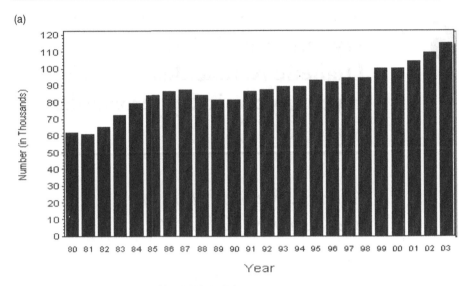

Fig. 1a. Incidence of DKA 1980–2003 (*ref. 2*).

(b)

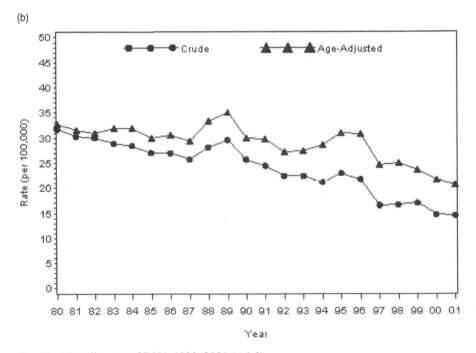

Fig. 1b. Mortality rate of DKA 1980–2001 (*ref. 2*).

HHS is less common than DKA, accounting for less than 1% of all diabetes-related admissions, but has a much higher mortality rate, currently on the order of 11% in the US but exceeding 40% in some series, in comparison to less than 5% in DKA patients *(3)*.

DKA can be described by three biochemical entities: hyperglycemia, ketosis, and metabolic acidosis (Fig. 2) *(4)*. The abbreviation HHS is used to replace the terms HHC (hyperglycemic hyperosmolar coma) and HHNS (hyperglycemic hyperosmolar non-ketotic state) in recognition of the fact that coma may occur in less than 50% of HHS patients despite a high serum osmolality, and that mild ketosis may be observed with HHS *(5)*. Both DKA and HHS are characterized by absolute or relative insulin deficiency and while they are usually considered separately, they represent different sites on a continuum of hyperglycemic medical emergencies. They are separated clinically by the more severe hyperglycemia and lack of appreciable ketosis or acidosis in HHS *(5)*. Whereas DKA most often is seen in patients with type 1 diabetes mellitus (DM 1), it may occur in patients with type 2 diabetes (DM 2), particularly in ethnic minorities. Recent investigation from many centers have reported presence of DKA cases in patients with African or Hispanic origin who present with DKA and require insulin therapy initially with transient impairment of ß cell function, but subsequently may be treated orally or by diet alone with 40% remaining non insulin dependent ten years following the initial episode of DKA *(6–10)*. These patients

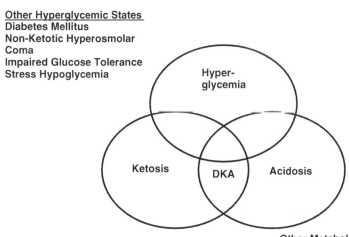

Fig. 2. Three components of DKA and related states from ref. *(4)*.

Table 1
Diagnostic criteria and typical total body deficits of water and electrolytes in Diabetic Ketoacidosis (DKA) and Hyperglycemic Hyperosmolar Syndrome (HHS)

	DKA			HHS
	Mild	*Moderate*	*Severe*	
Diagnostic criteria and classification				
Plasma glucose (mg/dl)	>250 mg/dl	>250 mg/dl	>250 mg/dl	>600 mg/dl
Arterial pH	7.25–7.30	7.00–<7.24	<7.00	>7.30
Serum bicarbonate (mEq/L)	15–18	10–<15	<10	>15
Urine ketone*	Positive	Positive	Positive	Small
Serum ketone*	Positive	Positive	Positive	Small
Effective Serum Osmolality**	Variable	Variable	Variable	>320 mOsm/kg
Anion Gap***	>10	>12	>12	<12
Mental Status	Alert	Alert/Drowsy	Stupor/Coma	Stupor/Coma
Typical deficits				
Total Water (L)	6			9
Water (ml/kg) δ	100			100–200
Na+ (mEq/kg)	7–10			5–13
Cl– (mEq/kg)	3–5			5–15
K+ (mEq/kg)	3–5			4–6
PO4 (mmol/kg)	5–7			3–7
Mg++ (mEq/kg)	1–2			1–2
Ca++ (mEq/kg)	1–2			1–2

*Nitroprusside reaction method
**Calculation: Effective serum osmolality: $2[\text{measured } Na^+ \text{ (mEq/L)}] + \text{glucose (mg/dl)}/18 = \text{mOsm/kg}$
***Calculation: Anion Gap:$[(Na^+)–(Cl^- + HCO3^- \text{ (mEq/L)})]$
δ Per Kg of body weight

$$2\left[Na + glu\right]/18$$

do not have the typical autoimmune laboratory findings of type 1 diabetes. Such patients have been labeled by different names such as Flat Bush diabetes, type 1 1/2 diabetes, or ketosis-prone type 2 diabetes *(11,12)*. Conversely, HHS is observed in DM2 and in older patients most frequently, but an extreme hyperosmolar state is seen occasionally in combination with DKA in DM1 *(13)*. Table 1 provides latest classification of and characterization of DKA and HHS as well as their total body deficits for water and electrolytes *(3)*.

PRECIPITATING CAUSES

DKA is the initial presentation in 20 to 30% of patients with DM1 *(6)*, whereas major underlying causes of DKA in known diabetic patients are infection and omission or inadequate dosing of insulin *(14)*. Other causes include silent myocardial infarction, pancreatitis, cerebrovascular accident, trauma, and drugs that affect carbohydrate metabolism such as corticosteroids, sympathomimetic agents, thiazides, and second generation antipsychotic agents *(15)*. Cocaine has also been associated with DKA, especially recurrent episodes *(16)*. Interruption of insulin delivery by continuous subcutaneous insulin infusion devices has also been a reported cause of DKA *(17)*, but mechanical improvements in pumps and devices for self glucose monitoring have greatly reduced its incidence. Recurrent DKA due to intentional omission of insulin has been cited in as many as 20% of DM1 women who have eating disorders *(18)*. There are even case reports of patients with DKA as the primary manifestation of acromegaly *(19–22)* as well as case report of DKA with a low carbohydrate diet *(23)*. A summary of major precipitating factors for DKA are presented in Table 2 *(15)*.

PATHOGENESIS OF DIABETIC KETOACIDOSIS AND HYPERGLYCEMIC HYPEROSMOLAR STATE

The underlying causes of DKA are better understood than that of HHS, but in both conditions there is a reduction in the net effective action of circulating insulin along with an elevation of counterregulatory hormones – glucagon, catecholamines, cortisol, and growth hormone - which impair the entrance of glucose into insulin sensitive tissues (muscle, adipocytes, and liver) *(5)*.

Diabetic Ketoacidosis

DKA is characterized by severe derangements of carbohydrate, lipid, and protein metabolism, with hyperglycemia, increased lipolysis, increased gluconeogenesis, and ketogenesis all contributing to the metabolic imbalance *(24)*.

GLUCOSE METABOLISM

The three sources of glucose in the blood are ingestion, glycogenolysis, and gluconeogenesis, whereas glucose is metabolized via oxidation, lipogenesis, and glycogen synthesis *(4)*. Hyperglycemia in DKA results from increased glycogenolysis and gluconeogenesis and decreased glucose utilization by liver,

Table 2
Precipitating factors for DKA

Study location/dates	Number of cases	infection	Cardiovascular disease	Noncompliance	New onset	Other conditions	Unknown
Frankfurt, Germany Petzold et al. 1971	472	19	6	38	+	+	+
Birmingham, UK Soler et al. 1968–72	258	28	3	23	+	+	+
Erfurt, Germany Panzram 1970–71	133	35	4	21	+	+	+
Basel, Switzerland Berger et al. 1968–78	163	56	5	31	+	+	+
Rhode Island Faich et al. 1975–79	152	43	–	26	+	+	+
Memphis, TN Kitabchi et al. 1974–85	202	38	–	28	22	10	4
Atlanta, GA Umpierez et al. 1993–94	144	28	–	41	17	10	4
Bronx, NY Nyenwe et al. 2001–04	219	25	3	44	25	12	15

Data are % of all cases except in Nyenwe et al, where new onset disease was not included in the percentage + complete data on these items were not given, therefore, the total is less than 100%. Adopted with modification from ref. (5, 15).

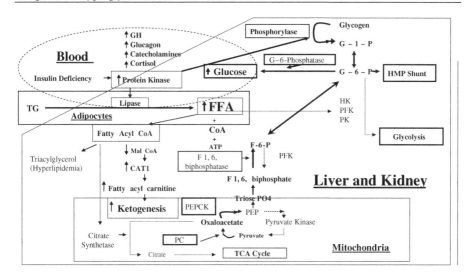

Fig. 3. Proposed Biochemical Alterations in Diabetic Ketoacidosis Leading to Increased Gluconeogenesis, Lipolysis, Ketogenesis and Decreased Glycolysis [adopted from ref. *(24)*].

muscle, and adipose tissue. Insulin deficiency combined with elevated cortisol produces diminished protein synthesis and increased proteolysis with release of amino acids (alanine and glutamine) that provide substrates for increased gluconeogenesis *(25)*. Insulinopenia along with increased levels of glucagon, catecholamines, and cortisol stimulate gluconeogenic enzymes, in particular phosphoenolpyruvate carboxykinse (PEPCK) *(5,24–27)*. Glucose utilization is further diminished by increased circulating levels of catecholamines and free fatty acids (FFA) as demonstrated in Fig. 3 *(24,25,27)*.

LIPID METABOLISM

Catecholamine excess and insulinopenia stimulate breakdown of triglycerides to FFA and glycerol (lipolysis), the former providing substrate for ketone body formation, and the latter the carbon skeleton for gluconeogenesis *(25–28)*. The elevated FFA lead to production of ketone bodies via beta oxidation and the production of very low-density lipoprotein (VLDL) in the liver. Increased levels of chylomicrons and VLDL may be manifested clinically by lipemia retinalis *(5,27)*. The importance of glucagon in the production of hyperglycemia and ketoacidosis in DKA was demonstrated in the following studies. In the first one, by preventing glucagon release with somatostatin infusion, the rate of rise in serum glucose was markedly attenuated after discontinuing insulin in a patient with type 1 diabetes *(29)*. In a second investigation, the extent of this effect was demonstrated in patients who had had total pancreatectomies and therefore made neither insulin nor glucagon. Four such patients were compared to six individuals with DM1. All were fasted and maintained on intravenous insulin for 24 hours. When insulin was withdrawn, the patients with DM1 had a brisk increase in glucagon and had significantly greater increases in blood glucose (225 versus 139 mg/dl [12.5 versus 7.7 mmol/L] and blood ketone concentration (4.1 versus 1.8 meq/L at 12 hours) compared to the pancreatectomized patients *(30)*.

Carnitine palmitoyl acyltransferase (CPTI), the rate-limiting enzyme of ketogenesis, is inhibited by malonyl coenzyme A (CoA). In DKA there are decreased amounts of malonyl CoA as result of the increased ratio of glucagon to insulin. That leads to stimulation of CPTI and an increase in ketogenesis *(27,28)* (Fig. 3). Ketonemia is also enhanced in DKA by a decreased clearance of ketone bodies *(29)*.

OXIDATIVE STRESS AND HYPERGLYCEMIC CRISES

Recent studies in adult patients with hyperglycemic crises of DKA or non ketotic hyperglycemia have demonstrated elevated levels of proinflammatory cytokines (TNFα, 1Lß, 1L6, and 1L8), a marker of oxidative stress, lipid peroxidation, cardiovascular risk factors such as CRP, plasminogen activator inhibitor -1, and free fatty acids *(31)*. All of these parameters return to near normal values with insulin therapy and hydration within 24 hours (Fig. 4). These events are also associated with increased levels of counter-regulatory

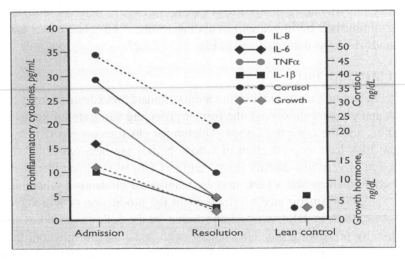

Fig. 4. Serum levels of proinflammatory cytokines, cortisol, and growth hormone in lean patients with diabetic ketoacidosis on admission and after resolution of diabetic ketoacidosis with insulin therapy, data from ref. *(31)*.

Table 3
Admission biochemical data in patients with HHS and DKA

Parameters measured	HHS	DKA
Glucose (mg/dl)	930 ± 83	616 ± 36
Na (mEq/l)	149 ± 3.2	134 ± 1.0
K(mEq/l)	3.9 ± 0.2	4.5 ± 0.13
BUN (mg/dl)	61 ± 11	32 ± 3
Creatinine (mg/dl)	1.4 ± 0.1	1.1 ± 0.1
pH	7.3 ± 0.03	7.12 ± 0.04
Bicarbonate(mEq/l)	18 ± 1.1	9.4 ± 1.4
B-hydroxybutyrate(mmol/l)	1.0 ± 0.2	9.1 ± 0.85
Total osmolality (mosm/kg)	380 ± 5.7	323 ± 2.5
IRI (nmol/l)	0.08 ± 0.01	0.07 ± 0.01
C-peptide (nmol/l)	1.14 ± 0.1	0.21 ± 0.03
FFA (nmol/l)	1.5 ± 0.19	1.6 ± 0.16
Human growth hormone (ng/l)	1.9 ± 0.2	6.1 ± 1.2
Cortisol (ng/l)	570 ± 49	500 ± 61
Glucagon(pg/l)	689 ± 215	580 ± 147
Cathecholamines (ng/l)	0.28 ± 0.09	1.78 ± 0.4
Anion Gap	11	17

Data are presented as mean ± SEM. Adapted from ref. *(5,24)*.

hormones and leukocytosis. The pro-coagulant and inflammatory states may be non-specific phenomena due to stress and may partially explain the association of hyperglycemic crises with a hypercoagulable state.

Hyperglycemic Hyperosmolar State

While the pathogenesis of DKA and HHS are similar, they differ in that with HHS there is *(1)* greater dehydration, *(2)* sufficient insulin to prevent excessive lipolysis (suppression of lipolysis requires one-tenth the amount of insulin necessary to promote glucose uptake), and *(3)* counterregulatory hormones are variable and there is no clear difference between DKA and HHS *(5,32,33)* (Table 3) (Fig. 5).

FLUID AND ELECTROLYTE ABNORMALITIES

Moderate to severe water and electrolyte imbalance occurs with DKA and HHS as a result of insulin deficiency, hyperglycemia, and hyperketonemia. Hyperglycemia causes osmotic diuresis which promotes loss of minerals and electrolytes including sodium, potassium, calcium, magnesium, chloride, and phosphate. The classical studies of Atchley et al and Butler et al provided the

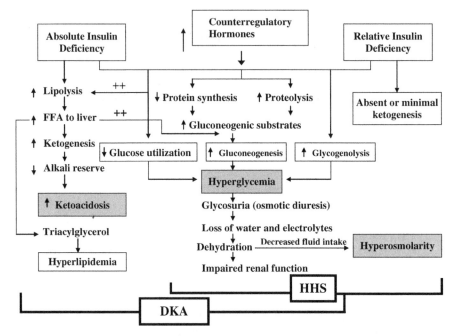

Fig. 5. Pathogenesis of DKA and HHS stress, infection and/or insufficient insulin [modified from ref. *(3)*.

first detailed studies of electrolyte balance in DKA *(34,35)*, and as they and others noted, while sodium, potassium, and chloride can be rapidly replaced during treatment other minerals may take weeks for full restoration *(36,37)*. Loss of water in DKA averages 5 to 6 L, with an average sodium and potassium loss of 400 to 700 meq *(37)* and 250 to 700 meq *(38)*, respectively. The fluid lost in DKA resembles hypotonic more closely than isotonic saline since there is a greater loss of water than sodium *(39,40)*. The excretion of ketoanions, which forces urinary cation excretion, also contributes to the derangement of electrolytes *(36)*. Insulin deficiency may directly contribute to renal losses of water and electrolytes due to lack of the effect of insulin on water and salt resorption in the renal tubule *(37,38)*. There is a shift of water out of cells due to increased plasma tonicity from hyperglycemia and water loss. An associated movement of potassium from cells to the extracellular compartment is aggravated by acidosis and the breakdown of intracellular protein *(41)*. In addition, potassium entry into cells is impaired by lack of effective insulin action. Excessive fluid losses may also be caused by vomiting, fever, diarrhea, and diuretic use. A combination of older age, more severe dehydration, and the presence of comorbid states in patients with HHS accounts for the higher mortality observed in this condition *(42)*.

Diagnosis

CLINICAL PRESENTATION

The symptoms of DKA usually evolve rapidly over a day or less. In our experience nearly one-quarter of patients presenting in DKA were newly diagnosed with diabetes *(24)*. Conversely, HHS may develop insidiously over days to weeks *(42)*. Common to both are symptoms of hyperglycemia including polyuria, polydypsia, and polyphagia, weakness and weight loss. Physical signs of dehydration include dry mucous membranes, poor skin turgor, sunken eyeballs, tachycardia, hypotension, and in severe cases shock. DKA patients may exhibit nausea, vomiting, Kussmaul respiration, acetone breath, and occasionally abdominal pain, the latter correlating with the degree of acidosis *(43)*. This may be sufficiently severe to be confused with an acute abdominal crisis. Normal body temperature or even mild hypothermia may be observed in some patients despite the presence of infection *(5)*. Approximately 30% of patients with DKA present with hyperosmolality *(13)*. The state of consciousness in adults is related to serum osmolality and most patients who present with an effective osmolality greater than 330 mOsm/kg are obtunded or comatose *(13)* (Fig. 6). A recent study in children suggests that other parameters such as pH and biocarbonate

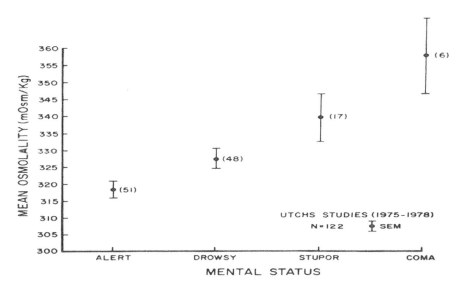

Fig. 6. Calculated serum osmolality in 122 patients with diabetic ketoacidosis with relation to mental status. About one third of patients with hyperglycemic crises may present with altered mental status *(13)*. This can be correlated to serum osmolality but needs to be differentiated from various clinical conditions associated with altered mental status or coma which may present in diabetic patients. [*Adopted from Kitabchi and Fisher (13)*].

Table 4

Admission clinical and biochemical profile and response to therapy of comatose versus noncomatose patients with DKA

	Noncomatosen=35	Comatosen=13	P values
Age (yr)	36.1 ± 3.9	50.2 ± 6.8	<0.02
Glucose (mg/dL)	577.5 ± 42.5	988 ± 175.15	<0.01
HCO⁻₃(meq/L)	8.6 ± 0.72	6.1 ± 0.9	<0.02
pH	7.19 ± 0.25	7.10 ± 0.45	NS
BUN (mg/dL)	24.1 ± 1.2	54.5 ± 5.2	<0.01
Osmolality(mOsmol/kg)	313.6 ± 2.2	365 ± 15.2	<0.01
Ketones (mM)	13.7 ± 0.76	14.3 ± 1.4	NS
Hours to Recovery			
Glucose ≤250(mg/dl)	5.2 ± 0.6	9.5 ± 2.5	<.05
HCO⁻₃≥15(meq/L)	10.6 ± 1.7	12.9 ± 2.7	NS
pH≥7.3	6.6 ± 1	10.15 ± 2.8	NS
Mentally alert	NA	7.78 ± 4.2	NA

may also correlate with mental status *(44)*. In our earlier studies of 48 patients with DKA using low dose versus high dose insulin therapy *(45)*, we evaluated the initial biochemical values of patients with stupor/coma versus non comatose patients *(46)*. Table 4 shows that only age, glucose, bicarbonate, blood urea nitrogen (BUN), and osmolality, but not pH, or ketones are significantly different between non-comatose and comatose patients. Conversely, patients with an effective osmolality less than 320 mOsm/kg are usually alert. Thus patients who are obtunded but have a normal or only mildly elevated osmolality should be evaluated for other co-morbidities such as cerebrovascular accident or other conditions. In every case, clues should be sought for underlying causes of DKA and HHS by a rapid but thorough history and physical examination.

LABORATORY EVALUATION

After the history and physical examination, the initial laboratory studies should include plasma glucose, blood urea nitrogen, creatinine, and electrolytes [with calculated anion gap], plasma osmolality and urine ketones by dipstick, serum ketones (if urine ketones are present), arterial blood gas, complete blood count with differential, and urinalysis. Ancillary investigations include electrocardiogram, chest x-ray, and culture of body fluids as indicated clinically. The diagnostic criteria for DKA and HHS are shown in Table 1. DKA is classified as mild, moderate, or severe based on the severity of the acidosis and the mental status *(3)*. More than a third of patients have features of both DKA and HHS

(4,13,45). By definition, patients with HHS typically have a pH greater than 7.30, bicarbonate level greater than 20 mEq/L, and negative ketone bodies in plasma and urine. Leukocytosis is common in both conditions *(5,14,47)*. The leukocytosis may be related to increased level of cortisol and catecholamines secondary to stress of hyperglycemia and dehydration. This may be a non specific phenomenon, as a similar level of leukocytosis may be seen in normal subjects undergoing stress of insulin-induced hypoglycemia *(48)*. However when leukocytes are greater than 25,000/μL evaluation for possible infection should be initiated *(49)*. The initial serum sodium is usually low due to the osmotic movement of water from the intracellular to extracellular space secondary to hyperglycemia. Therefore, the presence of hypernatremia and hyperglycemia indicates severe dehydration. Alternately, in the presence of lipemic serum from a high chylomicron concentration (which may be diagnosed clinically by lipemic retinalis or the presence of lactescent serum), pseudonormoglycemia and pseudohyponatremia may occur in DKA *(50,51)*. Because insulin deficiency may elevate serum potassium secondary to extracellular shift of potassium, the presence of a low-normal or frankly low potassium on admission with DKA suggests severe total body potassium deficit. In that instance, more vigorous potassium replacement should take place along with cardiac monitoring for possible arrhythmias. Total body potassium deficiency in DKA is usually on the order of 3 to 5 meq/kg body weight, but has been noted as high as10 meq/kg *(34,52)*. An elevated serum amylase may occur in up to 25% of DKA patients, but can arise from non-pancreatic tissue such as the parotid glands *(53,54)*. For that reason pancreatic enzymes may not be reliable to diagnose pancreatitis in the setting of DKA. Another source of laboratory error is the artificial elevation of serum creatinine, either because of dehydration or interference from ketone bodies if a colorimetric method is used for determination *(55)*. Most laboratory tests for ketone bodies use the nitroprusside method which detects acetoacetate but not beta hydroxybuterate (BOHB), which is the more abundant ketone body *(56)*. When newer meters that have the capacity to measure BOHB are not utilized, the use of ketone bodies to follow progress of DKA treatment is not advocated since BOHB is converted to acetoacetate during therapy and the ketone test may show high values, mistakenly suggesting a deterioration of ketonemia (Fig. 7) *(24)*. Another source of error are drugs, such the angiotensin-converting enzyme inhibitor captopril, which have sulfhydryl groups that may react with the agent in the nitroprusside test and give a false-positive reaction *(57)*. Therefore clinical judgment and other biochemical tests will be required in patients suspected of ketoacidosis who are receiving such medications. An alternative to measurement of venous pH and BOHB is monitoring of the serum bicarbonate and calculated anion gap. The anion gap [Serum anion gap = Serum sodium – (serum chloride + bicarbonate)] gives an estimate of the major unmeasured anions in

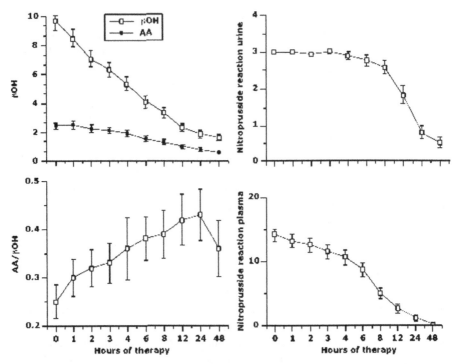

Fig. 7. Comparative data in 37 patients with diabetic ketoacidosis with regard to plasma acetoacetic acid (AA) and -hydroxybutyric acid (βOH) (*top left*); ratio of AA to βOH (*bottom left*); and ketone bodies (nitroprusside reaction) in the urine (*top right*) and plasma (*bottom right* before and during low-dose intravenous infusion of insulin for 48 hours. Reproduced with permission from ref. *(24)*.

plasma which in DKA are principally ketoacids. Normalization of the anion gap in DKA reflects correction of the ketoacidosis as ketoacid anions are removed from the blood.

Differential Diagnosis

Although there are many causes of acidosis, few are a source of confusion with DKA. Metabolic causes of acidosis and coma are shown in Table 5 *(58)*.

ALCOHOLIC AND FASTING KETOACIDOSIS

Acidosis can be fairly severe in alcoholic ketoacidosis (AKA), but the lack of hyperglycemia in AKA serves to eliminate DKA as a consideration. Rarely, modest elevations of blood glucose have been reported in AKA *(59)*, perhaps reflecting underlying unrecognized diabetes or a catecholamine stimulated

Table 5
Laboratory evaluation of metabolic causes of acidosis and coma

	Starvation or high fat intake	DKA	Lactic acidosis	Uremic acidosis	Alcoholic Ketosis	Salicylate intoxication	Methanol or ethyleneglycol intoxication	Hyper-osmolar coma	Hypo-Glycemic coma	Rhabdomyolysis	Isopropyl alcohol
pH	Normal	↓	↓	Mild ↓	↓↑	↓↑↑	↓	Normal	Normal	Mild ↓ Maybe↓↓	Normal
Plasma glucose	Normal	↑	Normal	Normal	↓ Or Normal	Normal or ↓	Normal	↑↑ >500 mg/dl	↓↓ <30 mg/dl	Normal	→
Total plasma Ketones*	Slight ↑	↑↑	Normal	Normal	Slight to Moderate ↑	Normal	Normal	Normal or slight ↑	Normal or slight ↑	Normal	↑↑
Anion gap	Slight ↑	↑	↑	Slight ↑	↑	↑	↑	Normal	Normal or Slight ↑	↑↑	Normal
Osmolality	Normal	↑	Normal	↑	Normal	Normal	↑↑	↑↑↑ >330 mOsm/kg	Normal	Normal or slight ↑	↑
Uric Acid	Mild ↑										Normal
Glycosuria^	Negative	++ False +	Negative	Negative	Negative	Negative †	Negative	++	Negative	Negative	Negative
Miscellaneous			lactate >7 mmol/l	Serum BUN> 200 mg/dl		Salicilate serum levels +	+ serum levels			Myoglobin-Uria Hemoglobin-Uria	

+, positive; *Acetest and Ketostix measure acetoacetic acid only: thus, misleading low values may be obtained because the majority of "ketone bodies" are β-hydroxybutyrate:

†respiratory alkalosis/metabolic acidosis; ^may get false-positive or false-negative urinary glucose caused by the presence of salicylate or its metabolites; Adopted from ref. (58).

rise from stress. After prolonged fasting alone ketoacid levels do not exceed 10 meq/L and serum bicarbonate is typically greater than 14 meq/L *(56)*.

ANION GAP ACIDOSIS

DKA must also be differentiated from other causes of high anion gap metabolic acidosis. These include lactic acidosis which can be induced by metformin, (but rarely in the absence of renal failure); aspirin, methanol, and ethylene glycol; and advanced renal failure. None of these disorders, however, causes ketoacidosis.

Treatment

THERAPEUTIC OBJECTIVES

The treatment of hyperglycemic crises, whether DKA of HHS, has several goals:

(a) restoration of circulatory volume and tissue perfusion; (b) steady but gradual reduction of serum glucose and plasma olmolality; (c) correction of electrolyte imbalances; (d) resolution of ketoacidosis in DKA; and (e) recognition and treatment of any precipitating causes or comorbid conditions.

MONITORING

Serum glucose values must be checked every 1–2 hours during treatment, and serum electrolytes, phosphate, and venous pH should be assessed every 2–6 hours depending on the clinical condition and response of the patient. Venous blood samples for pH, which is about 0.03 units lower, may be substituted for arterial blood and the pain and potential complications of arterial puncture avoided *(60)*. Figure 8 provides a detailed algorithm for management of DKA and HHS, in adults. A flow sheet (Fig. 9) is extremely valuable in organizing care and documenting treatment *(24)*.

REPLACEMENT OF FLUID AND ELECTROLYTES

As noted earlier, loss of water in DKA averages 5 to 6 L and in HHS may be as high as 9 L *(3,5,32)*. The severity of deficits is determined by a number of factors but primarily by the duration of hyperglycemia, the level of renal function, the balance of oral intake of solute and water with vomiting or loss by diarrhea, and presence of fever or high ambient temperature. Our initial choice of fluid is isotonic saline infused at a rate of 1 to 1.5 L the first hour to rapidly expand extracellular and interstitial compartments *(40)*. The optimal rate of infusion is dependent on the clinical state of the patient. In patients who are in shock it should be infused as quickly as possible. This is followed during the next 2 hours by either 0.45% or 0.9% NaCl given at 500–1000 ml/hour with

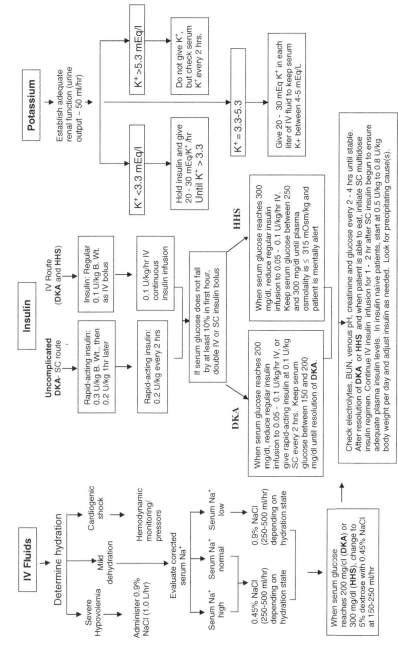

Fig. 8. Protocol for management of adult patients with DKA or HHS [adopted from ref. (3)].

DKA / HHS FLOWSHEET

Height: ________
Weight:
0° ________
24° ________

	DATE: HOUR:	ER												
	MENTAL STATUS*													
	TEMPERATURE													
	PULSE													
	RESPIRATION/DEPTH**													
	BLOOD PRESSURE													
	SERUM GLUCOSE (MG/DL)													
	SERUM "KETONES"													
	URINE "KETONES"													
ELECTROLYTES	SERUM Na^+ (mEq/L)													
ELECTROLYTES	SERUM K^+ (mEq/L)													
ELECTROLYTES	SERUM CL^- (mEq/L)													
ELECTROLYTES	SERUM HCO_3^- (mEq/L)													
ELECTROLYTES	SERUM BUN (mg/dl)													
ELECTROLYTES	EFFECTIVE OSMOLALITY 2 [measured Na (mEq/L)] + Glucose (mg/dl)/18													
ELECTROLYTES	ANION GAP													
A.B.G.	pH VENOUS(V) ARTERIAL (A)													
A.B.G.	pO_2													
A.B.G.	pCO_2													
A.B.G.	O_2 SAT													
INSULIN	UNITS PAST HOUR													
INSULIN	ROUTE													
INTAKE FLUID/METABOLITES	0.45% NaCl (ml) PAST HOUR													
INTAKE FLUID/METABOLITES	0.9% NaCl (ml) PAST HOUR													
INTAKE FLUID/METABOLITES	5% DEXTROSE (ml) PAST HOUR													
INTAKE FLUID/METABOLITES	KCL (mEq) PAST HOUR													
INTAKE FLUID/METABOLITES	PO_4 (mMOLES) PAST HOUR													
INTAKE FLUID/METABOLITES	OTHER													
OUTPUT	URINE (ml)													
OUTPUT	OTHER													

* A-ALERT D-DROWSY S-STUPOROUS C-COMATOSE
** D-DEEP S-SHALLOW N-NORMAL

Adopted by permission from Kitabchi, et. al., In: Joslin's Diabetes mellitus. 1994 (24).

Fig. 9. Adopted by permission from Kitabchi, et. al., In: Joslin's Diabetes mellitus. 1994 *(24)*.

subsequent fluid replacement dependent on the status of hydration, serum electrolyte levels, and urinary output. The goal should be to replace the estimated water deficit over the first 36 hours. As intravascular volume is restored, even in the absence of insulin treatment, there will be a decrease in counterregulatory hormones and blood glucose *(61)*. In patients with renal or cardiac compromise, frequent monitoring must be performed to avoid iatrogenic fluid overload *(14,40,61)*.

POTASSIUM

As noted previously, most patients with DKA and HHS have a significant and sometimes profound potassium deficit at the time of presentation due to urinary and in some instances gastrointestinal losses. This may be masked, however, by the shift of potassium out of cells so that serum potassium may be elevated on admission. With insulin therapy, fluid replacement, and correction of acidosis, hypokalemia will likely ensue if potassium therapy is delayed, but potassium repletion should not begin until serum potassium falls to less than 5.3 meq/L and urine output is at least 50 ml/hour. The use of one-half isotonic saline may be influenced by the need for potassium infusion since potassium is as osmotically active as sodium. The addition of 40 meq of potassium to a liter of one-half isotonic saline provides a solution that contains 117 meq of cation (77 meq of sodium and 40 meq of potassium) which is equivalent to approximately three-quarters isotonic saline. By contrast, if potassium is added to isotonic saline a hypertonic solution is produced that will not correct hyperosmolality.

INSULIN

Unless the episode of DKA is mild and uncomplicated, regular insulin by continuous intravenous infusion is the preferred treatment. The only reason for delaying insulin therapy would be initial serum potassium below 3.3 meq/L since insulin would worsen the hypokalemia by driving potassium into cells which could trigger a cardiac arrhythmia. The therapy should begin with an intravenous bolus of regular insulin (0.1 U/kg body weight) followed by a continuous infusion of low-dose regular insulin at a concentration of 0.1 U/kg per hour. The importance of the intravenous bolus was demonstrated in an investigation of the optimal route of insulin administration in DKA. Although the total time for resolution of DKA was the same in patients receiving insulin by intravenous, subcutaneous, or intramuscular routes, those who received intravenous insulin showed a more rapid decline in both glucose and ketone bodies during the first two hours (62). The same insulin dose is used for DKA and HHS.

With this approach to therapy, serum glucose will usually decrease by 50 to 70 mg/dl (2.8 to 3.9 mmol/L) per hour or more. If the serum glucose does not fall by 10% of the initial value in the first hour, the initial intravenous bolus should be repeated hourly until a steady decline in glucose is achieved. If glucose levels fail to decline with treatment, the intravenous access must be checked to insure that the insulin is being delivered and that there are no filters interposed that could bind insulin.

As already pointed out, glucose may decline considerably with fluid replacement alone due to hemodilution and increased glycosuria as renal perfusion is improved (61). Patients with HHS are usually more dehydrated and their rate of decline in serum glucose with therapy may be even more pronounced than in DKA patients.

When serum glucose reaches a level of 200 mg/dl (11.1 mmol/L) in DKA or 300 mg/dl in HHS, the intravenous solution should be changed to dextrose in saline, and the insulin infusion rate usually may be decreased to 0.05 U/kg per hour. Thereafter the rate of insulin and glucose infusion should be adjusted to maintain the blood glucose between 150 and 200 mg/dl in DKA and 250 to 300 mg/dl in HHS until the hyperglycemic crisis is over (in DKA) and effective osmolality is <320 mOsm/kg and patient is alert (in HHS). Effective osmolality is calculated by following formula: 2 (Na+) + glucose (mg/dl)/18 = mOsm/kg.

ALTERNATIVE TREATMENT WITH FAST-ACTING INSULIN ANALOGS

Two recent prospective randomized trials investigated the use of the rapid-acting insulin analogs aspart and lispro in treating DKA (63,64). A total of 95 patients with mild to moderate DKA were randomly assigned to receive intravenous regular insulin or a short-acting analog. The outcome of therapy was indistinguishable between the groups, but the lispro and aspart groups were managed on regular hospital wards or intermediate care units whereas the intravenous group was admitted to ICU. As a result, the cost of hospitalization was 39% higher for the latter group even though length of hospital stay was no different (Table 6).

BICARBONATE THERAPY

Since diabetic ketoacidosis usually corrects with insulin treatment and fluid replacement, most current reviews do not recommend bicarbonate use in DKA, although the subject remains controversial (65). In a randomized trial of 30 DKA patients with a pH between 6.90 and 7.10 on admission, morbidity and mortality was not changed by bicarbonate therapy (66). This study was small, however, and there was no difference in the rate of rise in serum bicarbonate or arterial pH between the bicarbonate and placebo arms of the study. There have been no prospective randomized trials of bicarbonate therapy in DKA patients with an admission pH less than 6.9. There are several potential concerns with the use of alkali in treating DKA:

- Use of alkali, particularly in large amounts, may cause a rapid rise in pCO2 by diminishing the acidemic stimulus to hyperventilation. That might result in a paradoxical fall in cerebral pH since the lipid-soluble CO_2 can rapidly cross the blood-brain barrier. Although neurological impairment has been reported in this setting, it is probably a rare event (67).
- The rate of recovery of ketosis may be decreased by alkali treatment. In one study of seven patients, the three patients given bicarbonate had an increase in serum ketoacid levels during bicarbonate infusion and a six hour delay in

Table 6
Comparative Effects of Subcutaneous (SC) Fast-acting Insulin vs IV Regular Insulin in DKA. [Data Adopted from ref. *(63,64)*]

	Aspartate* SC-2 hr.	Lispro* SC-1 hr.	Regular** IV.	P values
Length of hospital stay (days)	3.9 ± 1.5	4 ± 2	4.5 ± 3.0	NS
Duration of therapy until BG<250 mg/dl (hrs)	6.1 ± 1	7 ± 1	7.1 ± 1	NS
Duration of therapy until resolution of DKA (hrs)	10.7 ± 0.8	10 ± 1	11 ± 0.7	NS
Amount of insulin until resolution of DKA (units)	94 ± 32	84 ± 32	82 ± 28	NS
Episodes of Hypoglycemia	1	1	1	NS
Cost of Hospitalization	$10,173 \pm 1738	$9,816 \pm 4981	$17,030 \pm 1753	<0.01

Data are means $\pm$ SE, NS=Not Significant,

*treated in general medical wards

**Treated in ICU Insulin dose 0.2–0.3 U/Kg SC initially followed one hour later by 0.1 U/Kg/H or 0.2 U/Kg/2 h SC

ketosis resolution *(68)*. In the randomized trial cited above, however, treatment with bicarbonate had no effect on the rate of decline of serum ketone levels *(66)*.

- Post-treatment metabolic alkalosis may be caused by alkali therapy since the metabolism of ketoacid anions induced by insulin treatment promotes regeneration of bicarbonate and correction of most of the metabolic acidosis.
- Bicarbonate therapy may increase the risk of hypokalemia *(65)*.

Despite these caveats, because of the potential deleterious effects of severe acidosis including decreased myocardial contractility, in adult patients with a pH between 6.9 and 7.0 it may be prudent to give 50 mmol of bicarbonate (1 ampule) in 200 ml of sterile water with 10 mEq of potassium chloride over 2 hours. If the pH is <6.9, 100 mmol of bicarbonate (2 ampules) in 400 ml sterile water with 20 mEq potassium chloride should be administered at the rate of 200 ml/hour over 2 hours. Venous pH should be checked every two hours, and bicarbonate administered as above until the pH rises above 7.0.

PHOSPHATE

Although whole body phosphate deficiency is common in DKA, the serum phosphate may be normal or increased before initiation of therapy due to phosphate movement out of cells *(69,70)*. As observed with potassium balance, phosphate depletion is quickly apparent with institution of insulin treatment. Hypophosphatemia which occurs acutely during treatment of DKA is self-limited, and usually not severe or associated with adverse effects. Frank rhabdomyolysis with myoglobinuria and hemolysis has been reported in this situation, but is quite rare *(71–73)*.

Several prospective randomized trials of phosphate replacement in DKA have failed to demonstrate a benefit *(74–76)*. Furthermore, phosphate therapy can produce both hypocalcemia and hypomagnesemia *(74–78)*. In view of these comments, the routine use of phosphate replacement in the treatment of DKA is not recommended. There may be rare instances, however, where phosphate therapy might be of benefit. Since cardiac and skeletal weakness and respiratory depression has been associated with severe hypophosphatemia, patients with a serum phosphate less than 1.0 mg/dL (0.32 mmol/L), especially those with hemolytic anemia, cardiac dysfunction, or respiratory depression, should be considered for therapy *(79)*. Potassium phosphate, 20 to 30 meq/L can be added to replacement fluids.

RESOLUTION OF DKA AND HHS

When the following goals are met, the hyperglycemic crisis is considered to be resolved:

- Cessation of ketoacidosis is achieved, as evidenced by normalization of the serum anion gap to less than 12 meq/L or the absence of beta-hydroxybutyric acid by direct testing. Ketonemia and ketonuria may last for more than 36 hours because of the slower removal of acetone, in part through the lungs *(80)*. Acetone is biochemically neutral, however, so such patients are no longer in ketoacidosis.
- Patients with HHS have effective osmolality below 320 mOsmol/kg and are mentally alert.
- The patient is able to eat.

ADA guidelines suggest that intravenous insulin may be tapered and a multiple dose subcutaneous insulin schedule started in patients who meet the following goals, the last three applying only to DKA:

- Serum glucose less than 200 mg/ml in DKA or 250 to 300 mg/kg in HHS
- Serum anion gap < 12 meq/L (or less than upper normal limit for the local laboratory)
- Serum bicarbonate >18 meq/L
- Venous pH >7.30

Whenever rapid-acting or regular subcutaneous insulin in started, intravenous insulin infusion should be allowed to overlap for one to two hours in order to prevent a rebound of ketoacidosis or hyperglycemia. If the patient is unable to resume oral nutrition, it is preferable to continue intravenous insulin to allow more flexibility in glucose control.

COMPLICATIONS

Before the era of low-dose insulin treatment of DKA and HHS it was not unusual to give as much as 100 units per hour for several hours with hypoglycemia and hypokalemia frequent sequelae. These iatrogenic problems that resulted from excessive insulin, and often bicarbonate as well, seldom occur with current treatment protocols *(45)*. A brief hyperchloremic non-anion gap acidosis is seen often in the recovery phase of DKA, but is usually of no clinical consequence *(81,82)*. This results from the loss of large quantities of ketoanions in the urine during the development of DKA, limiting the regeneration of bicarbonate from the metabolism of ketoanions during recovery. In addition the excessive administration of chloride containing fluids and the intracellular shifts of $NaHCO_3$ contribute to this phenomena *(83,84)*.

Cerebral edema is a rare but highly fatal complication of DKA that occurs principally in children with newly diagnosed diabetes, but occasionally in children with known diabetes and in young adults *(85,86)*. The etiology of cerebral edema is unknown, but a recent study utilizing magnetic resonance imaging of 14 children in DKA suggested that increased cerebral perfusion from a vasogenic mechanism rather than osmotic cell swelling may be the underlying cause *(87)*. Cerebral edema in adults with DKA or HHS is extremely uncommon, and there have been no prospective studies to guide preventive measures or therapy. It would appear prudent to replace sodium and water deficits gradually in hyperosmolar patients, and to add dextrose to the hydrating solution once the blood glucose reaches 200 mg/dl in DKA or 300 mg/dl in HHS. In HHS it is recommended that a glucose level of 250–300 mg/dl be maintained until hyperosmolality and mental status has improved and the patient is clinically stable *(3)*.

Reduction in colloid osmotic pressure leading to increased lung water content and decreased lung compliance has been suggested as a cause of hypoxemia in DKA.

Rarely, non-cardiac pulmonary edema may be seen in this situation *(14)*.

PREVENTION

As early as 1980 it was shown that frequent follow up of adult diabetic patients in outpatient diabetic clinic could reduce incidence of recurrent DKA by about 60% *(88)*. In more recent studies similar results were obtained in children *(89)*. Educational programs in the proper use of medication and access to medical care also play pivotal roles in prevention of hyperglycemic crises *(90)*.

PROSPECTIVES AND FUTURE STUDIES

In spite of many advances in the diagnosis and treatment of hyperglycemic crises, there are major controversies in both DKA and HHS that deserve further study. Following are examples of such topics:

1. **The use of bicarbonate in DKA**. Limited studies suggest that for pH >7.0 bicarbonate does not provide any advantage *(66)*, but studies for pH <6.9 were limited and a larger number of subjects are necessary to settle the issue *(65,67,68)*. On the other hand *no* prospective randomized studies are available to establish efficacy of the use of bicarbonate in DKA for pH <6.9 *(91)*. Additionally the status of cardiac function in such severe acute acidotic states is not known *(91)*.
2. **Priming dose of insulin**. Although the use of priming dose of insulin in DKA during intravenous infusion of insulin is the recommended method in the most recent ADA Consensus Report *(3)*, in the pediatric group the use of bolus method has not been recommended in the ADA Consensus Report *(92)*. Furthermore our earlier study on pediatric patients clearly showed that 0.1 U/kg of body weight per hour of insulin infusion will result in orderly recovery of such patients *(93)*. Therefore the need for the use of priming or bolus dose of insulin in adult DKA requires further investigation.
3. **The mechanism for lack of ketosis in HHS**. In spite of the fact that recent studies suggest fatty acids and counter regulatory hormones are comparable in the two groups comparative studies are lacking. It also would appear that additional studies are needed to confirm the presence of higher concentration of C-peptide in HHS than DKA (Table 2), especially when C-peptide in ketosis-prone diabetes may be comparable to some of the patients with HHS *(7,8,12)*.
4. **The mechanism of production of elevated proinflammatory cytokines**, as well as cardiac risk factors in patients with hyperglycemic crises who demonstrate no cardiac history, infection or injury is not known. Interestingly these elevated values return to near normal levels with insulin therapy and hydration within 24 hours *(31)*. This non-specific effect of stress requires further investigation.
5. **The subcutaneous use of regular insulin in DKA**. We have demonstrated that the use of fast acting insulin analogues by the subcutaneous route in general wards (in mild or moderate DKA) is as effective as the use of regular insulin by the IV route in the ICU, with cost savings of about 39% *(63,64)*. However it is not known if a similar result could be obtained with standard regular insulin given every 2 hours by the subcutaneous route in general wards to such patients.

The use of regular insulin, if found effective, could certainly save additional money as the cost of insulin analogues is at least two to three fold higher than regular insulin.

REFERENCES

1. Johnson DD, Palumbo PJ, Chu CP. Diabetic ketoacidosis in a community-based population. Mayo Clinic Proceedings 1980; 55(2): 83–8.
2. Centers for Disease Control and Prevention Diabetes Surveillance System Atlanta. US Department of Health and Human Services, 2003. Available at: www.cecgov/diabetes/ statistics/indexhtm Accessed July 17, 2007.
3. Kitabchi AE, Umpierrez GE, Murphy MB, Kreisberg RA. Hyperglycemic crises in adult patients with diabetes: a concensus statement from the American Diabetes Association. Diabetes Care 2006; 29(12): 2739–48.
4. Kitabchi AE, Fisher JN. Diabetes Mellitus. In: Glew RA, Peters SP, ed. Clinical Studies in Medical Biochemistry. New York: Oxford University Press; 1987: 102–17.
5. Kitabchi AE, Umpierrez GE, Murphy MB, et al. Management of hyperglycemic crises in patients with diabetes. Diabetes Care 2001; 24(1): 131–53.
6. Umpierrez G, Fisher JN. Diabetic ketoacidosis and hyperosmolar hyperglycemic state. In: Rakel RE BE, ed. Conn's Current Therapy. Philadelphia: Saunders; 2003.
7. Umpierrez GE, Kelly JP, Navarrete JE, Casals MM, Kitabchi AE. Hyperglycemic crises in urban blacks. Arch Intern Med 1997; 157(6): 669–75.
8. Umpierrez GE, Woo W, Hagopian WA, Isaacs SD, Palmer JP, Gaur LK, Nepom GT, Clark WS, Mixon PS, Kitabchi AE. Immunogenetic analyses suggest different pathogenesis between obese and lean African-Americans with diabetic ketoacidosis. Diabetes Care 1999; 22: 1517–23.
9. Maldonado M, Hampe CS, Gaur LK, et al. Ketosis-prone diabetes: dissection of a heterogeneous syndrome using an immunogenetic and beta-cell functional classification, prospective analysis, and clinical outcomes. J Clin Endocrinol Metab 2003; 88: 5090–8.
10. Mauvais-Jarvis F, Sobngwi E, Porcher R, et al. Ketosis-prone type 2 diabetes in patients of sub-Saharan African origin: clinical pathophysiology and natural history of beta-cell dysfunction and insulin resistance. Diabetes 2004; 53: 645–53.
11. Kitabchi AE. Ketosis-prone diabetes–a new subgroup of patients with atypical type 1 and type 2 diabetes? J Clin Endocrinol Metab 2003; 88(11): 5087–9.
12. Umpierrez GE, Smiley D, Kitabchi AE. Ketosis-prone type 2 diabetes mellitus. Ann Intern Med 2006; 144: 350–7.
13. Kitabchi AE, Fisher JN. Insulin therapy of diabetic ketoacidosis: Physiologic versus pharmacologic doses of insulin and their routes of administration. In (Brownlee M, ed). Handbook of Diabetes Mellitus, 5: 95–149, New York, Garland ATPM Press, 1981.
14. Kitabchi AE, Umperrez GE, Murphy MB. Diabetic ketoacidosis and hyperglycemic hyperosmolar state. In: DeFronzo RA, Rerrannini E, Keen H, Zimmet P, ed. International Textbook of Diabetes Mellitus. 3rd ed. Chichester (UK): John Wiley & Sons; 2004: 1101–19.
15. Kitabchi AE, Nyenwe EA. Hyperglycemic crises in diabetes mellitus: diabetic ketoacidosis and hyperglycemic hyperosmolar state. Endocrinol Metab Clin North Am 2006; 35(4): 725–51.
16. Nyenwe EA, Loganathan RS, Blum S, et al. Active use of cocaine: an independent risk factor for recurrent diabetic ketoacidosis in a city hospital. Endocr Pract 2007; 13(1): 22–9.

17. Peden NR, Braaten JT, McKendry JB. Diabetic ketoacidosis during long-term treatment with continuous subcutaneous insulin infusion. Diabetes Care 1984; 7(1): 1–5.

18. Polonsky WH, Anderson BJ, Lohrer PA, Aponte JE, Jacobson AM, Cole CF. Insulin omission in women with IDDM. Diabetes Care 1994; 17(10): 1178–85.

19. Vidal Cortada J, Conget Donlo JI, Navarro Tellez MP, Halperin Rabinovic I, Vilardell Latorre E. Diabetic ketoacidosis as the first manifestation of acromegaly. An Med Interna 1995; 12(2): 76–8.

20. Katz JR, Edwards R, Khan M, Conway GS. Acromegaly presenting with diabetic ketoacidosis. Postgrad Med J 1996; 72(853): 682–3.

21. Szeto CC, Li KY, Ko GT, et al. Acromegaly in a woman presenting with diabetic ketoacidosis and insulin resistance. International journal of clinical practice 1997; 51(7): 476–7.

22. Soveid M, G. R-O. Ketoacidosis as the primary manifestation of acromegaly. Arch Iranian Med 2005; 8: 326–8.

23. Shah P, Isley WL. Ketoacidosis during a low carbohydrate diet. N Engl J Med 2006; 354: 97–8.

24. Kitabchi AE, Fisher JN, Murphy MB, et al. Diabetic ketoacidosis and the hyperglycemic hyperosmolar non-ketotic state. In: Kahn CR WG, ed. Joslin's Diabetes Mellitus. 13th ed. Philadelphia: Lea & Febiger; 1994: 738–70.

25. Exton JH. Mechanisms of hormonal regulation of hepatic glucose metabolism. Diabetes Metab Rev 1987; 3(1): 163–83.

26. Kitabchi AE, Umpierrez GE, Murphy MB, et al. Hyperglycemic crises in diabetes. Diabetes Care 2004; 27 Suppl 1: S94–102.

27. McGarry JD, Woeltje KF, Kuwajima M, Foster DW. Regulation of ketogenesis and the renaissance of carnitine palmitoyltransferase. Diabetes Metab Rev 1989; 5(3): 271–84.

28. Reichard GA, Jr., Skutches CL, Hoeldtke RD, Owen OE. Acetone metabolism in humans during diabetic ketoacidosis. Diabetes 1986; 35(6): 668–74.

29. Unger RH, Orci L. Glucagon and the α cell: physiology and pathophysiology (first two parts). N Engl J Med 1981; 304(25): 1518–24.

30. Barnes AJ, Bloom SR, Goerge K, et al. Ketoacidosis in pancreatectomized man. N Engl J Med 1977; 296(22): 1250–3.

31. Stentz FB, Umpierrez GE, Cuervo R, Kitabchi AE. Proinflammatory cytokines, markers of cardiovascular risks, oxidative stress, and lipid peroxidation in patients with hyperglycemic crises. Diabetes 2004; 53(8): 2079–86.

32. Matz R. Management of the hyperosmolar hyperglycemic syndrome. Am Fam Physician 1999; 60(5): 1468–76.

33. Kitabchi AE, Murphy MB. Hyperglycemic crises in adult patients with diabetes mellitus. In: Wass JA SS, Amiel SA, ed. Oxford Textbook of Endocrinology. New York: Oxford University Press; 2002: 1734–47.

34. Atchley DW, Loeb RE, Jr RD, et al. A detailed study of electrolyte balances following the withdrawal and reestablishment of insulin therapy. J Clin Invest 1933; 12: 297–326.

35. Butler AM, Talbot NB, Burnett CH, et al. Metabolic studies in diabetic coma. Trans Assoc Am Physicians 1947; 60: 102–9.

36. DeFronzo RA, Cooke CR, Andres R, Faloona GR, Davis PJ. The effect of insulin on renal handling of sodium, potassium, calcium, and phosphate in man. The Journal of Clinical Investigation 1975; 55(4): 845–55.

37. Howard RL, Bichet DG, RW. S. Hypernatremic polyuric states. In: The Kidney: Physiology and Pathophysiology. New York: Raven Press; 1991: 1578.

38. Marten HE, Smith K, ML W. The fluid and electrolyte therapy of severe diabetic acidosis and ketosis. Am J Med 1958; 24: 376–89.

39. Keller U. Diabetic ketoacidosis: Current views on pathogenesis and treatment. Diabetologia 1986; 29(2): 71–7.
40. Hillman K. Fluid resuscitation in diabetic emergencies—a reappraisal. Intensive Care Medicine 1987; 13(1): 4–8.
41. Castellino P, Luzi L, Simonson DC, Haymond M, DeFronzo RA. Effect of insulin and plasma amino acid concentrations on leucine metabolism in man. Role of substrate availability on estimates of whole body protein synthesis. The Journal of Clinical Investigation 1987; 80(6): 1784–93.
42. Wachtel TJ. The diabetic hyperosmolar state. Clinics in Geriatric Medicine 1990; 6(4): 797–806.
43. Umpierrez G, Freire AX. Abdominal pain in patients with hyperglycemic crises. J Crit Care 2002; 17: 63–7.
44. Edge JA, Roy Y, Bergomi A, Murphy NP, Ford-Adams MS, Ong KK, Dunger DB. Conscious level in children with diabetic ketoacidosis is related to severity of acidosis and not to blood glucose concentration. Pediatr Diabetes 2006; 7: 11–15.
45. Kitabchi AE, Ayyagari V, Guerra SM. The efficacy of low-dose versus conventional therapy of insulin for treatment of diabetic ketoacidosis. Ann Intern Med 1976; 84(6): 633–8.
46. Morris LR, Kitabchi AE. Efficacy of low dose insulin therapy for severely obtunded patients in diabetic ketoacidosis. Diabetes Care 1980; 3(1): 53–6.
47. Ennis ED, Stahl E, RA K. The hyperosmolar hyperglycemic syndrome. Diabetes Rev 1994; 2: 115–26.
48. Nematollahi LR, Taheri E, Larijana B, Mahajeri M, Gozashti M, Wan JY, Kitabchi AE. Catecholamine-induced leukocytosis in acute hypoglycemic stress. J Investig Med 2007: 55 pS262 Abstract 95.
49. Slovis CM, Mork VG, Slovis RJ, Bain RP. Diabetic ketoacidosis and infection: Leukocyte count and differential as early predictors of serious infection. Am J Emerg Med 1987; 5(1): 1–5.
50. Kaminska ES, Pourmotabbed G. Spurious laboratory values in diabetic ketoacidosis and hyperlipidemia. Am J Emerg Med 1993; 11(1): 77–80.
51. Rumbak MJ, Hughes TA, Kitabchi AE. Pseudonormoglycemia in diabetic ketoacidosis with elevated triglycerides. Am J Emerg Med 1991; 9(1): 61–3.
52. Beigelman PM. Potassium in severe diabetic ketoacidosis. Am J Med 1973; 54(4): 419–20.
53. Vinicor F, Lehrner LM, Karn RC, Merritt AD. Hyperamylasemia in diabetic ketoacidosis: sources and significance. Ann Intern Med 1979; 91(2): 200–4.
54. Yadav D, Nair S, Norkus EP, Pitchumoni CS. Nonspecific hyperamylasemia and hyperlipasemia in diabetic ketoacidosis: incidence and correlation with biochemical abnormalities. The American Journal of Gastroenterology 2000; 95(11): 3123–8.
55. Gerard SK, Khayam-Bashi H. Characterization of creatinine error in ketotic patients. A prospective comparison of alkaline picrate methods with an enzymatic method. American Journal of Clinical Pathology 1985; 84(5): 659–64.
56. Reichard GA, Jr., Owen OE, Haff AC, Paul P, Bortz WM. Ketone-body production and oxidation in fasting obese humans. The Journal of Clinical Investigation 1974; 53(2): 508–15.
57. Csako G, Elin RJ. Unrecognized false-positive ketones from drugs containing free-sulfhydryl group(s). JAMA 1993; 269(13): 1634.
58. Morris LR, Kitabchi AE. Coma in the Diabetic. In (Schnatz JD, ed), Diabetes Mellitus: Problems in Management. Menlo Park CA, Addison-Wesley Pub. Co, 234–251, 1982.
59. Wrenn KD, Slovis CM, Minion GE, Rutkowski R. The syndrome of alcoholic ketoacidosis. Am J Med 1991; 91(2): 119–28.

60. Middleton P, Kelly AM, Brown J, Robertson M. Agreement between arterial and central venous values for pH, bicarbonate, base excess, and lactate. Emerg Med J 2006; 23(8): 622–4.

61. Waldhausl W, Kleinberger G, Korn A, Dudczak R, Bratusch-Marrain P, Nowotny P. Severe hyperglycemia: Effects of rehydration on endocrine derangements and blood glucose concentration. Diabetes 1979; 28(6): 577–84.

62. Fisher JN, Shahshahani MN, Kitabchi AE. Diabetic ketoacidosis: Low-dose insulin therapy by various routes. N Engl J Med 1977; 297(5): 238–41.

63. Umpierrez GE, Cuervo R, Karabell A, Latif K, Freire AX, Kitabchi AE. Treatment of diabetic ketoacidosis with subcutaneous insulin aspart. Diabetes Care 2004; 27(8): 1873–8.

64. Umpierrez GE, Latif K, Stoever J, Cuervo R, Park L, Freire AX, Kitabchi AE. Efficacy of subcutaneous insulin lispro versus continuous intravenous regular insulin for the treatment of patients with diabetic ketoacidosis. Am J Med 2004; 117(5): 291–6.

65. Viallon A, Zeni F, Lafond P, et al. Does bicarbonate therapy improve the management of severe diabetic ketoacidosis? Critical Care Medicine 1999; 27(12): 2690–3.

66. Morris LR, Murphy MB, Kitabchi AE. Bicarbonate therapy in severe diabetic ketoacidosis. Ann Intern Med 1986; 105(6): 836–40.

67. Narins RG, Cohen JJ. Bicarbonate therapy for organic acidosis: The case for its continued use. Ann Intern Med 1987; 106(4): 615–8.

68. Okuda Y, Adrogue HJ, Field JB, Nohara H, Yamashita K. Counterproductive effects of sodium bicarbonate in diabetic ketoacidosis. J Clin Endocrinol Metab 1996; 81(1): 314–20.

69. Rose B, Post T. Clinical Physiology of Acid-Base and Electrolyte Disorders. 5th ed. New York: McGraw-Hill; 2001.

70. Kebler R, McDonald FD, Cadnapaphornchai P. Dynamic changes in serum phosphorus levels in diabetic ketoacidosis. Am J Med 1985; 79(5): 571–6.

71. Rainey RL, Estes PW, Neely CL, Amick LD. Myoglobinuria following diabetic acidosis with electromyographic evaluation. Arch Intern Med 1963; 111: 564–71.

72. Casteels K, Beckers D, Wouters C, Van Geet C. Rhabdomyolysis in diabetic ketoacidosis. Pediatric Diabetes 2003; 4(1): 29–31.

73. Shilo S, Werner D, Hershko C. Acute hemolytic anemia caused by severe hypophosphatemia in diabetic ketoacidosis. Acta Haematologica 1985; 73(1): 55–7.

74. Fisher JN, Kitabchi AE. A randomized study of phosphate therapy in the treatment of diabetic ketoacidosis. J Clin Endocrinol Metab 1983; 57(1): 177–80.

75. Keller U, Berger W. Prevention of hypophosphatemia by phosphate infusion during treatment of diabetic ketoacidosis and hyperosmolar coma. Diabetes 1980; 29(2): 87–95.

76. Wilson HK, Keuer SP, Lea AS, Boyd AE, 3rd, Eknoyan G. Phosphate therapy in diabetic ketoacidosis. Arch Intern Med 1982; 142(3): 517–20.

77. Barsotti MM. Potassium phosphate and potassium chloride in the treatment of DKA. Diabetes Care 1980; 3(4): 569.

78. Winter RJ, Harris CJ, Phillips LS, Green OC. Diabetic ketoacidosis. Induction of hypocalcemia and hypomagnesemia by phosphate therapy. Am J Med 1979; 67(5): 897–900.

79. Kreisberg RA. Phosphorus deficiency and hypophosphatemia. Hospital practice 1977; 12(3): 121–8.

80. Sulway MJ, Malins JM. Acetone in diabetic ketoacidosis. Lancet 1970; 2(7676): 736–40.

81. Adrogue HJ, Wilson H, Boyd AE, 3rd, Suki WN, Eknoyan G. Plasma acid-base patterns in diabetic ketoacidosis. N Engl J Med 1982; 307(26): 1603–10.

82. Wall BM JG, Kaminska E, Fisher JN, Kitabchi AE, Cooke, C. R. Causes of hyperchloremic acidosis during treatment of diabetic ketoacidosis. Clin Res 1990; 38: 960A.

83. Oh MS, Carroll HJ, Uribarri J. Mechanism of normochloremic and hyperchloremic acidosis in diabetic ketoacidosis. Nephron 1990; 54(1): 1–6.

84. Fleckman AM. Diabetic ketoacidosis. Endocrinology and Metabolism Clinics of North America 1993; 22(2): 181–207.

85. Duck SC, Wyatt DT. Factors associated with brain herniation in the treatment of diabetic ketoacidosis. J Pediatr 1988; 113(1 Pt 1): 10–14.

86. Glaser N, Barnett P, McCaslin I, et al. Risk factors for cerebral edema in children with diabetic ketoacidosis. The Pediatric Emergency Medicine Collaborative Research Committee of the American Academy of Pediatrics. N Engl J Med 2001; 344(4): 264–9.

87. Glaser NS, Wootton-Gorges SL, Marcin JP, et al. Mechanism of cerebral edema in children with diabetic ketoacidosis. J Pediatr 2004; 145(2): 164–71.

88. Runyan JW Jr, Zwaag RV, Joyner MB, Miller ST. The Memphis Diabetes Continuing Care Program. Diabetes Care 1980; 3: 382–6.

89. Vanelli M, Chiari G, Ghizzoni L, Costi G, Giacalone T, Chiarelli F. Effectiveness of a prevention program for diabetic ketoacidosis in children: An 8-year study in schools and private practices. Diabetes Care 1999; 22: 7–9.

90. Kitabchi AE. Editorial. Hypergycemic Crises: Improving prevention and management. Am Fam Physician 2005; 71: 1659–60.

91. Latif KA, Freire AX, Kitabchi AE, Umpierrez GE, Qureshi N. The use of alkali therapy in severe diabetic ketoacidosis (DKA). Diabetes Care 2002; 25: 2113–2114.

92. Wolfsdorf J, Glaser N, Sperling MA. American Diabetes Association. Diabetic ketoacidosis in infants, children, and adolescents: A consensus statement from the American Diabetes Association. Diabetes Care 2006; 29(5): 1150–9.

93. Burghen GA, Etteldorf JN, Fisher JN, Kitabchi AE. Comparison of high-dose to low-dose insulin by continuous intravenous infusion in the treatment of diabetic ketoacidosis in children. Diabetes Care 1980; 3: 15–20.

7 Hypoglycemia: An Endocrine Emergency

Jean-Marc Guettier, MD
and Phillip Gorden, MD

Contents

BACKGROUND

Pathophysiology

Conceptually, hypoglycemia results from an absolute or relative imbalance between the rate of appearance and disappearance of circulating glucose. Excess glucose utilization favors disappearance and is usually due to inappropriately high circulating insulin concentration; in rare cases, it may result from antibodies or incompletely processed insulin-like growth factors that act on insulin receptors. Increased consumption of glucose by tissues as seen in intense exercise, weight loss, sepsis, or pregnancy also favors disappearance of circulating glucose and can lead to hypoglycemia when glucose is not

From: *Contemporary Endocrinology: Acute Cause to Consequence*
Edited by: G. Van den Berghe, DOI: 10.1007/978-1-60327-177-6_7,
© Humana Press, New York, NY

replenished as quickly as it is used. Hypoglycemia in this setting is most frequently observed when compounded to disorders that compromise endogenous glucose production (see below). The rate of glucose appearance is determined by oral intake of substrate and in the fasting state by the rate of endogenous glucose production provided by glycogenolysis and gluconeogenesis. Diseases associated predominantly with compromised endogenous glucose production include; malnutrition, liver failure, renal failure, endocrine deficiencies, and enzymatic defects in glyco-metabolic pathways.

Hypoglycemia, the Brain, and Counterregulation

In the non-fasting state, glucose is the preferred substrate for the brain. The brain relies on a continuous external supply of glucose to meet its energy requirements as it lacks the capacity to store large amounts or produce this substrate *de novo*. When plasma levels of glucose fall below the transport maximum (Tm) for glucose across the blood brain, transport becomes rate limiting for energy production and consequently for brain function. Redundant mechanisms to counter insulin's glucose lowering action have evolved to ensure a continuous supply of glucose to the non-fasting brain. The counter-regulatory response (glucose-raising) involves both behavioral (e.g., hunger and food-seeking behavior) and physiological mediators. The latter include hormones, the autonomic nervous system and glucose itself. The central nervous system plays an important role in processing and coordinating the response to an acute drop in systemic blood glucose. Hormonal mechanisms that orchestrate the hypoglycemic response have been well characterized *(1,2)* and involve a decrease in the secretion of insulin (decreased glucose uptake from insulin dependent tissue and increased glycogenolysis) followed by a concomitant rise in systemic glucagon (increased glycogenolysis), epinephrine (increased glycogenolysis, increased gluconeogenesis, decreased glucose uptake from insulin dependent tissue, and decreased insulin secretion) growth hormone and cortisol. In concert, these mechanisms limit glucose utilization and increase glucose production with resultant recovery from hypoglycemia. Drugs (e.g., subcutaneously administered insulin, beta-blockers) or disease states (e.g., diabetes, liver or renal failure) can overwhelm and/or modulate behavioral (e.g., autonomic failure resulting in decreased or absent symptoms) or physiological elements (e.g., absence of glucagon, decreased sympathetic response) of the counter-regulatory response and impair recovery from hypoglycemia. The phenomenon of 'hypoglycemia unawareness' that follows frequent, recurrent hypoglycemic episodes in the setting of tightly controlled diabetes *(3)* or insulinoma *(4)* is an example of such modulation. The dysregulation of the counter-regulatory response in diabetes has been extensively studied and recently reviewed *(5,6)*.

DEFINITION, SYMPTOMS, RISK FACTORS, AND CLASSIFICATION

Definition of Hypoglycemia

Both biochemical and clinical features are needed to define pathologic forms of hypoglycemia. Hypoglycemic symptoms are non-specific and conditions other than low plasma glucose can present with similar symptoms. Thus, documentation of a plasma glucose level below the normal range is essential. Though evidence of low plasma glucose is necessary, relying solely on this criterion to define hypoglycemia can be misleading. Indeed, plasma glucose values below the normal range do not always differentiate between normal and pathologic forms of hypoglycemia (7). Furthermore, artifactual hypoglycemia caused by specimen mishandling or glycolysis within the collected sample, as seen in cases of severe erythrocytosis or leukocytosis, can lead to an erroneous diagnosis. With these caveats in mind, the definition proposed by Whipple in 1938 (8) remains the most useful. It defines pathologic hypoglycemia as a triad of low plasma glucose, hypoglycemic symptoms, and resolution of symptoms with correction of the blood sugar.

Symptoms of Hypoglycemia

Symptoms caused by a sudden drop in blood glucose (9,10) result from increased autonomic nervous system outflow and central nervous system (CNS) glucose deprivation. Classic adrenergic symptoms include anxiety, tremulousness, pallor, and palpitations. Whereas sweating, tingling, nausea, and hunger fall under cholinergic symptoms. Neuroglycopenic symptoms, which include weakness, fatigue, confusion, seizures, focal neurological deficit, and coma; denote compromised brain function due to insufficient glucose.

Risk Factors

Though many conditions predispose to hypoglycemia, it is most often observed in patients receiving hypoglycemic medications for the treatment of diabetes (11–14). Due to the high prevalence of diabetes, hypoglycemia is the most frequent endocrine emergency in both the ambulatory and inpatient care settings (11,14–17). In the Diabetes Control and Complications Trial (DCCT) the risk of suffering one hypoglycemic episode requiring third party assistance for treatment in one year of conventional or intensive treatment was estimated to be 19% and 62% respectively (18). Previous hypoglycemic episodes, lower glycosylated hemoglobin levels, and intensive therapy predicted hypoglycemic events in this population. In the first 10 years of the United Kingdom Prospective Diabetes Study (UKPDS), hypoglycemic episodes requiring third party intervention occurred at an incidence of 1.2% for type-2 patients treated with insulin *(19)*. More recent studies suggest an incidence of severe hypoglycemia in type 2 diabetes approximating that of type 1 *(12,20)*. In a retrospective analysis of an elderly population with type 2 diabetes, recent hospitalization, advanced age, African American ancestry and use of five or more medications independently predicted hypoglycemia *(21)*. As recognition of benefits derived from intensive therapy and subsequent implementation of such practice extend to the general medical community, an increase in incidence of hypoglycemic events can be expected *(13,18,19)*. Hypoglycemia is less common in the non-diabetic population (Reviewed in *(22)*) and its etiological basis and risk factors differ. In the non-diabetic hospitalized patient, the risk of developing hypoglycemia is associated with malnutrition, malignancy, renal disease, congestive heart failure, and sepsis *(15,23)*. In ambulatory patients, predisposing factors may not be readily apparent. In this population the clinician should be aware of risk factors such as poly-pharmacy, advanced age, ingestion of specific foods (e.g., unripened ackee fruit), undiagnosed underlying psychiatric disorder, or previous gastrointestinal surgery.

Classification of Hypoglycemia

The hypoglycemic syndromes can be divided into two categories; fasting (also termed post-absorptive) hypoglycemia and reactive (also termed postprandial) hypoglycemia. Fasting hypoglycemia occurs in the post-absorptive period ($\geq$ 4 hours after a meal) and reactive hypoglycemia occurs in relation to ingestion of either a mixed meal or a glucose load. Fasting hypoglycemia is a manifestation of a major health problem that necessitates diagnostic and therapeutic intervention.

Reactive hypoglycemia is a more controversial entity. While many patients are told they have reactive hypoglycemia, low plasma glucose is not often observed at the times of symptoms *(24,25)*. In addition, low post-prandial plasma glucose levels alone are not sufficient to define pathologic reactive hypoglycemia. Indeed, an estimated 10–30 % of normal individuals undergoing oral glucose tolerance testing have plasma glucose levels <50 mg/dL at the end of the test without ever developing symptoms *(26–28)*. That being said; any patient that has suffered a severe adverse event (loss of consciousness, traumatic injury, or accident) attributed to post-prandial hypoglycemia requires further work-up. One of the least disputed causes of reactive hypoglycemia is termed alimentary hypoglycemia and was most commonly observed in patients following gastrectomy for peptic ulcer disease *(29)*. The pathophysiology of this disorder involves disruption of controlled gastric emptying that results in decreased transit time of aliments from the stomach to the small intestine, which causes a rapid elevation in plasma glucose that triggers a fast and exaggerated insulin response. The abnormal insulin response can cause a precipitous drop in blood glucose with consequent adrenergic and neuroglycopenic symptoms. Alimentary hypoglycemia is most frequently observed two hours after a meal and has been described as a late component of the dumping syndrome. An ongoing debate over the etiological basis for reactive hypoglycemia following Roux-en-Y surgery for morbid obesity exists. Nesidioblastosis or islet hyperplasia has been proposed by some as causative *(30,31)* others consider it a consequence of the well established dumping syndrome *(32)*.

ETIOLOGY OF FASTING HYPOGLYCEMIA IN ADULTS

Drugs

Drugs account for the most frequent cause of hypoglycemia in adults. The most commonly implicated drugs are insulin, sulfonylurea, and ethanol *(11,14–17)*.

INSULIN

Insulin-induced hypoglycemia usually occurs in patients with diabetes treated with insulin. Factors to consider in assessing hypoglycemia in a patient with diabetes include: errors in the type, dose or timing of insulin injection; failure to account for changes in nutrition, affecting the peripheral action (e.g., weight loss, exercise), or clearance of insulin (e.g., renal failure); and altered counter-regulation as a result of underlying disease or drugs (e.g., beta-blockers). Some patients with psychiatric illness inject insulin surreptitiously, thereby inducing hypoglycemia. These patients have usually acquired their familiarity with insulin either through a relative with insulin treated diabetes or through employment as health care workers *(33)*.

SULFONYLUREA

As with insulin, sufonylurea associated hypoglycemia can occur as a result of volitional or inadvertent overdose *(34)*, surreptitious use *(35,36)* or criminally intended administration *(37,38)*. Risk factors associated with inadvertent overdose in patient taking sulfonylurea to treat diabetes include; advanced age, drug-drug interaction, and decreased renal (e.g., chlorpropamide) or hepatic clearance (e.g., tolbutamide, glipizide and glyburide) *(21,34)*. Accidental overdoses can also occur in patient patients unknowingly taking a sulfonylurea as a result of dispensing error *(39,40)*.

ETHANOL

Ethanol inhibits gluconeogenesis *(41)*. This phenomenon has been attributed to consumption of a rate-limiting co-factor (e.g., Nicotinamide Adenine

Dinucleotide (NAD+)) essential for gluconeogenesis as a result of ethanol metabolism *(42–44)*. Ethanol induced hypoglycemia occurs after glycogen stores have been depleted (12–72 hours) when levels of circulating glucose reflect *de novo* synthesis from alternate substrate. Ethanol levels in plasma may be normal or no longer detectable at the time of hypoglycemia. Hypoglycemia should be excluded before attributing impaired cognition to inebriation in the setting of ethanol ingestion.

OTHER DRUGS

Many other drugs have been reported to cause hypoglycemia. High dose salicylates *(44–46)*, beta-blockers *(47)*, and sulfa-based drugs *(48)* are commonly implicated. Pentamidine at doses used to treat *pneumocystis carinnii* pneumonia can also cause hypoglycemia *(49)*. Quinine *(50,51)* and antiarrythmics (e.g., quinidine *(52)*, disopyramide *(53)*) have been associated with hypoglycemia. Quinolone antibiotics *(54,55)* (e.g., gatifloxacin and levofloxacin) have received recent attention for their propensity to cause dysglycemias. Increased insulin secretion is postulated as the underlying mechanism behind pentamidine, quinine derivatives (including quinolones) and anti-arrythmic induced hypoglycemia.

Organ Failure

LIVER FAILURE

The liver, through glycogenolysis and gluconegenesis, supplies most of the glucose to the circulation in the fasting state. The normal liver has a large functional reserve *(56)* and it is estimated that as little as 20% residual function would suffice to prevent hypoglycemia. This large reserve likely accounts for the fact that most patients with liver disease never develop hypoglycemia. Liver diseases most commonly associated with hypoglycemia include hepatocellular carcinoma *(57)* and fulminant hepatitis caused by hepatotoxic agents or viruses *(58)*. Genetic defects in glyco-metabolic pathways can also lead to hypoglycemia as a consequence of deficient hepatic glycogenolysis and gluconeogenesis and most will be diagnosed in childhood. Finally, liver dysfunction can contribute to hypoglycemia through compromised drug metabolism (e.g., tolbutamide, glyburide, glipizide).

RENAL FAILURE

The kidney is second only to the liver as a gluconeogenic organ *(59)*. Factors associated with renal disease that predispose to hypoglycemia include: caloric deprivation from anorexia, vomiting or protein restriction; depletion of gluconegenic substrate from the latter or hemodialysis treatment; use of glucose-free dialysate; and decreased clearance of renally excreted drugs or their metabolites (e.g., insulin, chlorpropamide, and metabolite of glyburide)

ENDOCRINE FAILURE

Deficiencies in cortisol and growth hormone, have been causally linked to hypoglycemia *(60–65)*. Though these hormones do not play a major role in the recovery from acute hypoglycemia, they support the process of gluconeogenesis *(66–69)*. Hypoglycemia, in this setting, will usually develop after a period of fasting when *de novo* synthesis of glucose is the major contributor to circulating levels. Pituitary disease that results in combined ACTH and growth hormone deficiency particularly predispose to the development of hypoglycemia.

Cancer

NON ISLET CELL TUMORS

Mesenchymal tumors, hepatocellular carcinoma, adrenocortical tumors, carcinoid, leukemia, and lymphomas are tumors most commonly associated with hypoglycemia. These tumors cause hypoglycemia by secreting a factor with insulin-like action that is chemically distinct from insulin *(70,71)*. An incompletely processed Insulin Like Growth Factor-II (IGF) molecule termed 'Big' IGF-II *(72–74)* with decreased affinity to IGF binding protein is thought to cause hypoglycemia in some tumors *(75,76)*. A case *(77)* of reactive hypoglycemia caused by a tumor secreting both glucagon-like peptide 1 (GLP-1) and somatostatin has also been reported. Finally, ectopic insulin secretion from tumors is a rare phenomenon. Though sporadic case reports exist in the literature, very few reports *(78–80)* have conclusively excluded the possibility of a concomitant insulinoma.

INSULINOMA

Pancreatic beta-cell tumors are rare and can cause hypoglycemia by secreting insulin autonomously. The majority of these tumors are small, solitary and benign (<10% are malignant) *(81,82)*. The central defect is an inability of insulinoma cells to appropriately suppress insulin secretion in response to a decreasing circulating glucose concentration. This relative excess of insulin in relation to glucose leads to fasting hypoglycemia. Although development of hypoglycemia in the post-prandial period does not rule out the presence of an insulinoma, a negative supervised fast does; as virtually all patients with insulinomas develop hypoglycemia after a 48-hour supervised fast *(83)*. Thus, demonstrating fasting hypoglycemia is essential for the diagnosis of insulinoma.

ISLET HYPERPLASIA

In adults, a variety of histologic patterns in islets have been linked to hypoglycemia. This condition has been termed nesidioblastosis, diffuse islet hyperplasia, or coined syndrome of non-insulinoma pancreatogenous hyperinsulinism *(30,31,84,85)*. There is no doubt that these histological patterns exist but their relationship to hypoglycemia is controversial. Adding to the confusion is the fact that similar histological patterns are observed in cases of persistent hyperinsulinemic hypoglycemia of infancy (PHHI). However, in contrast to adults, many of these infants have an identifiable genetic basis for their hyperinsulinemia in the form of sulfonylurea receptor 1 (SUR1) *(86,87)* postassium channel Kir6.2 *(88,89)*, glucokinase *(90)*, or glutamate dehydrogenase *(91)* mutations. Finally, nesidioblastosis as a cause of hypoglycemia following bariatric surgery is confounded by the fact that gastric surgery can result in alimentary hypoglycemia.

AUTO-IMMUNE CAUSES

Anti-insulin Receptor Antibody

Rarely hypoglycemia is caused by auto-antibodies that bind the insulin receptor and mimic the biological action of insulin *(92,93,94)* (Reviewed in *(95)*). Most patients with this syndrome have an antecedent diagnosis of autoimmune disease. In some patients, an elevated erythrocyte sedimentation rate or positive anti-nuclear antibody titer may be the only finding suggestive of an autoimmune cause.

Anti-insulin Antibody

Development of hypoglycemia has also been associated to auto-antibodies directed against insulin itself *(95–98)*. These antibodies bind free circulating plasma insulin when its concentration is high and release insulin when the concentration of free plasma insulin drops. Release of insulin at inappropriate times can cause hypoglycemia. Hypoglycemia in this setting is typically observed in the post-prandial period but fasting hypoglycemia has been reported.

DIAGNOSIS

Documenting Fasting Hypoglycemia

The first step in the diagnosis is to establish the presence of fasting hypoglycemia. The supervised fast is used for this purpose. This test is performed in the hospital setting to mitigate the risk to the patient if hypoglycemia develops. The patient is fasted and monitored from 48 to 72 hours for biochemical and symptomatic evidence of hypoglycemia. A retrospective review of surgically proven insulinomas showed that in 95% *(83)* of cases hypoglycemia develops within the first 48 hours of the fast.

Determining The Cause

HISTORY

Once fasting hypoglycemia has been established, the next step is to identify the cause. The history provides the clinical context (e.g., liver failure, sepsis, autoimmune disease, neoplasm, or no past health problems), should be reviewed for a potential drug etiology (including ethanol) and may be suggestive of dispensing error as a cause especially if a recent refill precedes the onset of symptoms.

BIOCHEMICAL EVALUATION

Biochemical tests to assess for potential liver, renal, adrenal, and anterior pituitary dysfunction should be obtained. In patients with pituitary insufficiency, growth hormone and cortisol levels in the normal range at the time of hypoglycemia are not uncommon; in particular when the problem has been longstanding. Hormonal deficiency as a cause should be established using the appropriate stimulation tests (e.g., cosyntropin or insulin tolerance test). Blood and urine should be screened for the presence of hypoglycemic agents to rule out surreptitious use. A positive screen should be confirmed by a repeat test to rule out the presence of substances that may cross-react with the assay. The presence of insulin antibodies suggests that the patient has received insulin by injection but in rare cases may represent autoantibodies directed against insulin. The highly purified insulin preparations currently used for the treatment of diabetes are far less immunogenic than in the past. Thus, the absence of insulin antibodies does not reliably exclude surreptitious injection of insulin.

DIAGNOSIS OF INSULINOMA

If the initial evaluation fails to reveal a cause for the hypoglycemia, the possibility of insulinoma should next be considered. Several different approaches to demonstrate the presence of an insulinoma exist but the most useful is the 48-hour supervised fast with measurement of plasma insulin and proinsulin. Demonstrating abnormal insulin suppression at the time the patient develops fasting hypoglycemia makes the diagnosis of insulinoma. This test is based on the premise that insulin secretion in normal beta-cells is suppressed prior to the onset of symptoms at a plasma glucose level of 40–50 mg/dL. In contrast, the threshold for insulin suppression in insulinoma may be absent or shifted to a lower plasma glucose and symptoms arise prior to insulin suppression. Thus, a plasma insulin level that fails to suppress to <6 µU/mL at the time of hypoglycemia strongly suggests the presence of an insulin secreting tumor *(81)*. A plasma insulin level that suppresses to <6 µU/mL, in contrast, favors a different etiology. The sensitivity of this test is not 100% and in rare cases suppression of plasma insulin levels to <5 µU/mL is observed in patients with an insulin secreting tumor. Presumably, the tumors in these patients have retained some glucose sensing ability. In addition, newer more specific insulin assays no longer measure insulin precursors. When compared to the old assay used to establish the 6 µU/mL cutoff, these new assays would be expected to yield lower values. In these rare patients, measurement of proinsulin at the termination of the fast is extremely useful. An elevated fasting proinsulin level in this setting strongly suggests a diagnosis of insulinoma. A study using a gel filtration radioimmunoassay to measure proinsulin plasma levels in insulinoma, found that in 87% *(99)* of cases proinsulin made up 25% or more of the total immunoreactive insulin. Only two other conditions, easily distinguishable from insulinoma, present with a similarly high proinsulin to total measured insulin ratio; familial hyperproinsulinemia *(100)* and hyperglycemia. For the newer commercially available direct proinsulin sandwich assay, a fasting proinsulin plasma level above the assays normal range is seen in 85% *(99)* of insulinoma cases (≈22 pmol or 0.2 ng/mL) and in the fasting state is specific for the presence of an insulinoma. This test should be reserved to patients with equivocal plasma insulin levels.

C-PEPTIDE LEVELS

Measurement of the plasma c-peptide level at the time of hypoglycemia is useful to diagnose patients injecting insulin surreptitiously. The distinguishing biochemical features in these patients are low c-peptide levels accompanied by high insulin levels. A similar pattern may be seen in patients with autoantibodies directed against the insulin receptor. In these patients, antibodies interfere with insulin binding to its receptor thereby affecting its clearance from the circulation. Since c-peptide clearance is unaffected, these patients can present with elevated insulin levels and low c-peptide levels.

INSULIN-LIKE GROWTH FACTOR II LEVELS

It has been suggested that at least 50% of non-islet cell tumors that cause hypoglycemia produce an incompletely processed insulin like growth factor II ('Big IGF-2') and that IGF-II is directly responsible for causing hypoglycemia. The correlation between circulating IGF-II levels and IGF-II hypoglycemic activity is complex. The interaction between circulating IGF-II and specific binding proteins is believed to determine IGF-II hypoglycemic activity. Protein profiles that permit egress of IGF-II from the circulation and allow tissue entry are postulated to result in hypoglycemia. Measurement of circulating IGF-II levels in isolation is thus not a useful routine diagnostic test. The cause of hypoglycemia in these cases is recognized by the presence of a known, frequently large, tumor and appropriately suppressed circulating insulin levels at the time of hypoglycemia.

THERAPEUTIC PRINCIPLES

Administration of glucose in a quantity sufficient to maintain a plasma glucose level above 50 mg/dL is the first priority in the treatment of hypoglycemia. Oral carbohydrate replacement through frequent meals and snacks or intravenous glucose replacement can be used to this end. The second priority consists in addressing the underlying cause. Examples of interventions include removal or adjustment of the offending drug, appropriate hormone replacement for patients with deficiency, or confrontation and psychiatry referral for patients with factitious disorder. In the case of insulinoma, resection of the tumor is usually curative. For non-resectable malignant insulinoma, diazoxide may provide some benefit *(101)*. Hypoglycemia resulting from non-islet cell tumors is usually treated by interventions aimed at reducing tumor burden. If this cannot be achieved, glucose administration is the only therapy. The syndrome of autoantibodies against the insulin receptor can result in severe hypoglycemia and left untreated is associated with high mortality. This disorder is usually a self-limited condition that resolves over months in the majority of cases. Therapy consisting of high dose glucocorticoid (prednisone 60 mg/d) prevents hypoglycemia by inhibiting the insulinomimetic effect of the anti-receptor antibody but do not hasten their disappearance from plasma.

SUMMARY

Under physiologic conditions, glucose plays a critical role in providing energy to the central nervous system. A precipitous drop in the availability of this substrate results in dramatic symptoms that herald compromised brain function and warrant immediate therapy aimed at restoring plasma glucose to normal levels. A thorough and systematic review of the differential causes of hypoglycemia for a given clinical context will provide a clue as to the most likely etiology. This in turn , will guide further diagnostic and therapeutic interventions that address the specific underlying problem. In most cases this approach to diagnosis and therapy will be met with good outcome for the patient.

REFERENCES

1. Gerich J, Davis J, Lorenzi M, et al. Hormonal mechanisms of recovery from insulin-induced hypoglycemia in man. *Am J Physiol* 1979; 236(4): E380–5.
2. Cryer PE. Glucose counterregulation: prevention and correction of hypoglycemia in humans. *Am J Physiol* 1993; 264(2 Pt 1):E149–55.
3. Amiel SA, Sherwin RS, Simonson DC, Tamborlane WV. Effect of intensive insulin therapy on glycemic thresholds for counterregulatory hormone release. *Diabetes* 1988; 37(7): 901–7.
4. Mitrakou A, Fanelli C, Veneman T, et al. Reversibility of unawareness of hypoglycemia in patients with insulinomas. *N Engl J Med* 1993; 329(12):834–9.
5. Cryer PE. Diverse causes of hypoglycemia-associated autonomic failure in diabetes. *N Engl J Med* 2004; 350(22):2272–9.
6. Cryer PE, A. Kalsbeek. Hypoglycemia in diabetes: pathophysiological mechanisms and diurnal variation. In: Progress in Brain Research: Elsevier; 2006:361–5.
7. Merimee TJ, Tyson JE. Stabilization of plasma glucose during fasting; Normal variations in two separate studies. *N Engl J Med* 1974; 291(24):1275–8.
8. Whipple AO. The surgical therapy of hyperinsulinism. *J Int Chir* 1938; 3:237–76.
9. Hepburn DA, Deary IJ, Frier BM, Patrick AW, Quinn JD, Fisher BM. Symptoms of acute insulin-induced hypoglycemia in humans with and without IDDM. Factor-analysis approach. *Diabetes Care* 1991; 14(11):949–57.
10. Towler DA, Havlin CE, Craft S, Cryer P. Mechanism of awareness of hypoglycemia. Perception of neurogenic (predominantly cholinergic) rather than neuroglycopenic symptoms. *Diabetes* 1993; 42(12):1791–8.
11. Fischer KF, Lees JA, Newman JH. Hypoglycemia in hospitalized patients. Causes and outcomes. *N Engl J Med* 1986; 315(20):1245–50.
12. Holstein A, Plaschke A, Egberts EH. Incidence and costs of severe hypoglycemia. *Diabetes Care* 2002; 25(11):2109–10.
13. Johnson ES, Koepsell TD, Reiber G, Stergachis A, Platt R. Increasing incidence of serious hypoglycemia in insulin users. *J Clin Epidemiol* 2002; 55(3):253–9.
14. Hart SP, Frier BM. Causes, management and morbidity of acute hypoglycaemia in adults requiring hospital admission. *Qjm* 1998; 91(7):505–10.
15. Vriesendorp TM, van Santen S, DeVries JH, et al. Predisposing factors for hypoglycemia in the intensive care unit. *Crit Care Med* 2006; 34(1):96–101.
16. Su CC. Etiologies of acute hypoglycemia in a Taiwanese hospital emergency department. *J Emerg Med* 2006; 30(3):259–61.
17. Malouf R, Brust JC. Hypoglycemia: causes, neurological manifestations, and outcome. *Ann Neurol* 1985; 17(5):421–30.
18. Hypoglycemia in the Diabetes Control and Complications Trial. The Diabetes Control and Complications Trial Research Group. *Diabetes* 1997; 46(2):271–86.
19. Intensive blood-glucose control with sulphonylureas or insulin compared with conventional treatment and risk of complications in patients with type 2 diabetes (UKPDS 33). UK Prospective Diabetes Study (UKPDS) Group. *Lancet* 1998; 352(9131): 837–53.
20. Leese GP, Wang J, Broomhall J, et al. Frequency of severe hypoglycemia requiring emergency treatment in type 1 and type 2 diabetes: a population-based study of health service resource use. *Diabetes Care* 2003; 26(4):1176–80.

21. Shorr RI, Ray WA, Daugherty JR, Griffin MR. Incidence and risk factors for serious hypoglycemia in older persons using insulin or sulfonylureas. *Arch Intern Med* 1997; 157(15):1681–6.

22. Service FJ. Hypoglycemic disorders. *N Engl J Med* 1995; 332(17):1144–52.

23. Shilo S, Berezovsky S, Friedlander Y, Sonnenblick M. Hypoglycemia in hospitalized non-diabetic older patients. *J Am Geriatr Soc* 1998; 46(8):978–82.

24. Charles MA, Hofeldt F, Shackelford A, et al. Comparison of oral glucose tolerance tests and mixed meals in patients with apparent idiopathic postabsorptive hypoglycemia: absence of hypoglycemia after meals. *Diabetes* 1981; 30(6):465–70.

25. Palardy J, Havrankova J, Lepage R, et al. Blood glucose measurements during symptomatic episodes in patients with suspected postprandial hypoglycemia. *N Engl J Med* 1989; 321(21):1421–5.

26. Fariss BL. Prevalence of post-glucose-load glycosuria and hypoglycemia in a group of healthy young men. *Diabetes* 1974; 23(3):189–91.

27. Hofeldt FD. Reactive hypoglycemia. *Metabolism* 1975; 24(10):1193–208.

28. Lev-Ran A, Anderson RW. The diagnosis of postprandial hypoglycemia. *Diabetes* 1981; 30(12):996–9.

29. Hofeldt FD. Reactive hypoglycemia. *Endocrinol Metab Clin North Am* 1989; 18(1): 185–201.

30. Service GJ, Thompson GB, Service FJ, Andrews JC, Collazo-Clavell ML, Lloyd RV. Hyperinsulinemic hypoglycemia with nesidioblastosis after gastric-bypass surgery. *N Engl J Med* 2005; 353(3):249–54.

31. Patti ME, McMahon G, Mun EC, et al. Severe hypoglycaemia post-gastric bypass requiring partial pancreatectomy: evidence for inappropriate insulin secretion and pancreatic islet hyperplasia. *Diabetologia* 2005; 48(11):2236–40.

32. Meier JJ, Butler AE, Galasso R, Butler PC. Hyperinsulinemic Hypoglycemia After Gastric Bypass Surgery Is Not Accompanied by Islet Hyperplasia or Increased β-Cell Turnover. *Diabetes Care* 2006; 29(7):1554–9.

33. Grunberger G, Weiner JL, Silverman R, Taylor S, Gorden P. Factitious hypoglycemia due to surreptitious administration of insulin. Diagnosis, treatment, and long-term follow-up. *Ann Intern Med* 1988; 108(2):252–7.

34. van Staa T, Abenhaim L, Monette J. Rates of hypoglycemia in users of sulfonylureas. *J Clin Epidemiol* 1997; 50(6):735–41.

35. Duncan GG, Jenson W, Eberly RJ. Factitious hypoglycemia due to chlorpropamide. Report of a case, with clinical similarity to an islet cell tumor of the pancreas. *Jama* 1961; 175: 904–6.

36. Jordan RM, Kammer H, Riddle MR. Sulfonylurea-induced factitious hypoglycemia. A growing problem. *Arch Intern Med* 1977; 137(3):390–3.

37. Fernando R. Homicidal poisoning with glibenclamide. *Med Sci Law* 1999; 39(4):354–8.

38. Manning PJ, Espiner EA, Yoon K, Drury PL, Holdaway IM, Bowers A. An unusual cause of hyperinsulinaemic hypoglycaemia syndrome. *Diabet Med* 2003; 20(9): 772–6.

39. Sketris I, Wheeler D, York S. Hypoglycemic coma induced by inadvertent administration of glyburide. *Drug Intell Clin Pharm* 1984; 18(2):142–3.

40. Scala-Barnett DM, Donoghue ER. Dispensing error causing fatal chlorpropamide intoxication in a nondiabetic. *J Forensic Sci* 1986; 31(1):293–5.

41. Field JB, Williams HE, Mortimore GE. Studies on the mechanism of ethanol-induced hypoglycemia. *J Clin Invest* 1963; 42:497–506.

42. Lumeng L, Davis EJ. Mechanism of ethanol suppression of gluconeogenesis. Inhibition of phosphoenolpyruvate synthesis from glutamate and alpha-ketaglutarate. *J Biol Chem* 1970; 245(12):3179–85.

43. Zaleski J, Bryla J. Ethanol-induced impairment of gluconeogenesis from lactate in rabbit hepatocytes: correlation with an increased reduction of mitochondrial NAD pool. *Int J Biochem* 1980; 11(3–4):237–42.

44. Madison LL, Lochner A, Wulff J. Ethanol-induced hypoglycemia. II. Mechanism of suppression of hepatic gluconeogenesis. *Diabetes* 1967; 16(4):252–8.

45. Arena FP, Dugowson C, Saudek CD. Salicylate-induced hypoglycemia and ketoacidosis in a nondiabetic adult. *Arch Intern Med* 1978; 138(7):1153–4.

46. Raschke R, Arnold-Capell PA, Richeson R, Curry SC. Refractory hypoglycemia secondary to topical salicylate intoxication. *Arch Intern Med* 1991; 151(3):591–3.

47. Hirsch IB, Boyle PJ, Craft S, Cryer PE. Higher glycemic thresholds for symptoms during beta-adrenergic blockade in IDDM. *Diabetes* 1991; 40(9):1177–86.

48. Poretsky L, Moses AC. Hypoglycemia associated with trimethoprim/sulfamethoxazole therapy. *Diabetes Care* 1984; 7(5):508–9.

49. Waskin H, Stehr-Green JK, Helmick CG, Sattler FR. Risk factors for hypoglycemia associated with pentamidine therapy for Pneumocystis pneumonia. *Jama* 1988; 260(3):345–7.

50. Taylor TE, Molyneux ME, Wirima JJ, Fletcher KA, Morris K. Blood glucose levels in Malawian children before and during the administration of intravenous quinine for severe falciparum malaria. *N Engl J Med* 1988; 319(16):1040–7.

51. Limburg PJ, Katz H, Grant CS, Service FJ. Quinine-induced hypoglycemia. *Ann Intern Med* 1993; 119(3):218–9.

52. Barbato M. Another problem with Kinidin. *Med J Aust* 1984; 141(10):685.

53. Goldberg IJ, Brown LK, Rayfield EJ. Disopyramide (Norpace)-induced hypoglycemia. *Am J Med* 1980; 69(3):463–6.

54. Graumlich JF, Habis S, Avelino RR, et al. Hypoglycemia in inpatients after gatifloxacin or levofloxacin therapy: nested case-control study. *Pharmacotherapy* 2005; 25(10):1296–302.

55. Park-Wyllie LY, Juurlink DN, Kopp A, et al. Outpatient gatifloxacin therapy and dysglycemia in older adults. *N Engl J Med* 2006; 354(13):1352–61.

56. Chiolero R, Tappy L, Gillet M, et al. Effect of major hepatectomy on glucose and lactate metabolism. *Ann Surg* 1999; 229(4):505–13.

57. Luo JC, Hwang SJ, Wu JC, et al. Paraneoplastic syndromes in patients with hepatocellular carcinoma in Taiwan. *Cancer* 1999; 86(5):799–804.

58. Felig P, Brown WV, Levine RA, Klatskin G. Glucose homeostasis in viral hepatitis. *N Engl J Med* 1970; 283(26):1436–40.

59. Gerich JE, Meyer C, Woerle HJ, Stumvoll M. Renal gluconeogenesis: its importance in human glucose homeostasis. *Diabetes Care* 2001; 24(2):382–91.

60. Sovik O, Oseid S, Vidnes J. Ketotic hypoglycemia in a four-year-old boy with adrenal cortical insufficiency. *Acta Paediatr Scand* 1972; 61(4):465–9.

61. Artavia-Loria E, Chaussain JL, Bougneres PF, Job JC. Frequency of hypoglycemia in children with adrenal insufficiency. *Acta Endocrinol Suppl* (Copenh) 1986; 279:275–8.

62. Pia A, Piovesan A, Tassone F, et al. A rare case of adulthood-onset growth hormone deficiency presenting as sporadic, symptomatic hypoglycemia. *J Endocrinol Invest* 2004; 27(11):1060–4.

63. Nadler HL, Neumann LL, Gershberg H. Hypoglycemia, Growth Retardation, and Probable Isolated Growth Hormone Deficiency in a 1-Year-Old Child. *J Pediatr* 1963; 63: 977–83.

64. LaFranchi S, Buist NR, Jhaveri B, Klevit H. Amino acids as substrates in children with growth hormone deficiency and hypoglycemia. *Pediatrics* 1981; 68(2):260–4.
65. Wolfsdorf JI, Sadeghi-Nejad A, Senior B. Hypoketonemia and age-related fasting hypoglycemia in growth hormone deficiency. *Metabolism* 1983; 32(5):457–62.
66. De Feo P, Perriello G, Torlone E, et al. Demonstration of a role for growth hormone in glucose counterregulation. *Am J Physiol* 1989; 256(6 Pt 1):E835–43.
67. De Feo P, Perriello G, Torlone E, et al. Contribution of cortisol to glucose counterregulation in humans. *Am J Physiol* 1989; 257(1 Pt 1):E35–42.
68. Khani S, Tayek JA. Cortisol increases gluconeogenesis in humans: its role in the metabolic syndrome. *Clin Sci* (Lond) 2001; 101(6):739–47.
69. Boyle PJ, Cryer PE. Growth hormone, cortisol, or both are involved in defense against, but are not critical to recovery from, hypoglycemia. *Am J Physiol* 1991; 260(3 Pt 1):E395–402.
70. Megyesi K, Kahn CR, Roth J, Gorden P. Hypoglycemia in association with extrapancreatic tumors: demonstration of elevated plasma NSILA-s by a new radioreceptor assay. *J Clin Endocrinol Metab* 1974; 38(5):931–4.
71. Gorden P, Hendricks CM, Kahn CR, Megyesi K, Roth J. Hypoglycemia associated with non-islet-cell tumor and insulin-like growth factors. *N Engl J Med* 1981; 305(24):1452–5.
72. Daughaday WH, Emanuele MA, Brooks MH, Barbato AL, Kapadia M, Rotwein P. Synthesis and secretion of insulin-like growth factor II by a leiomyosarcoma with associated hypoglycemia. *N Engl J Med* 1988; 319(22):1434–40.
73. Daughaday WH, Kapadia M. Significance of abnormal serum binding of insulin-like growth factor II in the development of hypoglycemia in patients with non-islet-cell tumors. *Proc Natl Acad Sci U S A* 1989; 86(17):6778–82.
74. Daughaday WH, Trivedi B. Measurement of derivatives of proinsulin-like growth factor-II in serum by a radioimmunoassay directed against the E-domain in normal subjects and patients with nonislet cell tumor hypoglycemia. *J Clin Endocrinol Metab* 1992; 75(1): 110–5.
75. Wu JC, Daughaday WH, Lee SD, et al. Radioimmunoassay of serum IGF-I and IGF-II in patients with chronic liver diseases and hepatocellular carcinoma with or without hypoglycemia. *J Lab Clin Med* 1988; 112(5):589–94.
76. Ishida S, Noda M, Kuzuya N, et al. Big insulin-like growth factor II-producing hepatocellular carcinoma associated with hypoglycemia. *Intern Med* 1995; 34(12):1201–6.
77. Todd JF, Stanley SA, Roufosse CA, et al. A tumour that secretes glucagon-like peptide-1 and somatostatin in a patient with reactive hypoglycaemia and diabetes. *Lancet* 2003; 361(9353):228–30.
78. Shetty MR, Boghossian HM, Duffell D, Freel R, Gonzales JC. Tumor-induced hypoglycemia: a result of ectopic insulin production. *Cancer* 1982; 49(9):1920–3.
79. Morgello S, Schwartz E, Horwith M, King ME, Gorden P, Alonso DR. Ectopic insulin production by a primary ovarian carcinoid. *Cancer* 1988; 61(4):800–5.
80. Seckl MJ, Mulholland PJ, Bishop AE, et al. Hypoglycemia due to an insulin-secreting small-cell carcinoma of the cervix. *N Engl J Med* 1999; 341(10):733–6.
81. Service FJ, Dale AJ, Elveback LR, Jiang NS. Insulinoma: clinical and diagnostic features of 60 consecutive cases. *Mayo Clin Proc* 1976; 51(7):417–29.
82. Service FJ, McMahon MM, O'Brien PC, Ballard DJ. Functioning insulinoma – incidence, recurrence, and long-term survival of patients: a 60-year study. *Mayo Clin Proc* 1991; 66(7):711–9.
83. Hirshberg B, Livi A, Bartlett DL, et al. Forty-eight-hour fast: the diagnostic test for insulinoma. *J Clin Endocrinol Metab* 2000; 85(9):3222–6.

84. Service FJ, Natt N, Thompson GB, et al. Noninsulinoma pancreatogenous hypoglycemia: a novel syndrome of hyperinsulinemic hypoglycemia in adults independent of mutations in Kir6.2 and SUR1 genes. *J Clin Endocrinol Metab* 1999; 84(5):1582–9.

85. Thompson GB, Service FJ, Andrews JC, et al. Noninsulinoma pancreatogenous hypoglycemia syndrome: an update in 10 surgically treated patients. *Surgery* 2000; 128(6): 937–44;discussion 44–5.

86. Kane C, Shepherd RM, Squires PE, et al. Loss of functional KATP channels in pancreatic beta-cells causes persistent hyperinsulinemic hypoglycemia of infancy. *Nat Med* 1996; 2(12):1344–7.

87. Nestorowicz A, Wilson BA, Schoor KP, et al. Mutations in the sulonylurea receptor gene are associated with familial hyperinsulinism in Ashkenazi Jews. *Hum Mol Genet* 1996; 5(11):1813–22.

88. Thomas P, Ye Y, Lightner E. Mutation of the pancreatic islet inward rectifier Kir6.2 also leads to familial persistent hyperinsulinemic hypoglycemia of infancy. *Hum Mol Genet* 1996; 5(11):1809–12.

89. Nestorowicz A, Inagaki N, Gonoi T, et al. A nonsense mutation in the inward rectifier potassium channel gene, Kir6.2, is associated with familial hyperinsulinism. *Diabetes* 1997; 46(11):1743–8.

90. Glaser B, Kesavan P, Heyman M, et al. Familial hyperinsulinism caused by an activating glucokinase mutation. *N Engl J Med* 1998; 338(4):226–30.

91. Stanley CA, Lieu YK, Hsu BY, et al. Hyperinsulinism and hyperammonemia in infants with regulatory mutations of the glutamate dehydrogenase gene. *N Engl J Med* 1998; 338(19):1352–7.

92. Khokher MA, Avasthy N, Taylor AM, Fonseca VA, Dandona P. Insulin-receptor antibody and hypoglycaemia associated with Hodgkin's disease. *Lancet* 1987; 1(8534):693–4.

93. Moller DE, Ratner RE, Borenstein DG, Taylor SI. Autoantibodies to the insulin receptor as a cause of autoimmune hypoglycemia in systemic lupus erythematosus. *Am J Med* 1988; 84(2):334–8.

94. Arioglu E, Andewelt A, Diabo C, Bell M, Taylor SI, Gorden P. Clinical course of the syndrome of autoantibodies to the insulin receptor (type B insulin resistance): a 28-year perspective. *Medicine* (Baltimore) 2002; 81(2):87–100.

95. Taylor SI, Barbetti F, Accili D, Roth J, Gorden P. Syndromes of autoimmunity and hypoglycemia. Autoantibodies directed against insulin and its receptor. *Endocrinol Metab Clin North Am* 1989; 18(1):123–43.

96. Hirata Y, Tominaga M, Ito JI, Noguchi A. Spontaneous hypoglycemia with insulin autoimmunity in Graves' disease. *Ann Intern Med* 1974; 81(2):214–8.

97. Redmon B, Pyzdrowski KL, Elson MK, Kay NE, Dalmasso AP, Nuttall FQ. Hypoglycemia due to an insulin-binding monoclonal antibody in multiple myeloma. *N Engl J Med* 1992; 326(15):994–8.

98. Blackshear PJ, Rotner HE, Kriauciunas KA, Kahn CR. Reactive hypoglycemia and insulin autoantibodies in drug-induced lupus erythematosus. *Ann Intern Med* 1983; 99(2):182–4.

99. Gorden P, Skarulis MC, Roach P, et al. Plasma proinsulin-like component in insulinoma: a 25-year experience. *J Clin Endocrinol Metab* 1995; 80(10):2884–7.

100. Grupposo PA, Gorden P, Kahn CR, Cornblath M, Zeller WP, Schwartz R. Familial hyperproinsulinemia due to a proposed defect in conversion of proinsulin to insulin. *N Engl J Med* 1984; 311(10):629–34.

101. Hirshberg B, Cochran C, Skarulis MC, et al. Malignant insulinoma: spectrum of unusual clinical features. *Cancer* 2005; 104(2):264–72.

II ENDOCRINE DISTURBANCES CAUSED BY NON-ENDOCRINE CRITICAL ILLNESSES

8   The Dynamic Neuroendocrine Response to Critical Illness

Lies Langouche and Greet Van den Berghe

CONTENTS

INTRODUCTION
THE SOMATOTROPIC AXIS
THE THYROID AXIS
THE GONADAL AND LACTOTROPIC AXES
THE ADRENAL AXIS
CONCLUSIONS
REFERENCES

INTRODUCTION

Critical illness is characterized by a uniform dysregulation of all hypothalamic–anterior-pituitary axes. These neuroendocrine alterations contribute to the high risk of morbidity and mortality in the intensive care unit.

Through recent research, it has become clear that the neuroendocrine response is substantially different in the acute and prolonged phase of critical illness *(1,2)*. The acute phase is exemplified by low peripheral effector hormone levels, despite an actively secreting pituitary. In prolonged critical illness, a uniform suppression of the neuroendocrine axes, primarily of hypothalamic origin, contributes to the low levels of peripheral effector hormones.

The erroneously extrapolation of the changes observed in the acute-disease state to the chronic phase of critical illness has deluded investigators to use

From: *Contemporary Endocrinology: Acute Cause to Consequence*
Edited by: G. Van den Berghe, DOI: 10.1007/978-1-60327-177-6_8,
© Humana Press, New York, NY

certain endocrine treatments with an unexpectedly increased mortality in consequence *(3,4)*. Therefore, a thorough understanding of the pathophysiology underlying these neuroendocrine changes is essential. Moreover, before considering therapeutic intervention, it is important to differentiate between beneficial and harmful neuroendocrine responses to critical illness. The endocrine alterations in the acute phase of illness appear to direct to reduce energy and substrate expenditure, thereby pushing back costly anabolism and forcing the substrates released to vital tissues in order to improve survival. This hypercatabolic reaction is likely beneficial and, currently, there is no supportive evidence to intervene. In contrast, the chronic phase of critical illness suffers from persistent hypercatabolism despite feeding, which leads to substantial loss of lean body mass and often concomitant fatty infiltration of vital organs, which may compromise vital functions and delay recovery. Therefore, therapeutic interventions to correct these alterations may open perspectives to improved survival.

THE SOMATOTROPIC AXIS

Growth hormone (GH) is secreted by the somatotropes in the pituitary in a pulsatile fashion. It is essential for linear growth during childhood, but has many more functions throughout life, mostly anabolic. The regulation of the physiological pulsatile release of GH, with peaks followed by undetectable levels, is important for its metabolic effects *(5)*. Hypothalamic GH-releasing hormone (GHRH) stimulates and somatostatin inhibits GH secretion. Also several synthetic GH-releasing peptides (GHRPs) and non-peptide analogues with potent GH-releasing activity have been developed *(6)*. These GHRPs act via a G-protein-coupled receptor which is located in the hypothalamus and the pituitary *(7)*. The highly conserved ghrelin is an endogenous ligand for this receptor, and appears to be a third key factor in the physiological control of GH release *(8)*. The indirect actions of GH are regulated mainly through stimulation of insulin-like growth factor-I (IGF-I) production, of which the bio-activity in turn is controlled by several IGF-binding proteins (IGFBPs).

The Somatotropic Axis in Acute Illness

The acute phase of illness, in the first hours to days after an acute insult, is hallmarked by a dramatically changed GH profile. The number of GH bursts is increased, peak GH levels are elevated and inter-pulse concentrations are high *(1,9)*. Concurrently, a state of peripheral GH resistance develops, partly triggered by cytokines, such as TNF-α and interleukin-6 *(9,10)*. Despite the clear increase in GH secretion, serum concentrations of IGF-I, GH-dependent IGFBP-3, and acid-labile subunit (ALS) are low during the acute phase of critical illness *(9,11)*.

A reduced negative feedback inhibition with reduced expression of the GH receptor, and therefore low circulating IGF-I, has been suggested to be the primary event driving the abundant release of GH in the acute phase of illness (11,12). The elevated GH might theoretically enhance its direct lipolytic and insulin-antagonizing effects, resulting in increased fatty acid and glucose levels in the circulation, whereas indirect IGF-I-mediated somatotropic effects of GH would be attenuated. This would then result in postponing of costly anabolism, normally largely mediated by IGF-I, which seems appropriate in the struggle for survival. Clinical recovery is indeed also preceded by a rapid normalization of the somatotropic changes.

The Somatotropic Axis in Prolonged Illness

In prolonged critically ill patients, when recovery does not occur within a few days, the pulsatile release of GH becomes suppressed, whereas the non-pulsatile fraction of GH release remains somewhat elevated (13–15). Since the robust release of GH in response to GH secretagogues (5) excludes a possible inability of the somatotropes to synthesize GH, the relative hyposomatotropism probably originates within the hypothalamus. A hypothalamic deficiency or inactivity of endogenous GH secretagogues, not of GHRH, is a plausible mediator, as GH release in response to GHRH injection is less pronounced than to a GHRP-2 injection in prolonged critical illness (5). The combination of a ghrelin deficiency, together with a reduced somatostatin tone most likely brings about this secretory profile.

Circulating IGF-I, IGFBP-3, and ALS levels remain low and correlate positively with the pulsatile fraction of GH release, which suggests that the loss of pulsatile GH release contributes to these low levels (13–15). The administration of GH secretagogues increased IGF-I and IGFBP levels which indicates that GH responsiveness at least partially recovers in the chronic phase of critical illness (13,14).

The chronic GH deficiency, due to lack of pulsatile GH secretion, could contribute to the pathogenesis of the 'wasting syndrome' that characterizes prolonged critical illness. This is indicated by the tight relation between biochemical markers of impaired anabolism, such as low serum osteocalcin and leptin concentrations and the low circulating IGF-I and ternary-complex-binding proteins levels (15).

Therapeutic Interventions

Administration of pharmacological doses of GH, inspired by the assumption of sustained GH resistance in the prolonged phase of critical illness, unexpectedly increased morbidity and mortality (3). As it is now clear that peripheral GH sensitivity at least partially recovers in the chronic phase of critical illness, the administration of such high doses (up to 20-fold substitution dose) may have exposed the patients to toxic side effects. High doses of GH aggravate insulin resistance and induce hyperglycemia that usually develops during critical illness *(16)*. Hence, the glucose-counter-regulatory toxic side effects may have surpassed any possible benefits of these therapies. The combined administration of GH and IGF-I, additive in their anabolic actions, might be a better option, because they neutralize each other's side effects *(17)*.

Treatment with hypothalamic releasing factors to reactivate the pituitary may be more effective and safer than administration of pituitary or peripheral hormones. Indeed, infusions of GH secretagogues not only restored the pulsatile GH secretion, but also evoked an increase of IGF-I, IGFBP-3, and ALS, indicative of a restored peripheral responsiveness *(13,14)*.

THE THYROID AXIS

Thyroid hormones are essential for the regulation of energy metabolism and have profound effects on differentiation and growth *(18)*. At the level of the hypothalamus, thyrotropin-releasing hormone (TRH) is released and stimulates the pituitary thyrotropes to secrete thyroid-stimulating hormone (TSH). TSH in turn drives the thyroid gland to synthesize and secrete thyroid hormones. Although the thyroid gland predominantly produces T_4, the biological activity of thyroid hormones is largely exerted by T_3 *(18)*. Different types of deiodinases (D1-D3) are responsible for the peripheral activation of T_4 to either T_3 or to the biologically inactive reverse T_3 (rT_3) *(19,20)*. The thyroid hormones in their turn exert an inhibitory feedback control on both TRH and TSH secretion.

The Thyroid Axis in Acute Illness

The early response of the thyroid axis after the onset of severe physical stress consists of a rapid decline in the circulating levels of T_3 and a rise in rT_3 levels, predominantly because of altered peripheral conversion of T_4 *(21)*. TSH and T_4 levels are briefly elevated but subsequently return to normal levels, although T_4 levels may also decrease in the more severely ill *(22)*. Regardless of normal single-sample-TSH levels, the TSH profile is already affected in this acute phase of illness, as the normal nocturnal TSH surge is absent *(23)*. The low T_3 levels persevere beyond TSH normalization, a constellation referred to as 'the low T_3 syndrome', 'euthyroid sick syndrome' or 'non thyroidal illness'. The decrease in circulating T_3 during the first 24 hours after the insult reflects the severity of illness and correlates with mortality *(24,25)*.

Cytokines might play a role in the pathogenesis of the low T_3 syndrome, since they are able to mimic the acute stress response of the thyroid axis *(26,27)*. However, cytokine antagonists failed to restore normal thyroid function after endotoxemic challenge *(28,29)*. Other potential factors of the low T_3 syndrome at the tissue level include low concentrations of thyroid hormone binding proteins and inhibition of hormone binding, transport, and metabolism by elevated levels of free fatty acids and bilirubin *(30)*.

The observed alterations in the acute phase of critical illness are very similar to the ones observed in fasting. The immediate fall in circulating T_3 during starvation has been interpreted as an attempt of the body to reduce its energy expenditure, and prevent protein wasting *(31)*. It could be looked upon as a beneficial and adaptive response that does not warrant intervention. Whether this also applies to the reduced thyroid hormone action in the acute phase of critical illness remains controversial *(32)*.

The Thyroid Axis in Prolonged Critical Illness

Patients, who need prolonged intensive care, enter a more chronic phase of illness, during which in addition to the absent nocturnal TSH surge, a dramatically reduced pulsatile TSH secretion occurs. Furthermore, circulating T_4 and T_3 are low, but in particular the decline in T_3 correlates positively with the diminished pulsatile TSH release *(33)*. The prognostic value of the disturbed thyroid axis with regard to mortality is now illustrated by lower TSH, T_4, and T_3 and higher rT_3 levels in patients who ultimately die as compared with those surviving prolonged critical illness *(34)*. An impaired capacity of the thyrotropes to synthesize TSH, an alteration in set-point for feedback inhibition, inadequate TRH-induced stimulation of TSH or elevated somatostatin tone may explain these findings. Reduced hypothalamic TRH gene expression has been described in patients dying after chronic critical illness, indicating a predominantly central origin of the suppressed thyroid axis, similar to changes in the somatotropic axis *(35)*. The rise in TSH secretion and in peripheral thyroid hormone levels after TRH administration in prolonged critically ill patients further strengthens this interpretation *(14,15)*. Cytokines are less likely to be important at this stage of the disease, as circulating levels are usually much lower than in the acute phase *(36)*. Endogenous dopamine and/or hypercortisolism however, could be involved since they are known to provoke or severely aggravate hypothyroidism in critical illness *(37,38)*.

A disturbed peripheral metabolism of thyroid hormone also contributes to the low T_3 syndrome in the chronic phase of critical illness. This is illustrated by a reduced activity of type 1 deiodinase (D1), the enzyme mediating peripheral conversion of T_4 to T_3, and the induction of type 3 deiodinase (D3) activity, responsible for conversion of T_4 to inactive rT_3 *(39)*. Remarkably, type 2 deiodinase (D2) activity increases in the prolonged phase of critical illness and does not appear to play a role in the pathogenesis of the low T3 syndrome in prolonged critically ill patients *(40)*. Interestingly, concomitant infusion of TRH and GHRP-2 in critically ill patients, not only increased TSH, T_4, and T_3 levels but also prevented the rise in rT_3 seen with TRH alone *(14)*. This suggests that deiodinase activity may be affected by GHRP-2, either directly or indirectly through its effect on the somatotropic axis. Combined administration of TRH and GHRP-2 to a rabbit model of prolonged critical illness indeed decreased D3 activity whereas TRH infusion alone augmented D1 activity. This indicates that D1 suppression in critical illness is related to alterations within the thyroid axis, whereas D3 is increased under joint control of the somatotropic and thyroid axes *(41,42)*. Regulation of thyroid hormone action at the level of the thyroid hormone receptor also appears to be altered by critical illness, possibly causing an upregulated thyroid hormone sensitivity in response to low T_3 levels *(43)*.

Therapeutic Interventions

It remains controversial whether administration of thyroid hormone to critically ill patients is beneficial or harmful in prolonged critical illness. Administration of T_3 substitution doses to pediatric cardiac surgery patients has been associated with improved postoperative cardiac function, but these patients were treated with dopamine which induces hypothyroidism *(44)*. Treatment with T_4 failed to demonstrate a clinical benefit, although this could be partly due to impaired conversion of T_4 to T_3 *(45)*.

By continuous infusion of TRH in combination with a GH secretagogue, not only thyroid hormone levels were restored to physiological levels, but also markers of hypercatabolism were reduced *(14)*. This suggests that low thyroid hormone levels rather contribute to than protect from the hypercatabolism of prolonged critical illness.

THE GONADAL AND LACTOTROPIC AXES

The release of luteinizing hormone (LH) and follicle-stimulating hormone (FSH) from the gonadotropes in the pituitary is stimulated by the hypothalamic gonadotropin-releasing hormone (GnRH). In females, LH mediates ovarian androgen production, whereas FSH stimulates the aromatization of androgens to estrogens in the ovary. In men, LH stimulates androgen production by the testicular Leydig cells, whereas the combined action of FSH and testosterone on the Sertoli cells supports spermatogenesis. Sex steroids exert a negative feedback on GnRH and gonadotropin secretion. Several other hormones and cytokines are also involved in the complex regulation of the gonadal axis *(46)*.

Prolactin is produced and secreted by the lactotropes in the pituitary in a pulsatile and diurnal pattern. The main function of prolactin is to stimulate lactation, but is also known as stress hormone with immune-enhancing properties *(47)*. Physiological regulation of prolactin secretion is largely under the control of dopamine, but several other prolactin inhibiting and releasing factors can modulate prolactin secretion *(48)*.

The Gonadal and Lactotropic Axes in Acute Illness

Acute physical stress causes an immediate drop in the serum levels of testosterone, even though LH levels are elevated *(49–51)*. This suggests an immediate suppression of androgen production in Leydig cells which may be viewed as an attempt to reduce energy consumption and conserve substrates for more-vital functions. Although the exact cause remains unclear, cytokines are possibly involved *(52,53)*.

In response to acute stress, prolactin levels rise *(1,54)*. Vasoactive intestinal peptide, oxytocin, and dopaminergic pathways, but also cytokines may play a role. The rise in prolactin levels following acute stress are thought to play a part in the vital activation of the immune system early in the disease process, but this remains speculation.

The Gonadal and Lactotropic Axes in Prolonged Illness

More dramatic changes develop within the male gonadal axis when critical illness prolongs and hypogonadotropism ensues *(55,56)*. Circulating levels of testosterone become extremely low or even undetectable, in the presence of suppressed mean LH concentrations and pulsatile LH release *(57,58)*. Also total estradiol levels are relatively low, but since sex-hormone-binding globulin decreases simultaneously, the level of bio-available estradiol is probably maintained *(58)*. On the other hand, a remarkable rise in estrogen levels has been observed in several studies *(46,59,60)*. Since exogenous GnRH is only partially and transiently effective in correcting these abnormalities, they must result from combined central and peripheral defects within the male gonadal axis *(58)*. Indeed, aromatization of androgens to estrogens is enhanced in critically ill patients *(61)*. As testosterone is the most important endogenous anabolic steroid, the abnormalities in the gonadal axis could be important with regard to the catabolic state of critical illness.

The pulsatile fraction of prolactin release becomes suppressed in the prolonged phase of critical illness *(1, 33)*. Possibly, the blunted prolactin secretion contributes to the immune suppression or increased susceptibility to infection associated with prolonged critical illness. Endogenous dopamine may play a role, again hypothetically, since exogenous dopamine, a frequently used inotropic drug, not only further suppressed prolactin secretion, but also concomitantly aggravated T lymphocyte dysfunction and disturbed neutrophil chemotaxis *(37,62)*.

Therapeutic Interventions

No conclusive clinical benefit has been demonstrated for androgen treatment in prolonged critical illness *(63, 64)*. On the other hand, exogenous pulsatile GnRH administration partially overcomes the hypogonadotropic hypogonadism in prolonged critically ill men *(58)*.

THE ADRENAL AXIS

The corticotropes in the pituitary produce adrenocorticotropic hormone (ACTH, corticotropin), which stimulates the adrenal cortex to produce cortisol *(65)*. The hypothalamic corticotropin-releasing hormone (CRH) controls ACTH release. Cortisol itself exerts a negative feedback control on both hormones. In a stress-free healthy human, cortisol is released in a diurnal pattern. Although only free cortisol is biologically active, more than 90% of circulating cortisol is bound to binding proteins, predominantly corticosteroid-binding globulin (CBG) but also albumin *(66)*.

The Adrenal Axis in Acute Illness

In the early phase of critical illness, release of CRH and ACTH is increased, causing a rise in cortisol levels. The diurnal variation in cortisol secretion, however, is lost *(65)*. Moreover, CBG levels are substantially decreased, in part due to elastase-induced cleavage, resulting in proportionally much higher levels of free cortisol *(67–71)*. Cytokines might be involved in these alterations as they can modulate cortisol production and glucocorticoid receptor number and affinity in acute illness *(72)*.

Both very high and low cortisol levels have been associated with increased mortality *(73–78)*. High cortisol levels point to more-severe stress, whereas low levels indicate the inability to sufficiently respond to stress, labeled 'relative adrenal insufficiency'. An appropriate activation of the hypothalamic–pituitary–adrenal axis and cortisol response to critical illness are thus essential for survival, since it fosters the acute provision of energy by shifting carbohydrate, fat, and protein metabolism, protects against excessive inflammation by suppression of the inflammatory response and improves the hemodynamic status by induction of fluid retention and sensitization of the vasopressor response to catecholamines *(1,72)*.

The Adrenal Axis in Prolonged Illness

In the chronic phase of critical illness, ACTH levels decrease, whilst cortisol levels remain elevated *(79,80)*. Cortisol levels slowly decrease, only reaching normal levels in the recovery phase *(1)*. CBG levels recover in the chronic phase of illness *(69, 71)*. Whether the continued elevation in cortisol is beneficial in prolonged critical illness remains uncertain. It could theoretically be involved in the increased susceptibility to infectious complications associated with prolonged critical illness. On the other hand, an increased risk of 'relative adrenal failure' may predispose to adverse outcome *(81)*.

Therapeutic Interventions

Initial trials studying administration of high doses of glucocorticoids have clearly shown that this strategy is ineffective and perhaps even harmful *(4, 82)*. In contrast, studies using 'low-dose' glucocorticoid replacement therapy for relative adrenal insufficiency reported beneficial effects, at least in patients with septic shock *(77,82)*. The results of randomized controlled trials on hydrocortisone treatment, such as the CORTICUS study, are required to clarify this further *(83)*. However, administration of hydrocortisone in the so-called 'replacement dose' resulted in several fold higher total and free cortisol levels, indicating the need of a re-evaluation of the doses used *(71)*.

CONCLUSIONS

In conclusion, the anterior pituitary responds in two distinct phases to severe stress of illness and trauma. In the acute phase of critical illness, the pituitary is actively secreting, but target organs become resistant and concentrations of most peripheral effector hormones are low. These acute adaptations are probably beneficial in the struggle for short-term survival. In contrast, prolonged, intensive-care-dependent critical illness is characterized by a uniform suppression of the neuroendocrine axes, predominantly of hypothalamic origin, which contributes to low serum levels of the respective target-organ hormones. These chronic alterations may no longer be beneficial, as they participate in the general wasting syndrome of prolonged critical illness. Attempts to reverse these abnormalities with hormonal therapies have demonstrated that lack of pathophysiological insight holds danger, the choice of hormone and corresponding dosage are of crucial importance.

As most hypothalamic–pituitary axes show a decreased activity during prolonged critical illness, treatment with hypothalamic releasing factors to reactivate the pituitary may be more effective and safer than administration of pituitary or peripheral hormones. Indeed, infusions of GH secretagogues, TRH or GnRH have been shown to reactivate the corresponding pituitary axes, resulting in elevated levels of the peripheral effector hormones. Concomitant infusion of GHRP-2 and TRH reactivated both the somatotropic and thyrotropic axes, but avoided the rise of inactive rT_3 levels seen with TRH alone *(14)*. This combined intervention was associated with a reduced hypercatabolism and stimulated anabolism *(15)*. Additional co-activation of the gonadal axis by administering GnRH together with GHRP-2 and TRH in prolonged critically ill men at least partially restored the three pituitary axes and appeared to induce an even more distinct anabolic effect *(84)*.

These data emphasize the interactions between the different endocrine axes and the need for jointly correcting all hypothalamic–pituitary defects instead of a single hormone treatment. Moreover, overstimulation of the respective axes are avoided, thus preventing toxic side effects of high peripheral hormone levels since the endogenous negative feedback mechanisms remain intact *(14,15,84)*.

REFERENCES

1. Van den Berghe G, de Zegher F, Bouillon R. Clinical review 95: Acute and prolonged critical illness as different neuroendocrine paradigms. *J Clin Endocrinol Metab* 1998; 83(6): 1827–1834.
2. Weekers F, Van Herck E, Coopmans W et al. A novel in vivo rabbit model of hypercatabolic critical illness reveals a biphasic neuroendocrine stress response. *Endocrinology* 2002; 143(3):764–774.
3. Takala J, Ruokonen E, Webster NR et al. Increased mortality associated with growth hormone treatment in critically ill adults. *N Engl J Med* 1999; 341(11):785–792.
4. Roberts I, Yates D, Sandercock P et al. Effect of intravenous corticosteroids on death within 14 days in 10008 adults with clinically significant head injury (MRC CRASH trial): randomised placebo-controlled trial. *Lancet* 2004; 364(9442):1321–1328.
5. Van den Berghe G, Baxter RC, Weekers F, Wouters P, Bowers CY, Veldhuis JD. A paradoxical gender dissociation within the growth hormone/insulin-like growth factor I axis during protracted critical illness. *J Clin Endocrinol Metab* 2000; 85(1):183–192.
6. Bowers CY, Momany FA, Reynolds GA, Hong A. On the in vitro and in vivo activity of a new synthetic hexapeptide that acts on the pituitary to specifically release growth hormone. *Endocrinology* 1984; 114(5):1537–1545.
7. Howard AD, Feighner SD, Cully DF et al. A receptor in pituitary and hypothalamus that functions in growth hormone release. *Science* 1996; 273(5277):974–977.
8. Kojima M, Hosoda H, Date Y, Nakazato M, Matsuo H, Kangawa K. Ghrelin is a growth-hormone-releasing acylated peptide from stomach. *Nature* 1999; 402(6762):656–660.
9. Ross R, Miell J, Freeman E et al. Critically ill patients have high basal growth hormone levels with attenuated oscillatory activity associated with low levels of insulin-like growth factor-I. *Clin Endocrinol* (Oxf) 1991; 35(1):47–54.
10. Baxter RC, Hawker FH, To C, Stewart PM, Holman SR. Thirty-day monitoring of insulin-like growth factors and their binding proteins in intensive care unit patients. *Growth Horm IGF Res* 1998; 8(6):455–463.
11. Hermansson M, Wickelgren RB, Hammarqvist F et al. Measurement of human growth hormone receptor messenger ribonucleic acid by a quantitative polymerase chain reaction-based assay: demonstration of reduced expression after elective surgery. *J Clin Endocrinol Metab* 1997; 82(2):421–428.
12. Defalque D, Brandt N, Ketelslegers JM, Thissen JP. GH insensitivity induced by endotoxin injection is associated with decreased liver GH receptors. *Am J Physiol* 1999; 276(3 Pt 1): E565–E572.

13. Van den Berghe G, de Zegher F, Veldhuis JD et al. The somatotropic axis in critical illness: effect of continuous growth hormone (GH)-releasing hormone and GH-releasing peptide-2 infusion. *J Clin Endocrinol Metab* 1997; 82(2):590–599.

14. Van den Berghe G, de Zegher F, Baxter RC et al. Neuroendocrinology of prolonged critical illness: effects of exogenous thyrotropin-releasing hormone and its combination with growth hormone secretagogues. *J Clin Endocrinol Metab* 1998; 83(2):309–319.

15. Van den Berghe G, Wouters P, Weekers F et al. Reactivation of pituitary hormone release and metabolic improvement by infusion of growth hormone-releasing peptide and thyrotropin-releasing hormone in patients with protracted critical illness. *J Clin Endocrinol Metab* 1999; 84(4):1311–1323.

16. Langouche L, Vanhorebeek I, Van den Berghe G. Therapy insight: the effect of tight glycemic control in acute illness. *Nat Clin Pract Endocrinol Metab* 2007; 3(3):70–278.

17. Kupfer SR, Underwood LE, Baxter RC, Clemmons DR. Enhancement of the anabolic effects of growth hormone and insulin-like growth factor I by use of both agents simultaneously. *J Clin Invest* 1993; 91(2):391–396.

18. Yen PM. Physiological and molecular basis of thyroid hormone action. *Physiol Rev* 2001; 81(3):1097–1142.

19. Bianco AC, Salvatore D, Gereben B, Berry MJ, Larsen PR. Biochemistry, cellular and molecular biology, and physiological roles of the iodothyronine selenodeiodinases. *Endocr Rev* 2002; 23(1):38–89.

20. Friesema EC, Jansen J, Visser TJ. Thyroid hormone transporters. *Biochem Soc Trans* 2005; 33(Pt 1):228–232.

21. Michalaki M, Vagenakis AG, Makri M, Kalfarentzos F, Kyriazopoulou V. Dissociation of the early decline in serum T(3) concentration and serum IL-6 rise and TNFalpha in nonthyroidal illness syndrome induced by abdominal surgery. *J Clin Endocrinol Metab* 2001; 86(9): 4198–4205.

22. Van den Berghe G. Novel insights into the neuroendocrinology of critical illness. *Eur J Endocrinol* 2000; 143(1):1–13.

23. Romijn JA, Wiersinga WM. Decreased nocturnal surge of thyrotropin in nonthyroidal illness. *J Clin Endocrinol Metab* 1990; 70(1):35–42.

24. Rothwell PM, Lawler PG. Prediction of outcome in intensive care patients using endocrine parameters. *Crit Care Med* 1995; 23(1):78–83.

25. Rothwell PM, Udwadia ZF, Lawler PG. Thyrotropin concentration predicts outcome in critical illness. *Anaesthesia* 1993; 48(5):373–376.

26. Boelen A, Platvoet-ter Schiphorst MC, Bakker O, Wiersinga WM. The role of cytokines in the lipopolysaccharide-induced sick euthyroid syndrome in mice. *J Endocrinol* 1995; 146(3):475–483.

27. Van der Poll T, Romijn JA, Wiersinga WM, Sauerwein HP. Tumor necrosis factor: a putative mediator of the sick euthyroid syndrome in man. *J Clin Endocrinol Metab* 1990; 71(6): 1567–1572.

28. Van der Poll T, Van Zee KJ, Endert E et al. Interleukin-1 receptor blockade does not affect endotoxin-induced changes in plasma thyroid hormone and thyrotropin concentrations in man. *J Clin Endocrinol Metab* 1995; 80(4):1341–1346.

29. Van der Poll T, Endert E, Coyle SM, Agosti JM, Lowry SF. Neutralization of TNF does not influence endotoxininduced changes in thyroid hormone metabolism in humans. *Am J Physiol* 1999; 276(2 Pt 2):R357–R362.

30. Lim CF, Docter R, Visser TJ et al. Inhibition of thyroxine transport into cultured rat hepatocytes by serum of nonuremic critically ill patients: effects of bilirubin and nonesterified fatty acids. *J Clin Endocrinol Metab* 1993; 76(5):1165–1172.

31. Gardner DF, Kaplan MM, Stanley CA, Utiger RD. Effect of tri-iodothyronine replacement on the metabolic and pituitary responses to starvation. *N Engl J Med* 1979; 300(11): 579–584.

32. De Groot LJ. Dangerous dogmas in medicine: the nonthyroidal illness syndrome. *J Clin Endocrinol Metab* 1999; 84(1):151–164.

33. Van den Berghe G, de Zegher F, Veldhuis JD et al. Thyrotrophin and prolactin release in prolonged critical illness: dynamics of spontaneous secretion and effects of growth hormone-secretagogues. *Clin Endocrinol* (Oxf) 1997; 47(5):599–612.

34. Peeters RP, Wouters PJ, van Toor H, Kaptein E, Visser TJ, Van den Berghe G. Serum rT3 and T3/rT3 are prognostic markers in critically ill patients and are associated with post-mortem tissue deiodinase activities. *J Clin Endocrinol Metab* 2005; 90(8):4559–4565.

35. Fliers E, Guldenaar SE, Wiersinga WM, Swaab DF. Decreased hypothalamic thyrotropin-releasing hormone gene expression in patients with nonthyroidal illness. *J Clin Endocrinol Metab* 1997; 82(12):4032–4036.

36. Damas P, Reuter A, Gysen P, Demonty J, Lamy M, Franchimont P. Tumor necrosis factor and interleukin-1 serum levels during severe sepsis in humans. *Crit Care Med* 1989; 17(10): 975–978.

37. Van den Berghe G, de Zegher F, Lauwers P. Dopamine and the sick euthyroid syndrome in critical illness. *Clin Endocrinol* (Oxf) 1994; 41(6):731–737.

38. Faglia G, Ferrari C, Beck-Peccoz P, Spada A, Travaglini P, Ambrosi B. Reduced plasma thyrotropin response to thyrotropin releasing hormone after dexamethasone administration in normal subjects. *Horm Metab Res* 1973; 5(4):289–292.

39. Peeters RP, Wouters PJ, Kaptein E, van Toor H, Visser TJ, Van den Berghe G. Reduced activation and increased inactivation of thyroid hormone in tissues of critically ill patients. *J Clin Endocrinol Metab* 2003; 88(7):3202–3211.

40. Mebis L, Langouche L, Visser TJ, Van den Berghe G. The Type II Iodothyronine Deiodinase Is Up-Regulated in Skeletal Muscle during Prolonged Critical Illness. *J Clin Endocrinol Metab* 2007; 92(8):3330–3333.

41. Weekers F, Michalaki M, Coopmans W et al. Endocrine and metabolic effects of growth hormone (GH) compared with GH-releasing peptide, thyrotropin-releasing hormone, and insulin infusion in a rabbit model of prolonged critical illness. *Endocrinology* 2004; 145(1):205–213.

42. Debaveye Y, Ellger B, Mebis L et al. Tissue deiodinase activity during prolonged critical illness: effects of exogenous thyrotropin-releasing hormone and its combination with growth hormone-releasing peptide-2. *Endocrinology* 2005; 146(12):5604–5611.

43. Thijssen-Timmer DC, Peeters RP, Wouters P et al. Thyroid hormone receptor isoform expression in livers of critically ill patients. *Thyroid* 2007; 17(2):105–112.

44. Bettendorf M, Schmidt KG, Grulich-Henn J, Ulmer HE, Heinrich UE. Tri-iodothyronine treatment in children after cardiac surgery: a double-blind, randomised, placebo-controlled study. *Lancet* 2000; 356(9229):529–534.

45. Brent GA, Hershman JM. Thyroxine therapy in patients with severe nonthyroidal illnesses and low serum thyroxine concentration. *J Clin Endocrinol Metab* 1986; 63(1):1–8.

46. Spratt DI. Altered gonadal steroidogenesis in critical illness: is treatment with anabolic steroids indicated? *Best Pract Res Clin Endocrinol Metab* 2001; 15(4):479–494.

47. Russell DH. New aspects of prolactin and immunity: a lymphocyte-derived prolactin-like product and nuclear protein kinase C activation. *Trends Pharmacol Sci* 1989; 10(1):40–44.

48. Samson WK, Taylor MM, Baker JR. Prolactin-releasing peptides. *Regul Pept* 2003; 114(1):1–5.

49. Wang C, Chan V, Yeung RT. Effect of surgical stress on pituitary-testicular function. *Clin Endocrinol* (Oxf) 1978; 9(3):255–266.
50. Wang C, Chan V, Tse TF, Yeung RT. Effect of acute myocardial infarction on pituitary-testicular function. *Clin Endocrinol* (Oxf) 1978; 9(3):249–253.
51. Dong Q, Hawker F, McWilliam D, Bangah M, Burger H, Handelsman DJ. Circulating immunoreactive inhibin and testosterone levels in men with critical illness. *Clin Endocrinol* (Oxf) 1992; 36(4):399–404.
52. Rivier C, Vale W, Brown M. In the rat, interleukin-1 alpha and -beta stimulate adrenocorticotropin and catecholamine release. *Endocrinology* 1989; 125(6):3096–3102.
53. Guo H, Calkins JH, Sigel MM, Lin T. Interleukin-2 is a potent inhibitor of Leydig cell steroidogenesis. *Endocrinology* 1990; 127(3):1234–1239.
54. Noel GL, Suh HK, Stone JG, Frantz AG. Human prolactin and growth hormone release during surgery and other conditions of stress. *J Clin Endocrinol Metab* 1972; 35(6): 840–851.
55. Vogel AV, Peake GT, Rada RT. Pituitary-testicular axis dysfunction in burned men. *J Clin Endocrinol Metab* 1985; 60(4):658–665.
56. Woolf PD, Hamill RW, McDonald JV, Lee LA, Kelly M. Transient hypogonadotropic hypogonadism caused by critical illness. *J Clin Endocrinol Metab* 1985; 60(3):444–450.
57. Van den Berghe G, de Zegher F, Lauwers P, Veldhuis JD. Luteinizing hormone secretion and hypoandrogenaemia in critically ill men: effect of dopamine. *Clin Endocrinol* (Oxf) 1994; 41(5):563–569.
58. Van den Berghe G, Weekers F, Baxter RC et al. Five-day pulsatile gonadotropin-releasing hormone administration unveils combined hypothalamic-pituitary-gonadal defects underlying profound hypoandrogenism in men with prolonged critical illness. *J Clin Endocrinol Metab* 2001; 86(7):3217–3226.
59. Christeff N, Benassayag C, Carli-Vielle C, Carli A, Nunez EA. Elevated oestrogen and reduced testosterone levels in the serum of male septic shock patients. *J Steroid Biochem* 1988; 29(4):435–440.
60. Fourrier F, Jallot A, Leclerc L et al. Sex steroid hormones in circulatory shock, sepsis syndrome, and septic shock. *Circ Shock* 1994; 43(4):171–178.
61. Spratt DI, Morton JR, Kramer RS, Mayo SW, Longcope C, Vary CP. Increases in serum estrogen levels during major illness are caused by increased peripheral aromatization. *Am J Physiol Endocrinol Metab* 2006; 291(3):E631–E638.
62. Devins SS, Miller A, Herndon BL, O'Toole L, Reisz G. Effects of dopamine on T-lymphocyte proliferative responses and serum prolactin concentrations in critically ill patients. *Crit Care Med* 1992; 20(12):1644–1649.
63. Ferrando AA, Sheffield-Moore M, Wolf SE, Herndon DN, Wolfe RR. Testosterone administration in severe burns ameliorates muscle catabolism. *Crit Care Med* 2001; 29(10): 1936–1942.
64. Angele MK, Ayala A, Cioffi WG, Bland KI, Chaudry IH. Testosterone: the culprit for producing splenocyte immune depression after trauma hemorrhage. *Am J Physiol* 1998; 274(6 Pt 1):C1530–C1536.
65. Cooper MS, Stewart PM. Corticosteroid insufficiency in acutely ill patients. *N Engl J Med* 2003; 348(8):727–734.
66. Burchard K. A review of the adrenal cortex and severe inflammation: quest of the "eucorticoid" state. *J Trauma* 2001; 51(4):800–814.
67. Pemberton PA, Stein PE, Pepys MB, Potter JM, Carrell RW. Hormone binding globulins undergo serpin conformational change in inflammation. *Nature* 1988; 336(6196):257–258.

68. Hammond GL, Smith CL, Paterson NA, Sibbald WJ. A role for corticosteroid-binding globulin in delivery of cortisol to activated neutrophils. *J Clin Endocrinol Metab* 1990; 71(1): 34–39.

69. Beishuizen A, Thijs LG, Vermes I. Patterns of corticosteroid-binding globulin and the free cortisol index during septic shock and multitrauma. *Intensive Care Med* 2001; 27(10): 1584–1591.

70. Hamrahian AH, Oseni TS, Arafah BM. Measurements of serum free cortisol in critically ill patients. *N Engl J Med* 2004; 350(16):1629–1638.

71. Vanhorebeek I, Peeters RP, Vander PS et al. Cortisol response to critical illness: effect of intensive insulin therapy. *J Clin Endocrinol Metab* 2006; 91(10):3803–3813.

72. Marik PE, Zaloga GP. Adrenal insufficiency in the critically ill: a new look at an old problem. *Chest* 2002; 122(5):1784–1796.

73. Finlay WE, McKee JI. Serum cortisol levels in severely stressed patients. *Lancet* 1982; 1(8286):1414–1415.

74. Rothwell PM, Udwadia ZF, Lawler PG. Cortisol response to corticotropin and survival in septic shock. *Lancet* 1991; 337(8741):582–583.

75. Span LF, Hermus AR, Bartelink AK et al. Adrenocortical function: an indicator of severity of disease and survival in chronic critically ill patients. *Intensive Care Med* 1992; 18(2):93–96.

76. Annane D, Sebille V, Troche G, Raphael JC, Gajdos P, Bellissant E. A 3-level prognostic classification in septic shock based on cortisol levels and cortisol response to corticotropin. *JAMA* 2000; 283(8):1038–1045.

77. Annane D, Sebille V, Charpentier C et al. Effect of treatment with low doses of hydrocortisone and fludrocortisone on mortality in patients with septic shock. *JAMA* 2002; 288(7): 862–871.

78. Sam S, Corbridge TC, Mokhlesi B, Comellas AP, Molitch ME. Cortisol levels and mortality in severe sepsis. Clin Endocrinol (Oxf) 2004; 60(1):29–35.

79. Bornstein SR, Chrousos GP. Clinical review 104: Adrenocorticotropin (ACTH)- and non-ACTH-mediated regulation of the adrenal cortex: neural and immune inputs. *J Clin Endocrinol Metab* 1999; 84(5):1729–1736.

80. Vermes I, Beishuizen A. The hypothalamic-pituitary-adrenal response to critical illness. *Best Pract Res Clin Endocrinol Metab* 2001; 15(4):495–511.

81. Barquist E, Kirton O. Adrenal insufficiency in the surgical intensive care unit patient. *J Trauma* 1997; 42(1):27–31.

82. Minneci PC, Deans KJ, Banks SM, Eichacker PQ, Natanson C. Meta-analysis: the effect of steroids on survival and shock during sepsis depends on the dose. *Ann Intern Med* 2004; 141(1):47–56.

83. Annane D, Briegel J, Sprung CL. Corticosteroid insufficiency in acutely ill patients. *N Engl J Med* 2003; 348(21):2157–2159.

84. Van den Berghe G, Baxter RC, Weekers F et al. The combined administration of GH-releasing peptide-2 (GHRP-2), TRH and GnRH to men with prolonged critical illness evokes superior endocrine and metabolic effects compared to treatment with GHRP-2 alone. *Clin Endocrinol* (Oxf) 2002; 56(5):655–669.

9 Changes Within the GH/IGF-I/IGFBP Axis in Critical Illness

Dieter Mesotten, MD, PhD and Greet Van den Berghe, MD, PhD

THE SOMATOTROPIC AXIS

The peptide hormones of the anterior pituitary are essential for the regulation of growth and development, response to stress, and intermediary metabolism. Their synthesis and secretion are controlled by hypothalamic hormones (upstream) and by hormones from the peripheral endocrine organs (downstream). Hence, the complex interactions among the hypothalamus, the pituitary and the peripheral endocrine glands provide elegant examples of integrated feedback regulation. Seven major anterior pituitary hormones have been identified in humans. They can be divided in three classes: the somatotropic hormones [growth hormone (GH) and prolactin], the glycoprotein hormones [luteinizing hormone (LH), follicle-stimulating hormone (FSH), and thyroid-stimulating

From: *Contemporary Endocrinology: Acute Cause to Consequence*
Edited by: G. Van den Berghe, DOI: 10.1007/978-1-60327-177-6_9,
© Humana Press, New York, NY

hormone (TSH)] and the proopiomelanocortin-derived hormones [corticotropin (ACTH) and α-melanocyte-stimulating hormone]. Additionally, the posterior pituitary, also known as the neurohypophysis, releases arginine vasopressin and oxytocin.

Growth hormone, the most abundant anterior pituitary hormone, is synthesized and secreted by somatotrophs in a pulsatile fashion *(1)*. The normal nocturnal pattern of GH secretion consists of peaks, alternating with troughs in which GH levels are virtually undetectable. The amplitude of the secretory pulses is maximal at night and physiological stimuli of GH release include stress, exercise, fasting, and sleep. Daily GH secretion is high in children, reaches maximal levels during adolescence and then decreases in an age-related manner in adulthood.

Classically, two hypothalamic hormones control GH secretion: GH-releasing hormone (GHRH), which stimulates the production and release of GH, and

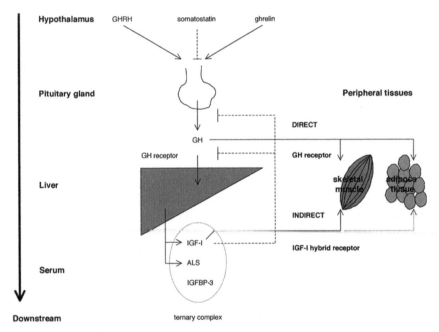

Fig. 1. Schematic overview of the somatotropic axis. Through a complex network, the GH/IGF-I/IGFBP axis exerts its effects on the peripheral tissues. In skeletal muscle GH will act via a direct (GHR) and indirect (IGF-I hybrid receptor) pathway. The liver and the adipose tissue barely have IGF-I receptors. Hence, direct GH effects will be dominant, resulting in increased heptic glucose output and lipolysis, respectively. The dual role of GH is tightly regulated by numerous feedback loops. → : stimulation, ⊥ : inhibition, *dashed* ⊥ : feedback inhibition

somatostatin, which exerts an inhibitory effect. Appreciation of a third component, however, arose from studies of synthetic GH-releasing peptides (GHRPs)
and non-peptide analogs *(2)* (Figure 1).

These GH secretagogues (GHS) exert their potent GH-releasing capacities
through a specific G-protein coupled receptor, distinct from the GHRH receptor
and located in the pituitary and in the hypothalamus *(3)*. The endogenous ligand
for the GHS-receptor has long been hypothetical until the discovery of ghrelin in 1999. This highly conserved 28-amino acid octanoylated peptide originates in the stomach and the hypothalamic arcuate nucleus *(4)*. It stimulates GH
release and appetite. Ghrelin's concentrations fall post-prandially and in obesity,
and rise during fasting and after weight loss. It basically acts as leptin's coun-
terpoise *(5)*. Now, ghrelin has emerged as a key factor alongside GHRH and
somatostatin, involved in the complex control of GH secretion. This ensemble
orchestrates serum GH concentrations to alternate between peaks and virtually
undetectable troughs, as observed in normal, healthy humans *(6)* (Figure 2).

All three peptidyl effectors are regulated by a reversible auto-feedback
enforced by GH and IGF-I, primarily aimed to maintain a physiological homeostasis. The GH auto-feedback and the feedback of insulin-like growth factor
1 (IGF-I) stimulate somatostatin and suppress GHRH secretion in the hypothalamus. However, the dominant feedback action of IGF-I occurs directly on the
pituitary gland.

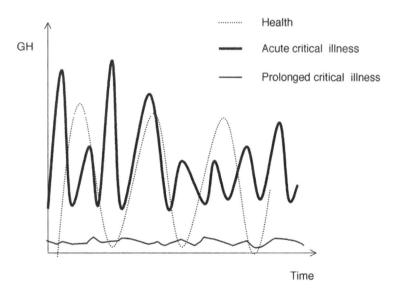

Fig. 2. Nocturnal serum concentration profiles of GH, illustrating the differences between
the acute and the prolonged phase of critical illness, in comparison with healthy subjects.

When GH secreted from the pituitary gland has reached the systemic circulation, it will exert its hormonal effects on the peripheral tissues, such as the liver, skeletal muscle, heart, and bone.

While GH encompasses cellular effects directly through the GH receptor (GHR), it essentially affects body growth and metabolism, indirectly, through stimulation of IGF-I production *(7)*. In the circulation of normal healthy individuals, roughly 99% of IGF-I is bound to binding proteins, with IGF binding protein 3 (IGFBP-3) the major one (Figure 3). Together with the acid labile subunit (ALS) they form the large 150 kDa ternary complex, which extends the half-life of IGF-I from about 14 minutes to 16 hours and regulates its hypoglycaemic potential *(8,9)*. IGFBP-5 can also form an alternative ternary complex with IGF-I and ALS *(10)*. Whereas IGFBP-3 is produced by many cell types, circulating IGF-I and ALS are almost exclusively liver-derived *(11,12)*.

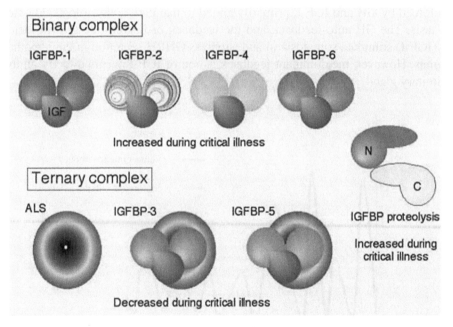

Fig 3. The insulin-like growth factor binding protein (IGFBP) family during critical illness The "smaller" IGFBPs (IGFBP-1, –2, –4, –6), which do not bind to the acid-labile subunit (ALS), form a binary complex with IGF-I. IGFBP-3, and –5 bind ALS in conjunction with IGF-I to form the ternary complex. During critical illness ternary complex proteins are decreased, circulating levels of the "smaller" IGFBPs are elevated and IGFBP-3 and –5 are proteolysed, phenomena that supposedly increase the bioavailability of IGF-I. (Artwork by RC Baxter).

The synthesis of the latter proteins is strongly stimulated by growth hormone at the transcriptional level *(13)*.

Hence, the circulating components of the ternary complex are often used as markers of peripheral GH effect *(14,15)*. Under normal circumstances, only a little fraction of IGF-I is bound by the other IGFBPs, notably IGFBP-1, –2, –4 and –6, in binary complexes *(16)*. As the latter binding proteins are unsaturated under normal conditions and the half-lives of their complexes with IGF-I come to 90 min, they function to regulate free IGF-I levels in the short term. IGF-I bound to these 'small' IGFBPs may also cross the endothelial barrier more easily, hence increasing its bioavailability *(17)*. On the contrary, the ternary complexes provide a stable reservoir of IGF-I in plasma. Nevertheless, bioavailability of IGF-I may also be increased by proteolysis of IGFBP-3, such as during pregnancy *(18)* and type 2 diabetes mellitus *(19)*.

GH SECRETION DURING CRITICAL ILLNESS

Critical illness involves a serious metabolic derangement *(20)*. When this critical illness persists for several days the muscle mass gradually melts away, while adipose tissue is maintained, despite adequate nutritional support *(21)*. It resembles the change of body mass composition in GH deficient subjects *(22)*. This protein hypercatabolism gives rise to functionally important complications such as prolonged immobilisation, delayed weaning from mechanical ventilation, impaired tissue repair and atrophy of the intestinal mucosa, together resulting in prolonged convalescence, conceivably with a higher cost burden *(23)*. The "wasting syndrome" boils down to a rerouting of amino acids, such as glutamine and alanine, from skeletal muscle to the liver for the synthesis of acute phase proteins and the gluconeogenesis. The main driving force is the systemic inflammation in combination with the metabolic derangement. As organ failure progresses, this reliance on amino acids as an energy source becomes even more pronounced *(24)*.

GH secretion is stimulated by stress, and the mean serum GH levels may be elevated in the course of early critical illness. However, studies examining the pulsatility of the GH secretion reveal a convoluted pattern. In patients who underwent major surgery *(25)* or were suffering from septic shock *(26)* early investigations pointed to raised GH concentrations between the secretory bursts, while mean GH levels did not differ from those in healthy controls. Deconvolution analysis confirmed that the number of GH bursts released by the somatotrophs is increased and the peak GH levels, as well as interpulse concentrations, are high *(27)*. The hypothalamic control of the changes during critical illness is still unclear. It may resemble situations of starvation during which elevated GHRH levels and more frequent absences of inhibitory somatostatin result in enhanced circulating GH concentrations *(28)*. In rats, plasma ghrelin levels are suppressed by lipopolysaccharide (LPS) injections in the first hours and are elevated after 2–5 days of repeated LPS injections *(29)*.

If clinical recovery does not occur, after about a week of critical illness, the pattern of GH secretion appears to be entirely different from that during the acute phase *(30–32)*. Now, it displays a generally reduced pulsatile fraction, a non-pulsatile fraction that is still somewhat elevated and a pulse frequency that remains high *(27,33–35)*. In addition, the GH pulses appeared to be less regular, as judged by an increase in the apparent entropic statistic. The result is a mean serum GH concentration that is low to normal. This relative suppression of GH release seems to be dependent more on length of time than on the type or severity of the critical condition. The combination of a deficiency of ghrelin, the endogenous ligand for the growth hormone-secretagogue receptor, together with a reduced somatostatin tone, and maintenance of some GHRH effect, most likely brings about this secretory profile. As this finding is not in line with the above mentioned animal data *(29)*, cohort studies in the critically ill patients are desirable.

RELATIONSHIP BETWEEN GH AND THE TERNARY COMPLEX DURING CRITICAL ILLNESS

Plasma IGF-I concentrations in critically ill patients are invariably low. During the acute phase of critical illness, the concurrence of elevated GH levels and low IGF-I levels *(36,37)* has been interpreted as resistance to GH, which may be related to decreased expression of the GH receptor *(38,39)* and/or post-receptor signal transduction *(40)*. The low serum concentrations of IGF-I are associated with low levels of IGFBP-3 and ALS, which are all regulated by GH, of which the latter at transcriptional level *(36,41)*. Because IGF-I and IGFBP-3 have greatly extended circulating half-lives when in complex with ALS, their circulating levels must to some extent reflect the concentration of the ternary complex rather than the rate of production of the individual components. During the course of critical illness, IGFBP-3 and ALS remain tightly related, corroborating the pivotal role of ALS *(36)*. In the acute phase of critical illness paediatric patients show similar changes in the somatotropic axis as adults, with elevated GH concentrations in combination with decreased IGF-I/IGFBP-3 levels *(42,43)*.

In the convalescent phase of critical illness, this coordinated behaviour of the ternary complex intact. If a patient is improving, his IGF-I levels will increase and IGFBP-3 and ALS will follow. On the contrary, when the patient does not recover and slips into the prolonged phase of critical illness, the components of the ternary complex will remain lowered or further decrease. In the background of reduced GH secretion, these changes do not support the notion of prolonged critical illness as a GH-resistant state, as reflected by a decreased GH over IGF-I ratio *(44)*. The reduced amount of GH that is released in the pulses correlates positively with low circulating levels of IGF-I, IGFBP-3, and ALS *(33–35)*. Intriguingly, a greater loss of pulsatility within the GH secretory pattern and lower IGF-I and ALS levels are observed in male compared with female patients, despite an indistinguishable total GH output *(45)*.

In protracted critically ill patients, the somatotropic axis can be reactivated by the administration of GHRH and GHRP-2. Here too, serum IGF-I and ALS levels show a strong correlation with the re-established pulsatile GH fraction *(45)*. The dependence of these proteins on GH is so strong that their serum levels decay as soon as the GHRP-2 infusion ceases. Hence, during prolonged critical illness the restoration of the pulsatile GH secretory pattern with infusion of GHSs, in conjunction with an increase in serum levels of the GH-dependent ternary complex proteins, can only be explained by a relative hyposomatotropism of essentially hypothalamic origin and preserved peripheral GH responsiveness *(46)*. The latter was corroborated by the increase in serum GHBP, reflecting GH receptor abundance, upon GHS administration *(45)*. This relative GH deficiency could contribute to the wasting syndrome as the often very low levels of IGF-I and ALS are closely related to biochemical markers of impaired anabolism such as low serum levels of osteocalcin *(35)* and leptin *(47)* during prolonged critical illness.

Serum concentrations of the other small IGF-binding proteins, such as IGFBP-1, –2, –4 and –6 are elevated *(36,48)*. They normally bind only a small amount of IGF-I compared with IGFBP-3. It is hard to speculate on the consequences of these IGFBP changes during critical illness. The decrease in IGFs in ternary complexes and redistribution into the more bio-available binary complexes may imply an enhanced IGF transport to the tissues. The increased proteolysis of IGFBP-3 during critical illness may further amplify the latter *(41, 49–51)*. Nevertheless, most downstream, the cellular effects of IGF-I in the peripheral tissues (the indirect GH action) during critical illness remain difficult to gauge.

Without exception, all other pituitary axes such as the thyrotropic, gonadotropic, adrenocortical, and lactotropic axes are characterized by the same biphasic response *(31,46)*. During acute critical illness the pituitary is activated with increased (pulsatile) levels of TSH, LH, ACTH, and prolactin. During the protracted phase of critical illness these pituitary-released hormones are decreased. Downstream, in the peripheral organs levels of T4 and T3, testosterone and cortisol decrease further as the patient passes into the protracted phase of critical illness.

Essentially, the latter embodies a totally different neuro-endocrine paradigm, which should be reflected in our therapeutic approach of these prolonged critically ill patients.

CLINICAL INTERVENTIONS REGARDING THE SOMATOTROPIC AXIS DURING CRITICAL ILLNESS

In light of the previous discussions, it would appear that IGF is exclusively regulated by GH. Among others, the nutritional status, insulin, oestrogens, androgens, T4, and cortisol are significantly contributing factors though *(52)*. Therapies involving these may provoke far-reaching and unpredictable effects as interference with the tiniest part can disrupt the multi-facetted GH system.

Growth Hormone

Inspired by the beneficial effects of recombinant human growth hormone in GH-deficient patients on lean body mass and bone remodelling, rhGH was proposed as a treatment for reversing the feeding-resistant wasting syndrome. Through a wide array of small, often uncontrolled and non-randomized, studies using surrogate markers of outcome, such as the nitrogen balance, human GH was generally perceived as an effective anabolic agent in critical illness *(53–57)*. However, the first large multi-centre prospective, double-blind, randomized, controlled trial on rhGH administration, with sufficient power to analyze mortality, revealed increased fatalities due to septic shock, and/or multiple organ failure in the therapeutic arm of the study *(58)*. It is crucial that in the latter study GH administration was started 5–8 days from admission and for a maximum of 3 weeks at a dosage of 0.1 mg/kg/day, consequently supra-physiological GH administration in prolonged critically ill patients. It is noteworthy to highlight that in the study the markers of GH responsiveness (IGF-I and IGFBP-3) were increased upon GH therapy, despite almost doubling the ICU mortality.

The lack of GH resistance *(59)*, the induction of insulin resistance, hallmarked by elevated IGFBP-1 levels, and hyperglycaemia by GH *(58)*, the modulation of the immune system *(60)*, the prevention of glutamine mobilization *(61)*, deterioration in the acid-base balance due to increased lipolysis with ketone body production as well as the exacerbation of the cholestatic potential of LPS *(62,63)*, have all been suggested as potential mechanisms for the excess mortality associated with GH therapy in long-stay ICU patients *(64)*. Hence the use of recombinant human GH in adult prolonged critically ill patients should be discouraged *(65)*. A more physiological GH administration (0.05 mg/kg/day divided into 8 boluses in combination with alanyl-glutamine supplementation) may be an alternative *(66)*. This mode of administration has less side-effects, but insulin resistance cannot be avoided and a clinical outcome benefit still has to be proven.

GH Secretagogues

Possibly, more upstream therapies for the somatotropic axis may be the obvious means in prolonged critically ill patients. Here the goal is the restoration of the relative hyposomatotropism of hypothalamic origin by a continuous infusion of GH secretagogues. While bolus administration of GHRP, compared to GHRH, resulted in much higher serum GH levels (67), the combination of them attains the most powerful stimulus of pituitary GH release. The restored IGF-I levels subsequently instigate a feedback inhibition of GH release, hence preventing over-treatment (35). The benefits would be similar to the direct administration of GH. GHS may inhibit the metabolic changes that produce a relative increase of visceral fat at the expanse of muscle and slow down the critical illness-related sarcopaenia with maintenance of muscle mass and strength.

Nevertheless, one should bear in mind that recent animal studies suggest that reducing GH and IGF-I increases longevity (68–70). Whether it also improves the quality of life, whether it can be extrapolated to animals under severe stress or to humans, is doubtful. Long-term stimulation of IGF-I may also increase tumour growth, but by using GHS, the IGFBPs, which inhibit the proliferative effects of IGF-I, rise concomitantly (71).

Thyroid Hormone and Sex Steroid Substitution

To fully normalize the somatotropic axis, stimulation of additional pituitary axes through the administration of thyrotropin-releasing hormone (TRH) and gonadotropin-releasing hormone (GnRH) seems vital (35,72). These co-infusions induce anabolism in peripheral lean tissues, reflected by elevated serum insulin, leptin, and osteocalcin levels (35,47). In statistical models, this improved anabolism could be linked to the restored somatotropic axis. On the other hand, the suppression of catabolic markers, such as the urea over creatinine ratio, appears to be merely explained by the reversal of the tertiary hypothyroidism. In non-critically ill patients, hypothyroidism results in low IGF-I levels. T4 replacement therapy returns GH and IGF-I concentrations to normal and enhances the pulsatile GH response to GHRH (73). Contrary, the influences of sex steroid hormones on the somatotropic axis are much more complicated (74). In general, oestrogens suppress the GH-stimulated IGF-I synthesis, while androgens increase the GH and IGF-I concentrations in primary hypogonadal patients. Paradoxically, the androgen effect on pulsatile GH secretion is mediated by the oestrogen receptor after aromatization of testosterone (75). During critical illness it has to be taken into account that serum testosterone levels are low due to this peripheral aromatization to oestrogen (76).

Intensive Insulin Therapy

Two large prospective RCTs, totalling 2748 patients in a surgical *(77)* and a medical ICU *(78)*, showed a significant decrease in mortality and morbidity through strict glycaemia control below 6.1 mmol/L (110 mg/dL) with intensive insulin therapy, as compared with the conventional approach which only recommended insulin therapy when blood glucose levels exceeded 12 mmol/L (220 mg/dL). The effect occurred particularly in the prolonged critically ill patient population, where an absolute risk reduction of 9% for mortality was described *(79)*.

In a sub-analysis of 363 critically ill patients with an ICU stay of more than seven days, mean GH levels were initially increased, before decreasing over time *(44)*. This is in line with the biphasic response during critical illness. Although insulin treatment in diabetes mellitus is known to inhibit GH secretion *(80)*, intensive insulin therapy compared to conventional treatment increased serum GH levels in critically ill patients. Contrary to expectation, intensive insulin therapy also prevented the recovery over time of the circulating levels of IGF-I, IGFBP-3, and ALS. The stimulation of GH secretion in combination with a suppression of the ternary complex proteins suggests an induction of GH resistance by intensive insulin therapy, as can be evidenced by diminished GHBP levels under the latter therapy. Surprisingly, intensive insulin therapy had no effect on IGFBP-1, the binding protein under direct suppression of insulin *(81)*. Intensive insulin therapy during the chronic phase of critical illness appears to convert prolonged critical illness back into a more 'acute phenotype'.

IGF-I

Although no large, randomized clinical trials have been established, IGF-I has been put forward as an anabolic agent for some time *(54)*. From a theoretical point of view it comprises several advantages. Firstly, IGF-I is mediator of the anabolic (indirect) effects of GH. Hence, upon IGF-I administration, the direct adverse effects of GH such as lipolysis and sodium retention could be avoided. Secondly, IGF-I is able to lower blood glucose levels. This has often been regarded as a serious disadvantage, but the latter view should be reconsidered in light of the Leuven insulin trials. Recent tissue-specific gene deletion experiments have emphasized the role of the somatotropic axis in intermediary metabolism. Mice with a liver-specific IGF-I gene deletion have minimal growth retardation, but show significant muscle insulin insensitivity *(82)*. This insulin resistance could be abrogated by the simultaneous deletion of IGF-I and ALS, probably due to maintenance of relatively high free IGF-I concentrations *(83)*. It strongly suggests that maintenance of normal serum IGF-I levels is required for normal insulin sensitivity.

The molecular mechanism by which IGF-I enhances insulin sensitivity hasn't been clearly delineated. However, IGF-I is capable of binding to the hybrid insulin/IGF receptors in skeletal muscle, resulting in stimulated glucose uptake. Other ways by which IGF-I lowers blood glucose levels include the inhibition of renal nocturnal gluconeogenesis and the suppression of GH-initiated hepatic glucose release. Hence, IGF-I treatment during acute critical illness may be interesting as it can lower blood glucose levels as well as suppress the increased GH concentrations *(84)*. A major drawback of this therapy emerged in a study in which patients with type 2 diabetes, receiving insulin therapy, were administered the rhIGF-I/rhIGFBP-3 complex. Its blood glucose lowering capacity was strongly self-limiting by suppression of ALS concentrations *(85)*.

Nutrition

Often the pivotal postion of the nutritional status in the IGF-I regulation is neglected. It has been known for a long time that caloric restriction reduces serum IGF-I concentrations *(86,87)* and that at least 700 kcal of carbohydrate must be ingested per day to maintain them *(88)*. This modulation of the somatotropic axis by nutrition presumably works through the variation of intra-portal insulin levels *(89)*. During fasting conditions, numbers of GHR decrease and consequently impair GH's ability to stimulate IGF-I synthesis, indicating liver and peripheral GH-resistance *(90)*. The resulting low levels of IGF-I give rise to increased GH secretion as the negative feedback loop on the pituitary is curtailed. The state of a high GH over IGF-I ratio amplifies the anti-insulin effects of GH, with increased glucose and free fatty acid availability *(91)*.

An observational 30-day study in critically patients demonstrated that nutritional markers (pre-albumin, transferrin, and retinol-binding protein) are robustly associated with ALS and the other components of the ternary complex *(36)*. Amino acids deprivation suppresses serum IGF-I and ALS *(92,93)*. Well controlled interventional studies examining the effects of amino acid/protein supplementation on the GH-IGF-I axis during critical illness are lacking.

As amino acids such as arginine provoke an enhanced GH release, one could assume that amino-acid supplemented parenteral nutrition may be an aid to restore the somatotropic axis during critical illness. Arginine is part of the so called "immunonutrition" as it plays a central role in the immune system. However, clinical trials with those feeds have been inconclusive *(94)*. Another interesting amino acid may be glutamine, formed in the muscle from the catabolism of branched amino acids. During critical illness it serves as a precursor for the gluconeogenesis in liver and kidney, and its levels drop significantly in muscle and serum. Nevertheless, glutamine supplementation in critically ill patients does not increase IGF-I concentrations nor improves patient survival *(95)*. At most it decreases critical illness-related infectious complications and insulin resistance *(96,97)*.

The somatotropic axis may also take part in the enteral versus parenteral feeding discussion as total enteral nutrition more effectively increases plasma ghrelin levels compared with TPN during LPS-induced sepsis in rats *(98)*. This was associated with a better preserved cardiac function. Involuntarily, feeding modus studies are often marred by differences in total caloric intake. Caloric restriction, as well as mutations in the GH-IGF-insulin signalling, has been shown to increase longevity in species from worms to humans *(99)*. The induction of GH resistance by a targeted disruption of the GHR, however, interferes with the beneficial actions of the caloric restriction *(100)*. Despite the fact that extensive trials on hypocaloric nutritional support during critical illness are still missing, preliminary data indicate that they could be beneficial.

SUMMARY

The neuro-endocrine features of the somatotropic axis that distinguish acute from prolonged critical illness have only recently been described. They hallmark a biphasic pattern in the hypothalamic-pituitary response to critical illness.

Early in critical illness, a transition occurs from stimulated GH secretion and peripheral resistance to pronounced pulsatile GH reduction together with an apparent reinstated GH sensitivity.

The complexity of the GH/IGF-I/IGFBP system in combination an evolution over time during critical illness may render therapeutic anabolic interventions rather daunting. This is well illustrated by the disastrous results of the multi-centre GH trial. Other strategies such as the use of GH secretagogues look promising but still need to show a clear advantage for the ICU patient. Unexpected avenues come into the spotlight through fascinating animal studies that link insulin, GH/IGF-I and nutritional manipulations to a survival benefit.

REFERENCES

1. Giustina A, Veldhuis JD. Pathophysiology of the neuroregulation of growth hormone secretion in experimental animals and the human. *Endocr Rev* 1998; 19:717–797.
2. Bowers CY, Momany FA, Reynolds GA, Hong A. On the in vitro and in vivo activity of a new synthetic hexapeptide that acts on the pituitary to specifically release growth hormone. *Endocrinology* 1984; 114:1537–45.
3. Howard AD, Feighner SD, Cully DF, et al. A receptor in pituitary and hypothalamus that functions in growth hormone release. *Science* 1996; 273:974–7.

4. Kojima M, Hosoda H, Date Y, Nakazato M, Matsuo H, Kangawa K. Ghrelin is a growth-hormone-releasing acylated peptide from stomach. *Nature* 1999; 402:656–60.

5. Kojima M, Kangawa K. Drug insight: The functions of ghrelin and its potential as a multi-therapeutic hormone. *Nat Clin Pract Endocrinol Metab* 2006; 2:80–8.

6. Veldhuis JD. A tripeptidyl ensemble perspective of interactive control of growth hormone secretion. *Horm Res* 2003; 60:86–101.

7. Berneis K, Keller U. Metabolic actions of growth hormone: direct and indirect. *Baillieres Clin Endocrinol Metab* 1996; 10:337–52.

8. Baxter RC. Insulin-like growth factor binding proteins as glucoregulators. *Metabolism Clin Exp* 1995; 44:12–7.

9. Baxter RC. Insulin-like growth factor (IGF)-binding proteins: interactions with IGFs and intrinsic bioactivities. *Am J Physiol Endocrinol Metab* 2000; 278:E967–76.

10. Twigg SM, Baxter RC. Insulin-like growth factor (IGF)-binding protein 5 forms an alternative ternary complex with IGFs and the acid-labile subunit. *J Biol Chem* 1998; 273:6074–9.

11. Yakar S, Liu JL, Stannard B, et al. Normal growth and development in the absence of hepatic insulin-like growth factor I. *Proc Natl Acad Sci USA* 1999; 96:7324–9.

12. Boisclair YR, Rhoads RP, Ueki I, Wang J, Ooi GT. The acid-labile subunit (ALS) of the 150 kDa IGF-binding protein complex: an important but forgotten component of the circulating IGF system. *J Endocrinol* 2001; 170:63–70.

13. Ooi GT, Cohen FJ, Tseng LY, Rechler MM, Boisclair YR. Growth hormone stimulates transcription of the gene encoding the acid-labile subunit (ALS) of the circulating insulin-like growth factor-binding protein complex and ALS promoter activity in rat liver. *Mol Endocrinol* 1997; 11:997–1007.

14. Brabant G. Insulin-like growth factor-I: marker for diagnosis of acromegaly and monitoring the efficacy of treatment. *Eur J Endocrinol* 2003; 148:S15–20.

15. Baxter RC. The binding protein's binding protein – clinical applications of acid-labile subunit (ALS) measurement. *J Clin Endocrinol Metab* 1997; 82:3941–3.

16. Wetterau LA, Moore MG, Lee KW, Shim ML, Cohen P. Novel aspects of the insulin-like growth factor binding proteins. *Mol Genet Metab* 1999; 68:161–81.

17. Baxter RC. The insulin-like growth factor (IGF)-IGF-binding protein axis in critical illness. *Growth Horm IGF Res* 1999; 9:67–9.

18. Lassarre C, Binoux M. Insulin-like growth factor binding protein-3 is functionally altered in pregnancy plasma. *Endocrinology* 1994; 134:1254–62.

19. Bang P, Brismar K, Rosenfeld RG. Increased proteolysis of insulin-like growth factor-binding protein-3 (IGFBP-3) in noninsulin-dependent diabetes mellitus serum, with elevation of a 29-kilodalton (kDa) glycosylated IGFBP-3 fragment contained in the approximately 130- to 150-kDa ternary complex. *J Clin Endocrinol Metab* 1994; 78:1119–27.

20. Wolfe RR, Martini WZ. Changes in intermediary metabolism in severe surgical illness. *World J Surg* 2000; 24:639–47.

21. Streat SJ, Beddoe AH, Hill GL. Aggressive nutritional support does not prevent protein loss despite fat gain in septic intensive care patients. *J Trauma-Injury Infect Critic Care* 1987; 27:262–6.

22. Haymond MW, Sunehag AL, Ellis KJ. Body composition as a clinical endpoint in the treatment of growth hormone deficiency. *Horm Res* 1999; 51:132–40.

23. Hadley JS, Hinds CJ. Anabolic strategies in critical illness. *Curr Opin Pharmacol* 2002; 2:700–7.

24. Cerra FB, Siegel JH, Coleman B, Border JR, McMenamy RR. Septic autocannibalism. A failure of exogenous nutritional support. *Ann Surg* 1980; 192:570–80.

25. Ross R, Miell J, Freeman E, et al. Critically ill patients have high basal growth hormone levels with attenuated oscillatory activity associated with low levels of insulin-like growth factor-I. *Clin Endocrinol* (Oxf) 1991; 35:47–54.

26. Voerman HJ, Strack van Schijndel RJ, Groeneveld AB, de Boer H, Nauta JP, Thijs LG. Pulsatile hormone secretion during severe sepsis: accuracy of different blood sampling regimens. *Metabolism* 1992; 41:934–40.

27. Van den Berghe G, de Zegher F, Lauwers P, Veldhuis JD. Growth hormone secretion in critical illness: effect of dopamine. *J Clin Endocrinol Metab* 1994; 79:1141–6.

28. Hartman ML, Veldhuis JD, Johnson ML, et al. Augmented growth hormone (GH) secretory burst frequency and amplitude mediate enhanced GH secretion during a two-day fast in normal men. *J Clin Endocrinol Metab* 1992; 74:757–65.

29. Hataya Y, Akamizu T, Hosoda H, et al. Alterations of plasma ghrelin levels in rats with lipopolysaccharide-induced wasting syndrome and effects of ghrelin treatment on the syndrome. *Endocrinology* 2003; 144:5365–71.

30. Van den Berghe G, de Zegher F, Bouillon R. Clinical review 95: Acute and prolonged critical illness as different neuroendocrine paradigms. *J Clin Endocrinol Metab* 1998; 83: 1827–34.

31. Van den Berghe G. Novel insights into the neuroendocrinology of critical illness. *Eur J Endocrinol* 2000; 143:1–13.

32. Weekers F, Van Herck E, Coopmans W, et al. A novel in vivo rabbit model of hyper-catabolic critical illness reveals a biphasic neuroendocrine stress response. *Endocrinology* 2002; 143:764–74.

33. Van den Berghe G, de Zegher F, Veldhuis JD, et al. The somatotropic axis in critical illness: effect of continuous growth hormone (GH)-releasing hormone and GH-releasing peptide-2 infusion. *J Clin Endocrinol Metab* 1997; 82:590–9.

34. Van den Berghe G, de Zegher F, Baxter RC, et al. Neuroendocrinology of prolonged critical illness: effects of exogenous thyrotropin-releasing hormone and its combination with growth hormone secretagogues. *J Clin Endocrinol Metab* 1998; 83:309–19.

35. Van den Berghe G, Wouters P, Weekers F, et al. Reactivation of pituitary hormone release and metabolic improvement by infusion of growth hormone-releasing peptide and thyrotropin-releasing hormone in patients with protracted critical illness. *J Clin Endocrinol Metab* 1999; 84:1311–23.

36. Baxter RC, Hawker FH, To C, Stewart PM, Holman SR. Thirty-day monitoring of insulin-like growth factors and their binding proteins in intensive care unit patients. *Growth Horm IGF Res* 1998; 8:455–63.

37. Lang CH, Pollard V, Fan J, et al. Acute alterations in growth hormone-insulin-like growth factor axis in humans injected with endotoxin. *Am J Physiol* 1997; 273:R371–8.

38. Hermansson M, Wickelgren RB, Hammarqvist F, et al. Measurement of human growth hormone receptor messenger ribonucleic acid by a quantitative polymerase chain reaction-based assay: demonstration of reduced expression after elective surgery. *J Clin Endocrinol Metab* 1997; 82:421–8.

39. Defalque D, Brandt N, Ketelslegers JM, Thissen JP. GH insensitivity induced by endotoxin injection is associated with decreased liver GH receptors. *Am J Physiol* 1999; 276: E565–72.

40. Mao Y, Ling PR, Fitzgibbons TP, et al. Endotoxin-induced inhibition of growth hormone receptor signaling in rat liver in vivo. *Endocrinology* 1999; 140:5505–5515.

41. Timmins AC, Cotterill AM, Hughes SC, et al. Critical illness is associated with low circulating concentrations of insulin-like growth factors-I and -II, alterations in insulin-like

growth factor binding proteins, and induction of an insulin-like growth factor binding protein 3 protease. *Crit Care Med* 1996; 24:1460–6.

42. Gardelis JG, Hatzis TD, Stamogiannou LN, et al. Activity of the growth hormone/insulin-like growth factor-I axis in critically ill children. *J Pediatr Endocrinol Metab* 2005; 18: 363–72.

43. de Groof F, Joosten KF, Janssen JA, et al. Acute stress response in children with meningo-coccal sepsis: important differences in the growth hormone/insulin-like growth factor I axis between nonsurvivors and survivors. *J Clin Endocrinol Metab* 2002; 87:3118–24.

44. Mesotten D, Wouters PJ, Peeters RP, et al. Regulation of the somatotropic axis by intensive insulin therapy during protracted critical illness. *J Clin Endocrinol Metab* 2004; 89: 3105–3113.

45. Van den Berghe G, Baxter RC, Weekers F, Wouters P, Bowers CY, Veldhuis JD. A paradoxical gender dissociation within the growth hormone/insulin-like growth factor I axis during protracted critical illness. *J Clin Endocrinol Metab* 2000; 85:183–92.

46. Van den Berghe G. Dynamic neuroendocrine responses to critical illness. *Front Neuroendocrinol* 2002; 23:370–91.

47. Van den Berghe G, Wouters P, Carlsson L, Baxter RC, Bouillon R, Bowers CY. Leptin levels in protracted critical illness: effects of growth hormone-secretagogues and thyrotropin-releasing hormone. *J Clin Endocrinol Metab* 1998; 83:3062–70.

48. Lang CH, Frost RA. Role of growth hormone, insulin-like growth factor-I, and insulin-like growth factor binding proteins in the catabolic response to injury and infection. *Curr Opin Clin Nutr Metab Care* 2002; 5:271–9.

49. Davies SC, Wass JA, Ross RJ, et al. The induction of a specific protease for insulin-like growth factor binding protein-3 in the circulation during severe illness. *J Endocrinol* 1991; 130:469–73.

50. Davenport ML, Isley WL, Pucilowska JB, et al. Insulin-like growth factor-binding protein-3 proteolysis is induced after elective surgery. *J Clin Endocrinol Metab* 1992; 75:590–5.

51. Cotterill AM, Mendel P, Holly JM, et al. The differential regulation of the circulating levels of the insulin-like growth factors and their binding proteins (IGFBP) 1, 2 and 3 after elective abdominal surgery. *Clin Endocrinol* (Oxf) 1996; 44:91–101.

52. Clemmons DR. Clinical utility of measurements of insulin-like growth factor 1. *Nat Clin Pract Endocrinol Metab* 2006; 2:436–46.

53. Raguso CA, Genton L, Kyle U, Pichard C. Management of catabolism in metabolically stressed patients: a literature survey about growth hormone application. *Curr Opin Clin Nutr Metab Care* 2001; 4:313–320.

54. Carroll PV. Protein metabolism and the use of growth hormone and insulin-like growth factor-I in the critically ill patient. *Growth Horm IGF Res* 1999; 9:400–413.

55. Gore DC, Honeycutt D, Jahoor F, Wolfe RR, Herndon DN. Effect of exogenous growth hormone on whole-body and isolated-limb protein kinetics in burned patients. *Arch Surg* 1991; 126:38–43.

56. Voerman HJ, van Schijndel RJ, Groeneveld AB, et al. Effects of recombinant human growth hormone in patients with severe sepsis. *Ann Surg* 1992; 216:648–655.

57. Wilmore DW. The use of growth hormone in severely ill patients. *Adv Surg* 1999; 33: 261–274.

58. Takala J, Ruokonen E, Webster NR, et al. Increased mortality associated with growth hormone treatment in critically ill adults. *N Engl J Med* 1999; 341:785–792.

59. Van den Berghe G. Increased mortality associated with growth hormone treatment in critically ill adults. *N Engl J Med* 2000; 342:135; author reply 135–6.

60. Zarkesh-Esfahani SH, Kolstad O, Metcalfe RA, et al. High-dose growth hormone does not affect proinflammatory cytokine (tumor necrosis factor-a, interleukin-6, and interferon-g) release from activated peripheral blood mononuclear cells or after minimal to moderate surgical stress. *J Clin Endocrinol Metab* 2000; 85:3383–3390.

61. Hinds CJ. Administration of growth hormone to catabolic patients. *Growth Horm IGF Res* 1999; 9:71–5.

62. Liao W, Rudling M, Angelin B. Growth hormone potentiates the in vivo biological activities of endotoxin in the rat. *Eur J Clin Invest* 1996; 26:254–258.

63. Mesotten D, Van den Berghe G, Liddle C, et al. Growth hormone modulation of the rat hepatic bile transporter system in endotoxin-induced cholestasis. *Endocrinology* 2003; 144:4008–17.

64. Ruokonen E, Takala J. Dangers of growth hormone therapy in critically ill patients. *Curr Opin Clin Nutr Metab Care* 2002; 5:199–209.

65. Carroll PV, Van den Berghe G. Safety aspects of pharmacological GH therapy in adults. *Growth Horm IGF Res* 2001; 11:166–72.

66. Duska F, Fric M, Pazout J, Waldauf P, Tuma P, Pachl J. Frequent intravenous pulses of growth hormone together with alanylglutamine supplementation in prolonged critical illness after multiple trauma: Effects on glucose control, plasma IGF-I and glutamine. *Growth Horm IGF Res* 2007; 18:18.

67. Van den Berghe G, de Zegher F, Bowers CY, et al. Pituitary responsiveness to GH-releasing hormone, GH-releasing peptide-2 and thyrotrophin-releasing hormone in critical illness. *Clin Endocrinol* 1996; 45:341–51.

68. Coschigano KT, Clemmons D, Bellush LL, Kopchick JJ. Assessment of growth parameters and life span of GHR/BP gene-disrupted mice. *Endocrinology* 2000; 141:2608–13.

69. Chen NY, Chen WY, Bellush L, et al. Effects of streptozotocin treatment in growth hormone (GH) and GH antagonist transgenic mice. *Endocrinology* 1995; 136:660–7.

70. Flyvbjerg A, Bennett WF, Rasch R, Kopchick JJ, Scarlett JA. Inhibitory effect of a growth hormone receptor antagonist (G120K-PEG) on renal enlargement, glomerular hypertrophy, and urinary albumin excretion in experimental diabetes in mice. *Diabetes* 1999; 48: 377–82.

71. Firth SM, Baxter RC. Cellular actions of the insulin-like growth factor binding proteins. *Endocr Rev.* 2002; 23:824–54.

72. Van den Berghe G, Baxter RC, Weekers F, et al. The combined administration of GH-releasing peptide-2 (GHRP-2), TRH and GnRH to men with prolonged critical illness evokes superior endocrine and metabolic effects compared to treatment with GHRP-2 alone. *Clin Endocrinol* (Oxf) 2002; 56:655–69.

73. Miell JP, Taylor AM, Zini M, Maheshwari HG, Ross RJ, Valcavi R. Effects of hypothyroidism and hyperthyroidism on insulin-like growth factors (IGFs) and growth hormone- and IGF-binding proteins. *J Clin Endocrinol Metab* 1993; 76:950–5.

74. Meinhardt UJ, Ho KK. Modulation of growth hormone action by sex steroids. *Clin Endocrinol* (Oxf). 2006; 65:413–22.

75. Keenan BS, Richards GE, Ponder SW, Dallas JS, Nagamani M, Smith ER. Androgen-stimulated pubertal growth: the effects of testosterone and dihydrotestosterone on growth hormone and insulin-like growth factor-I in the treatment of short stature and delayed puberty. *J Clin Endocrinol Metab* 1993; 76:996–1001.

76. Spratt DI, Morton JR, Kramer RS, Mayo SW, Longcope C, Vary CP. Increases in serum estrogen levels during major illness are caused by increased peripheral aromatization. *Am J Physiol Endocrinol Metab* 2006; 291:E631-8.

77. Van den Berghe G, Wouters P, Weekers F, et al. Intensive insulin therapy in critically ill patients. *N Engl J Med* 2001; 345:1359–1367.
78. Van den Berghe G, Wilmer A, Hermans G, et al. Intensive insulin therapy in the medical ICU. *N Engl J Med* 2006; 354:449–61.
79. Van den Berghe G, Wilmer A, Milants I, et al. Intensive insulin therapy in mixed medical/surgical intensive care units: benefit versus harm. *Diabetes* 2006; 55:3151–9.
80. Holt RI, Simpson HL, Sonksen PH. The role of the growth hormone-insulin-like growth factor axis in glucose homeostasis. *Diabet Med* 2003; 20:3–15.
81. Mesotten D, Delhanty PJD, Vanderhoydonc F, et al. Regulation of Insulin-like Growth Factor Binding Protein-1 during Protracted Critical Illness. *J Clin Endocrinol Metab* 2002; 87:5516–23.
82. Yakar S, Liu JL, Fernandez AM, et al. Liver-specific igf-1 gene deletion leads to muscle insulin insensitivity. *Diabetes* 2001; 50:1110–8.
83. Haluzik M, Yakar S, Gavrilova O, Setser J, Boisclair Y, LeRoith D. Insulin resistance in the liver-specific IGF-1 gene-deleted mouse is abrogated by deletion of the acid-labile subunit of the IGF-binding protein-3 complex: relative roles of growth hormone and IGF-1 in insulin resistance. *Diabetes* 2003; 52:2483–9.
84. Hartman ML, Clayton PE, Johnson ML, et al. A low dose euglycemic infusion of recombinant human insulin-like growth factor I rapidly suppresses fasting-enhanced pulsatile growth hormone secretion in humans. *J Clin Invest* 1993; 91:2453–62.
85. Clemmons DR, Sleevi M, Allan G, Sommer A. Effects of combined recombinant insulin-like growth factor (IGF)-I and IGF binding protein-3 in type 2 diabetic patients on glycemic control and distribution of IGF-I and IGF-II among serum binding protein complexes. *J Clin Endocrinol Metab* 2007; 92:2652–8.
86. Isley WL, Underwood LE, Clemmons DR. Dietary components that regulate serum somatomedin-C concentrations in humans. *J Clin Invest* 1983; 71:175–82.
87. Oster MH, Fielder PJ, Levin N, Cronin MJ. Adaptation of the growth hormone and insulin-like growth factor-I axis to chronic and severe calorie or protein malnutrition. *J Clin Invest* 1995; 95:2258–65.
88. Snyder DK, Clemmons DR, Underwood LE. Dietary carbohydrate content determines responsiveness to growth hormone in energy-restricted humans. *J Clin Endocrinol Metab* 1989; 69:745–52.
89. Hanaire-Broutin H, Sallerin-Caute B, Poncet MF, et al. Effect of intraperitoneal insulin delivery on growth hormone binding protein, insulin-like growth factor (IGF)-I, and IGF-binding protein-3 in IDDM. *Diabetologia* 1996; 39:1498–504.
90. Dominici FP, Turyn D. Growth hormone-induced alterations in the insulin-signaling system. *Exp Biol Med* 2002; 227:149–57.
91. Yuen KC, Dunger DB. Therapeutic aspects of growth hormone and insulin-like growth factor-I treatment on visceral fat and insulin sensitivity in adults. *Diabet Obes Metab* 2007; 9:11–22.
92. Kee AJ, Baxter RC, Carlsson AR, Smith RC. Parenteral amino acid intake alters the anabolic actions of insulin-like growth factor I in rats. *Am J Physiol* 1999; 277:E63–72.
93. Pao CI, Farmer PK, Begovic S, et al. Regulation of insulin-like growth factor-I (IGF-I) and IGF-binding protein 1 gene transcription by hormones and provision of amino acids in rat hepatocytes. *Mol Endocrinol* 1993; 7:1561–8.
94. Heyland DK, Novak F, Drover JW, Jain M, Su X, Suchner U. Should immunonutrition become routine in critically ill patients? A systematic review of the evidence. *JAMA* 2001; 286:944–53.

95. Jackson NC, Carroll PV, Russell-Jones DL, Sonksen PH, Treacher DF, Umpleby AM. Effects of glutamine supplementation, GH, and IGF-I on glutamine metabolism in critically ill patients. *Am J Physiol Endocrinol Metab* 2000; 278:E226–33.

96. Novak F, Heyland DK, Avenell A, Drover JW, Su X. Glutamine supplementation in serious illness: a systematic review of the evidence. *Crit Care Med* 2002; 30:2022–9.

97. Dechelotte P, Hasselmann M, Cynober L, et al. L-alanyl-L-glutamine dipeptide-supplemented total parenteral nutrition reduces infectious complications and glucose intolerance in critically ill patients: the French controlled, randomized, double-blind, multicenter study. *Crit Care Med* 2006; 34:598–604.

98. Hagiwara S, Iwasaka H, Matsumoto S, Noguchi T. Effect of Enteral Versus Parenteral Nutrition on LPS-Induced Sepsis in a Rat Model. *J Surg Res* 2007; 25:25.

99. Kenyon C. The plasticity of aging: insights from long-lived mutants. *Cell* 2005; 120: 449–60.

100. Bonkowski MS, Rocha JS, Masternak MM, Al Regaiey KA, Bartke A. Targeted disruption of growth hormone receptor interferes with the beneficial actions of calorie restriction. *Proc Natl Acad Sci USA* 2006; 103:7901–5. Epub 2006 May 8.

10 Changes Within the Thyroid Axis During the Course of Critical Illness

Liese Mebis, MSc, Lies Langouche, PhD and Greet Van den Berghe, MD, PhD

CONTENTS

INTRODUCTION

Thyroid hormones are indispensable for normal growth, development and metabolism of virtually every cell and organ *(1,2)*. The secretion of thyroid hormone is regulated by the hypothalamus-pituitary-thyroid (HPT) axis which functions as a classical feedback system. At the level of the hypothalamus, thyrotropin-releasing hormone (TRH) is released which stimulates the pituitary to secrete thyroid-stimulating hormone (thyrotropin or TSH). TSH in turn drives the thyroid gland to release the prohormone thyroxin (T4) into the circulation. Conversion of T4 in peripheral tissues produces the active hormone tri-iodothyronine (T3) and reverse T3 (rT3) which are thought to be metabolically inactive. T4 and T3 in turn exert a negative feedback control on the level of the hypothalamus and the pituitary.

From: *Contemporary Endocrinology: Acute Cause to Consequence*
Edited by: G. Van den Berghe, DOI: 10.1007/978-1-60327-177-6_10,
© Humana Press, New York, NY

Sepsis, surgery, myocardial infarction, and trauma are all examples of conditions that evoke an acute stress response. Already within a few hours after the onset of acute stress, circulating T3 levels drop and rT3 levels increase. At the same time, there is a brief rise in circulating levels of T4 and TSH *(3)*. These observed changes in circulating thyroid hormone levels during the acute phase of critical illness are largely explained by disturbances in peripheral thyroid hormone metabolism and binding.

When patients require prolonged intensive care therapy, they enter a chronic phase of illness during which T4 levels start to decline as well, and circulating T3 levels decrease even further *(4)*. Despite the major drop in serum T3 and in severe cases of T4, single-sample-TSH-levels do not rise but remain within the normal range *(4)* suggesting that in the chronic phase of critical illness, patients develop an additional neuroendocrine dysfunction.

Together, these changes are commonly referred to as the 'euthyroid sick syndrome'. More neutral terms, avoiding the assumption that patients are really euthyroid are 'low T3 syndrome' or 'Non Thyroidal Illness'. In this article, we will review the mechanisms behind the observed changes in the HPT axis in the acute phase and the chronic phase of critical illness.

PERIPHERAL CHANGES DURING CRITICAL ILLNESS

Peripheral transport, metabolism, and receptor binding of thyroid hormones are essential steps for normal thyroid hormone action. During critical illness and particularly in the acute phase of critical illness, alterations occur in thyroid hormone metabolism which plays a major role in the pathogenesis of the low T3 syndrome. In prolonged critical illness, these alterations continue to persist, but here a neuroendocrine dysfunction leading to a decline of thyroidal T4 release is superimposed on the peripheral 'adaptations'.

Thyroid Hormone Deiodination

Iodothyronine deiodinases are selenoproteins that activate or inactivate thyroid hormone depending on whether they remove outer or inner ring iodines. Three types of deiodinases have been characterized (D1-D3) *(5)* and in general, each is expressed in a given cell type. D1 is expressed in the thyroid gland, liver, kidney, and pituitary and activates or inactivates T4 at the same rate. It was considered to be the main source of circulating T3; however, recently its role in health is questioned *(6,7)*. D2 is expressed in the brain, thyroid gland, skeletal muscle, and anterior pituitary and converts T4 into the active hormone T3 and rT3 into $3,3'$-diiodothyronine (T2). D2 is thought to contribute to circulating T3 *(7)* and is essential for local T3 production, especially in brain and pituitary *(8)*. D3 is the major inactivating enzyme: it catalyzes the conversion of T4 into rT3 and of T3 into T2 *(5,9)*. It is present in brain, skin, various fetal tissues, and in pregnant uterus and placenta where it protects the fetus against excess T3 concentrations, which are detrimental for normal development *(10)*.

The observed changes in circulating thyroid hormone parameters during critical illness, that is, low T3 and high rT3, suggests that decreased monodeiodination of T4 could be involved *(11,12)*. This would result in reduced conversion of T4 into active T3 and increased metabolisation of T4 into the inactive metabolite rT3. Peeters et al. indeed confirmed a decreased activation and an increased inactivation of thyroid hormone in critically ill patients *(13)*. A unique rabbit model for prolonged critical illness *(14, 15)* as well as a mouse model of acute illness *(16)* further elucidated the role of the deiodinases during critical illness.

Reduced D1 Activity During Critical Illness

D1 activity is regulated by T3 at the transcriptional level which results in a stimulation of D1 activity during hyperthyroidism and a decrease in D1 activity during hypothyroidism *(17)*. Critically ill patients indeed showed a marked reduction in liver D1 activity, measured in postmortem liver samples as compared with values previously observed in healthy individuals *(13)*. Furthermore, D1 activity correlated positively with the serum T3/rT3 ratio, a marker for the severity of illness *(13)*.

Decreased hepatic D1 expression and activity is likely mediated by cytokines as shown in a mouse model of acute illness and in primary cultures of rat hepatocytes *(18–20)*. Debaveye et al. were able to demonstrate that the drop in D1 activity is reversible by infusing critically ill rabbits with TRH *(14,21)*. This treatment restored hepatic D1 activity and brought serum T4 and T3 levels back within normal range *(14)*.

Increased D2 Activity During Critical Illness

D2 activity is controlled by thyroid status both at the pre- and posttranslational level: D2 is upregulated during hypothyroidism, whereas high T3 levels will lead to diminished D2 activity *(5)*. These characteristics make D2 an ideal player for regulating local T3 levels, demonstrated clearly in the rat brain *(22,23)*. Recently it was shown that skeletal muscle D2 may have a significant contribution to circulating T3 as well, particularly in the hypothyroid state *(7,24)*. It was therefore hypothesized that diminished D2 activity during critical illness played a role in the reduced activation of T4 into T3. However, analysis of postmortem obtained skeletal muscle biopsies from critically ill patients showed elevated D2 gene expression and activity levels, compared to acutely stressed patients and healthy controls *(25)*. Thus reduced D2 activity does not appear to play a role in the pathogenesis of the low T3 syndrome in prolonged critically ill patients. Acutely stressed patients showed no difference in D2 activity with healthy controls despite their lower T3 levels *(25)* indicating that D2 fails to compensate for the reduced T3 levels in the early phase of illness.

Increased D3 Activity During Critical Illness

D3 decreases local T3 concentrations and is particularly important during fetal development. It has been named an oncofetal protein since it has also been found in vascular tumors and malignant cell lines *(26)*. These D3-expressing tumors cause a massive inactivation of circulating thyroid hormone which leads to a condition called consumptive hypothyroidism *(27)*. Critically ill patients also showed increased D3 activity in liver and muscle leading to similar alterations in circulating thyroid hormone levels *(13,28)*. By continuously infusing TRH to prolonged ill rabbits, the increased D3 activity was diminished and T3 levels were normalized, while rT3 levels increased *(14)*. The addition of a growth hormone secretagogue to the infusion prevented the rise in rT3 *(14)*.

In addition to the down-regulation of D1, an induction of D3 activity in liver and muscle is likely to contribute to the low serum T3 and high serum rT3 levels seen in critically ill patients. D2 does not seem to play a role in the pathogenesis of the low T3 syndrome.

Thyroid Hormone Binding and Transport

THYROID HORMONE BINDING

A decrease in T4 binding proteins such as T4 binding globulin (TBG), albumin, and transthyretin (TTR) is shown to be involved in the decreased serum T4 levels observed during acute events as sepsis and cardiac bypass surgery *(28–30)*. It has also been suggested that a binding inhibitor may be present in the serum of critically ill patients *(31,32)*. Such a binding inhibitor would result in diminished uptake of thyroid hormone by cells or in a distortion of the normal interaction between thyroid hormone and its nuclear receptors. However, exogenous T4 administration to prolonged critically ill patients can easily increase circulating T4 levels, indicating that an inhibitor of binding is not the predominate cause of low serum T4 during critical illness *(33)*.

THYROID HORMONE TRANSPORT

Thyroid hormone must first be transported over the cell membrane before it can be converted by the selenocysteine deiodinases and interact with its receptor. During critical illness, T4 uptake in the liver is decreased which may contribute to lowered T3 production *(34,35)*. Furthermore, serum of critically ill patients can inhibit the uptake of T4 into cultured hepatocytes *(36–38)*. This observation has led to the identification of several inhibitors, such as indoxyl sulfate, nonesterified fatty acids (NEFAs), and bilirubin which circulate in increased concentrations during critical illness *(36,39)*. Inhibition of liver T4 uptake during critical illness can also be explained by an existing negative energy balance leading to hepatic ATP depletion *(40,41)*. This idea is supported by the observation that administration of fructose to healthy volunteers, transiently decreasing liver ATP levels, was followed by a temporary decrease in liver T4 uptake *(42)*

Thyroid hormone cannot enter the cell by simple passive diffusion through the cell lipid bilayer, but needs specific transmembrane transporters *(34)*. Monocarboxylate transporter 8 (MCT8, SLC16A2) is such an amino acid transporter which recently has been shown to be very active and specific for thyroid hormone *(43,44)*. Expression analysis in liver and muscle tissue of critically ill patients suggested that MCT8 is not crucial for transport of iodothyronines, at least not in these tissues *(45)*. Very recently, it was shown that MCT10 can transport thyroid hormone as well *(46)*. The precise role and regulation of MCT8 and MCT10 during acute and chronic critical illness remains to be addressed in future studies.

Tissue Levels of Thyroid Hormone and Interaction with its Receptors

It is still not clear whether the low concentrations of circulating thyroid hormone and the decreased tissue uptake of T4 actually result in reduced thyroid hormone levels in the tissue and thus a low bioactivity of thyroid hormone. The study by Arem et al. showed that, in general, T3 concentrations were decreased in the tissues of critically ill patients compared with tissues from patients who died acutely *(47)*. This is supported by the observation that circulating T3 levels correlate well with skeletal muscle and liver T3 content in critically ill patients *(45)*. In this larger study, the investigators also showed that in patients who had received thyroid hormone treatment, serum T3 concentrations were higher with concomitant higher skeletal muscle T3 concentrations *(45)*.

The bioactivity of thyroid hormone is not only dependent on its concentration in the cell; it can also be modulated at the level of its nuclear receptors. Nuclear thyroid hormone receptors (TR) exist in two isoforms: TRα and TRβ. By alternative splicing each gene can encode several proteins. TRα–1, TRβ-1, and TRβ-2 bind T3 with similar affinity. Upon binding, target genes are transcriptionaly activated or repressed. Importantly, in the absence of thyroid hormone, these receptors repress or silence basal transcription of positively regulated genes *(48)*. Of special interest is TRα-2 which is also encoded by the TRα gene. It lacks a functional ligand binding domain and acts as a dominant negative inhibitor of thyroid hormone action *(49)*. The ratio of the different splice variants could therefore have a marked influence on T3-regulated gene expression.

Analysis of post-mortem obtained liver biopsies from critically ill patients showed an inverse correlation between T3/rT3 ratio and the TRα-1/TRα-2 ratio *(50)*. Furthermore, sicker and older patients showed higher TRα-1/TRα-2 ratios as compared with the less sick and younger ones. Increasing the expression of the active form of the thyroid hormone receptor gene can be regarded as an adaptive response to the decreasing thyroid hormone levels during critical illness. On the other hand, experimental work on animals showed a decline in number and in occupancy of hepatic nuclear T3 receptors *(51,52)*.

Degradation of Thyroid Hormones

Sulfation is another important mechanism for thyroid hormone metabolism *(53)*. Sulfated iodothyronines do not bind to thyroid hormone receptors and are rapidly degraded by D1. Therefore, the concentrations of sulfated iodothyronines in serum are normally low *(54, 55)*. In one study, increased circulating concentrations of sulfated T4 (T4S) were found in prolonged critically ill patients as compared with healthy references *(56)*. These increased serum T4S levels showed a negative correlation with hepatic D1 activity suggesting that a decreased liver D1 activity plays an important role in the increase of T4S levels during critical illness. Contradicting results were obtained when analyzing serum T4S levels in children with meningococcal sepsis *(28)*. In these children, average T4S levels were decreased as compared to healthy controls.

NEUROENDOCRINE CHANGES DURING CRITICAL ILLNESS

In the prolonged phase of critical illness, the above-described peripheral changes persist but patients develop additional alterations in the central component of the HPT-axis. Some of these changes are already perceivable in the acute phase of illness. For example, TSH levels only rise very briefly (+/–2 hours) in face of declining T3 concentrations and even return to normal despite ongoing decline in T3 levels *(3,4)*. This can be indicative of an altered set-point for feedback inhibition. Acute critically ill patients also lack a nocturnal TSH surge as seen in healthy individuals *(3,57)*.

In the prolonged phase of critical illness, TSH release loses its pulsatility and correlates positively with the low circulating T3 and T4 levels *(4,58)*. Continuous infusion of TRH can increase TSH secretion and, concomitantly, the low circulating levels of T4 and T3 back to normal levels *(58)* which suggests a predominantly central origin of the suppressed thyroid axis *(59)*. This is further substantiated by the work of Fliers et al., who indeed showed reduced TRH gene expression in the hypothalamus of patients dying after chronic critical illness compared with those who died after a road accident or an acute illness *(60)*. Furthermore, a positive correlation was found between TRH mRNA levels and serum TSH and T3 *(60)*. An increase in circulating levels of TSH is also an early marker of recovery from severe illness *(61–63)*.

Role of Cytokines

The neuroendocrine pathophysiology behind these changes is incompletely understood. Endogenous dopamine and/or hypercortisolism could be involved since they are known to provoke or severely aggravate hypothyroidism in critical illness *(64,65)*. Also, cytokines may play a role since injection of tumor necrosis factor-α (TNF-α), interleukin (IL)-1 or IL-6, were able to mimic the acute stress-induced alterations in thyroid status *(18,66)*. Other studies question the role of cytokines in evoking the low T3 syndrome. First, in contrast to the acute phase, circulating cytokines are usually low in the chronic phase of severe illness *(67)*. Secondly, cytokine antagonism failed to restore normal thyroid function both in humans *(68)* and animals *(69)*. And thirdly, in a large group of hospitalized patients, cytokines were not withheld as independent determinants of the variability in circulating T3 *(70,71)*.

Central Hyperthyroidism?

It is intriguing that TRH gene expression is suppressed in face of low circulating thyroid hormone levels. This could be explained by a local hyperthyroid state, either by an increased activation of T3 by D2 or a decreased inactivation by D3. Several studies in rodents indeed showed an increase in D2 expression and activity in the mediobasal hypothalamus after injection with lipopolysacharide (LPS) *(16,72,73)*. This effect seemed not to be induced by hypothyroidism *(73)* but could be a direct effect of induced cytokines on D2 expressing tanycytes *(74–76)*. Decreased hypothalamic expression of D3 was also observed in chronic inflamed mice *(77)*. However, these data are in conflict with the observation that the hypothalamus of patients who died after chronic severe illness contained less then half the concentration of T3 as compared to patients who died from an acute trauma *(47)*. The fact that LPS injection induces an acute illness rather than a chronic illness could explain some of the discrepancies.

Role of Thyroid Hormone Transporters and Receptors

MCT8, a specific thyroid hormone transporter, and organic anion transporter OATP1C1, a high affinity T4 transporter, are both expressed in the hypothalamus *(78,79)*. Analysis of MCT8 null mice showed increased TRH expression levels in hypophysiotropic neurons despite their increased circulating T3 levels *(80)*. This shows that MCT8 is necessary for normal TRH feedback regulation. OATP1C1 is known to be regulated by thyroid state in the brain *(81)* but up until now, the regulation of these thyroid hormone transporters in the hypothalamus and their involvement in the altered hypothalamic set-point in critical illness has not been studied.

Expression of thyroid hormone receptor isoforms were also shown to be regulated by thyroid hormone status in the hypothalamus *(82)*, but their role in critical illness has not been studied so far.

Feedback by Neuronal Afferents

TRH neuron function can also be controlled by the melanocortin signaling system. This system consists of a group of neurons that synthesize alpha melanocyte stimulating hormone (α-MSH) and a group of neurons synthesizing agouti-related protein (AGRP). The first peptide has an activating effect on TRH neurons, while the latter suppresses TRH mRNA in the PVN (for review see *(83)*). The precise role of the melanocortin system in critical illness remains to be unraveled. Until now, most of the research has been done on LPS-induced inflammation models and starvation which has led to some puzzling results. During fasting, α-MSH expression decreases and AGRP increases in the PVN resulting in decreased TRH expression *(84)*. Inflammation in the rat also resulted in an overall suppression of TRH in the PVN, however, this was accompanied by an increased expression of α-MSH *(85)*. Neuropeptide Y (NPY) may be additionally involved since it potentiates the inhibitory effect of AGRP on TRH. In patients who died from severe illness, NPY expression was reduced and showed a positive correlation with TRH levels *(86)* while an inverse correlation was seen during starvation *(84)*.

TREATING THE LOW T3 SYNDROME

The pathophysiology of the low T3 syndrome is still not fully understood, and studying the underlying mechanisms should therefore be a priority before contemplating on treatment strategies. Research by Van den Berghe et al. has shown that there are important differences between the acute and the chronic phase of critical illness *(87–89)*. Patients from both groups are thus not likely to benefit from the same therapy.

The observed alterations in the acute phase of critical illness are very similar to the ones observed in fasting. In fasting, the reduced amounts of circulating T3 have been interpreted as an attempt of the body to reduce its energy expenditure, prevent protein wasting and to promote survival *(90,91)*. The acute changes in the thyroid axis during acute critical illness are so uniformly present in all types of acute illnesses that they could be looked upon as a beneficial and adaptive response that does not warrant intervention.

Prolonged critical illness is a relatively new condition arising from the development of modern intensive care medicine. It is an unnatural condition, which could not have been selected by nature, making it unlikely that it represents an adaptive response. These prolonged ill patients show high levels of biochemical markers of catabolism (urea production and bone degradation). When thyroid hormone is restored to physiological levels by continuous infusion of TRH in combination with a growth hormone (GH) secretagogue, these markers of hypercatabolism can be reduced *(92)*. This suggests that low thyroid hormone levels rather contribute to than protect from the hypercatabolism of prolonged critical illness. Importantly, the negative feedback inhibition, exerted by thyroid hormones on the thyroid gland to prevent overstimulation of the thyroid axis, can be maintained when infusing TRH in prolonged critical illness *(58,93)*.

It is still under debate whether these patients should be treated with direct administration of T3 and/or T4 to raise circulating T3 levels *(47,94)*. Treatment with T4 has yet failed to demonstrate a clinical benefit, although this could be in part due to the impaired conversion of T4 to T3 *(33,95)*. Administration of substitution doses of T3 after cardiac surgery in pediatric patients has been associated with improvements in postoperative cardiac function *(96)*. These patients however, were treated with dopamine which induces hypothyroidism and therefore this study does not provide evidence of clinical benefit of treating the non-iatrogenic low T3 levels characteristic of prolonged critical illness *(97,98)*.

Another possibility is to treat patients with hypothalamic releasing factors. This enables the body to use its normal feedback systems and protect itself against over-treatment. Infusion with TRH increased nonpulsatile TSH release and circulating T3 and T4 levels but rT3 levels increased as well. The combined infusion of TRH with growth hormone releasing peptide 2 (GHRP-2) prevented the rise in rT3 and also increased pulsatile TSH secretion *(58)*. Intriguingly, infusion of GHRP-2 alone, although accompanied by increases in GH secretion and in serum concentrations of insulin-like growth factor 1 (IGF-I), IGF-binding protein 3 (IGFBP-3), and its acid-labile subunit (ALS), did not induce any of the anabolic tissue responses which were evoked by the combined infusion of GHRP and TRH, *(93)*. Further studies should be undertaken to assess the clinical benefits on morbidity and mortality of TRH infusion alone or in combination with GH secretagogues in prolonged critical illness.

Acknowledgments This work was supported by the Fund for Scientific Research Flanders, Belgium (FWO)

REFERENCES

1. Larsen PR, Davies TF, Hay ID. The thyroid Gland. In: Wilson JD, Foster DW, Kronenberg HM, et al, editors. Williams Textbook of Endocrinology. 9th Edition. Philadelphia: WB Saunders; 1998 p. 389–515.

2. Yen PM. Physiological and molecular basis of thyroid hormone action. *Physiol Rev* 2001; 81(3): 1097–1142.

3. Michalaki M, Vagenakis AG, Makri M, Kalfarentzos F, Kyriazopoulou V. Dissociation of the early decline in serum T(3) concentration and serum IL-6 rise and TNFalpha in non-thyroidal illness syndrome induced by abdominal surgery. *J Clin Endocrinol Metab* 2001; 86(9): 4198–4205.

4. Van den Berghe G, de Zegher F, Veldhuis JD et al. Thyrotrophin and prolactin release in prolonged critical illness: dynamics of spontaneous secretion and effects of growth hormone-secretagogues. *Clin Endocrinol (Oxf)* 1997; 47(5): 599–612.

5. Bianco AC, Salvatore D, Gereben B, Berry MJ, Larsen PR. Biochemistry, Cellular and Molecular Biology, and Physiological Roles of the Iodothyronine Selenodeiodinases. *Endocr Rev* 2002; 23(1): 38–89.

6. Bianco AC, Kim BW. Deiodinases: implications of the local control of thyroid hormone action. *J Clin Invest* 2006; 116(10): 2571–2579.

7. Luiza Maia A, Kim BW, Huang SA, Harney JW, Larsen PR. Type 2 iodothyronine deiodinase is the major source of plasma T3 in euthyroid humans. *J Clin Invest* 2005; 115(9): 2524–2533.

8. Bianco AC, Larsen PR. Cellular and structural biology of the deiodinases. *Thyroid* 2005; 15(8): 777–786.

9. Leonard JL, Koehrle J. Intracellular pathways of iodothyronine metabolism. Philadelphia: Lippincott Williams & Wilkins; 2000.

10. Zimmerman D. Fetal and neonatal hyperthyroidism. *Thyroid* 1999; 9(7): 727–733.

11. Carter JN, Eastmen CJ, Corcoran JM, Lazarus L. Inhibition of conversion of thyroxine to triiodothyronine in patients with severe chronic illness. *Clin Endocrinol (Oxf)* 1976; 5(6): 587–594.

12. Chopra IJ, Chopra U, Smith SR, Reza M, Solomon DH. Reciprocal changes in serum concentrations of 3,3′,5-triiodothyronine (T3) in systemic illnesses. *J Clin Endocrinol Metab* 1975; 41(6): 1043–1049.

13. Peeters RP, Wouters PJ, Kaptein E, van Toor H, Visser TJ, Van den Berghe G. Reduced activation and increased inactivation of thyroid hormone in tissues of critically ill patients. *J Clin Endocrinol Metab* 2003; 88(7): 3202–3211.

14. Debaveye Y, Ellger B, Mebis L et al. Tissue Deiodinase Activity during Prolonged Critical Illness: Effects of Exogenous Thyrotropin-Releasing Hormone and Its Combination with Growth Hormone-Releasing Peptide-2. *Endocrinology* 2005; 146(12): 5604–5611.

15. Weekers F, Van Herck E, Coopmans W et al. A Novel in Vivo Rabbit Model of Hypercatabolic Critical Illness Reveals a Biphasic Neuroendocrine Stress Response. *Endocrinology* 2002; 143(3): 764–774.

16. Boelen A, Kwakkel J, Thijssen-Timmer DC, Alkemade A, Fliers E, Wiersinga WM. Simultaneous changes in central and peripheral components of the hypothalamus-pituitary-thyroid axis in lipopolysaccharide-induced acute illness in mice. *J Endocrinol* 2004; 182(2): 315–323.

17. O'Mara BA, Dittrich W, Lauterio TJ, St Germain DL. Pretranslational regulation of type I 5′-deiodinase by thyroid hormones and in fasted and diabetic rats. *Endocrinology* 1993; 133(4): 1715–1723.

18. Boelen A, Platvoet-ter Schiphorst MC, Bakker O, Wiersinga WM. The role of cytokines in the lipopolysaccharide-induced sick euthyroid syndrome in mice. *J Endocrinol* 1995; 146(3): 475–483.

19. Yu J, Koenig RJ. Regulation of Hepatocyte Thyroxine 5'-Deiodinase by T3 and Nuclear Receptor Coactivators as a Model of the Sick Euthyroid Syndrome. *J Biol Chem* 2000; 275(49): 38296–38301.

20. Yu J, Koenig RJ. Induction of type 1 iodothyronine deiodinase to prevent the nonthyroidal illness syndrome in mice. *Endocrinology* 2006; 147(7): 3580–3585.

21. Weekers F, Michalaki M, Coopmans W et al. Endocrine and metabolic effects of growth hormone (GH) compared with GH-releasing peptide, thyrotropin-releasing hormone, and insulin infusion in a rabbit model of prolonged critical illness. Endocrinology 2004; 145(1): 205–213.

22. Crantz FR, Silva JE, Larsen PR. An analysis of the sources and quantity of 3,5,3'-triiodothyronine specifically bound to nuclear receptors in rat cerebral cortex and cerebellum. *Endocrinology* 1982; 110(2): 367–375.

23. Larsen PR, Silva JE, Kaplan MM. Relationships between circulating and intracellular thyroid hormones: physiological and clinical implications. *Endocr Rev* 1981; 2(1): 87–102.

24. Salvatore D, Bartha T, Harney JW, Larsen PR. Molecular biological and biochemical characterization of the human type 2 selenodeiodinase. *Endocrinology* 1996; 137(8): 3308–3315.

25. Mebis L, Langouche L, Visser TJ, Van den Berghe G. The Type II Iodothyronine Deiodinase Is Up-Regulated in Skeletal Muscle during Prolonged Critical Illness. *J Clin Endocrinol Metab* 2007; 92(8): 3330–3333.

26. Richard K, Hume R, Kaptein E et al. Ontogeny of iodothyronine deiodinases in human liver. *J Clin Endocrinol Metab* 1998; 83(8): 2868–2874.

27. Huang SA, Tu HM, Harney JW et al. Severe hypothyroidism caused by type 3 iodothyronine deiodinase in infantile hemangiomas. *N Engl J Med* 2000; 343(3): 185–189.

28. den Brinker M, Joosten KF, Visser TJ et al. Euthyroid sick syndrome in meningococcal sepsis: the impact of peripheral thyroid hormone metabolism and binding proteins. *J Clin Endocrinol Metab* 2005; 90(10): 5613–5620.

29. Afandi B, Vera R, Schussler GC, Yap MG. Concordant decreases of thyroxine and thyroxine binding protein concentrations during sepsis. *Metabolism* 2000; 49(6): 753–754.

30. Afandi B, Schussler GC, Arafeh AH, Boutros A, Yap MG, Finkelstein A. Selective consumption of thyroxine-binding globulin during cardiac bypass surgery. *Metabolism* 2000; 49(2): 270–274.

31. Chopra IJ, Huang TS, Beredo A, Solomon DH, Chua Teco GN, Mead JF. Evidence for an inhibitor of extrathyroidal conversion of thyroxine to 3,5,3'-triiodothyronine in sera of patients with nonthyroidal illnesses. *J Clin Endocrinol Metab* 1985; 60(4): 666–672.

32. Kaptein EM. Thyroid hormone metabolism and thyroid diseases in chronic renal failure. *Endocr Rev* 1996; 17(1): 45–63.

33. Brent GA, Hershman JM. Thyroxine therapy in patients with severe nonthyroidal illnesses and low serum thyroxine concentration. *J Clin Endocrinol Metab* 1986; 63(1): 1–8.

34. Hennemann G, Krenning EP, Polhuys M et al. Carrier-mediated transport of thyroid hormone into rat hepatocytes is rate-limiting in total cellular uptake and metabolism. *Endocrinology* 1986; 119(4): 1870–1872.

35. Hennemann G, Everts ME, de Jong M, Lim CF, Krenning EP, Docter R. The significance of plasma membrane transport in the bioavailability of thyroid hormone. *Clin Endocrinol (Oxf)* 1998; 48(1): 1–8.

36. Lim CF, Docter R, Visser TJ et al. Inhibition of thyroxine transport into cultured rat hepatocytes by serum of nonuremic critically ill patients: effects of bilirubin and nonesterified fatty acids. *J Clin Endocrinol Metab* 1993; 76(5): 1165–1172.

37. Sarne DH, Refetoff S. Measurement of thyroxine uptake from serum by cultured human hepatocytes as an index of thyroid status: reduced thyroxine uptake from serum of patients with nonthyroidal illness. *J Clin Endocrinol Metab* 1985; 61(6): 1046–1052.

38. Vos RA, de Jong M, Bernard BF, Docter R, Krenning EP, Hennemann G. Impaired thyroxine and 3,5,3′-triiodothyronine handling by rat hepatocytes in the presence of serum of patients with nonthyroidal illness. *J Clin Endocrinol Metab* 1995; 80(8): 2364–2370.

39. Lim CF, Docter R, Krenning EP et al. Transport of thyroxine into cultured hepatocytes: effects of mild non-thyroidal illness and calorie restriction in obese subjects. *Clin Endocrinol (Oxf)* 1994; 40(1): 79–85.

40. Bodoky G, Yang ZJ, Meguid MM, Laviano A, Szeverenyi N. Effects of fasting, intermittent feeding, or continuous parenteral nutrition on rat liver and brain energy metabolism as assessed by 31P-NMR. *Physiol Behav* 1995; 58(3): 521–527.

41. Krenning EP, Docter R, Bernard B, Visser T, Hennemann G. Decreased transport of thyroxine (T4), 3,3′,5-triiodothyronine (T3) and 3,3′,5′-triiodothyronine (rT3) into rat hepatocytes in primary culture due to a decrease of cellular ATP content and various drugs. *FEBS Lett* 1982; 140(2): 229–233.

42. de Jong M, Docter R, Bernard BF et al. T4 uptake into the perfused rat liver and liver T4 uptake in humans are inhibited by fructose. *Am J Physiol* 1994; 266(5 Pt 1): E768–E775.

43. Friesema EC, Ganguly S, Abdalla A, Manning Fox JE, Halestrap AP, Visser TJ. Identification of monocarboxylate transporter 8 as a specific thyroid hormone transporter. *J Biol Chem* 2003; 278(41): 40128–40135.

44. Friesema EC, Kuiper GG, Jansen J, Visser TJ, Kester MH. Thyroid hormone transport by the human monocarboxylate transporter 8 and its rate-limiting role in intracellular metabolism. *Mol Endocrinol* 2006; 20(11): 2761–2772.

45. Peeters RP, van der Geyten S, Wouters PJ et al. Tissue Thyroid Hormone Levels in Critical Illness. *J Clin Endocrinol Metab* 2005; 90(12): 6498–6507.

46. Friesema EC, Jachtenberg W, Jansen J, Kester MH, Visser TJ. Human monocarboxylate transporter 10 does transport thyroid hormone. *Thyroid* 16, 913. 2006. Ref Type: Abstract

47. Arem R, Wiener GJ, Kaplan SG, Kim HS, Reichlin S, Kaplan MM. Reduced tissue thyroid hormone levels in fatal illness. *Metabolism* 1993; 42(9): 1102–1108.

48. Brent GA, Dunn MK, Harney JW, Gulick T, Larsen PR, Moore DD. Thyroid hormone aporeceptor represses T3-inducible promoters and blocks activity of the retinoic acid receptor. *New Biol* 1989; 1(3):329–336.

49. Koenig RJ, Lazar MA, Hodin RA et al. Inhibition of thyroid hormone action by a non-hormone binding c-erbA protein generated by alternative mRNA splicing. *Nature* 1989; 337(6208):659–661.

50. Thijssen-Timmer DC, Peeters RP, Wouters P et al. Thyroid hormone receptor isoform expression in livers of critically ill patients. *Thyroid* 2007; 17(2): 105–112.

51. Carr FE, Seelig S, Mariash CN, Schwartz HL, Oppenheimer JH. Starvation and hypothyroidism exert an overlapping influence on rat hepatic messenger RNA activity profiles. *J Clin Invest* 1983; 72(1): 154–163.

52. Thompson P, Jr., Burman KD, Lukes YG et al. Uremia decreases nuclear 3,5,3′-triiodothyronine receptors in rats. *Endocrinology* 1980; 107(4): 1081–1084.

53. Visser TJ, Kaptein E, Glatt H, Bartsch I, Hagen M, Coughtrie MW. Characterization of thyroid hormone sulfotransferases. *Chem Biol Interact* 1998; 109(1–3): 279–291.

54. Chopra IJ, Wu SY, Teco GN, Santini F. A radioimmunoassay for measurement of 3,5,3′-triiodothyronine sulfate: studies in thyroidal and nonthyroidal diseases, pregnancy, and neonatal life. *J Clin Endocrinol Metab* 1992; 75(1): 189–194.

55. Eelkman Rooda SJ, Kaptein E, Visser TJ. Serum triiodothyronine sulfate in man measured by radioimmunoassay. *J Clin Endocrinol Metab* 1989; 69(3): 552–556.

56. Peeters RP, Kester MH, Wouters PJ et al. Increased thyroxine sulfate levels in critically ill patients as a result of a decreased hepatic type I deiodinase activity. *J Clin Endocrinol Metab* 2005; 90(12): 6460–6465.

57. Wellby ML, Kennedy JA, Barreau PB, Roediger WE. Endocrine and cytokine changes during elective surgery. *J Clin Pathol* 1994; 47(11): 1049–1051.

58. Van den Berghe G, de Zegher F, Baxter RC et al. Neuroendocrinology of Prolonged Critical Illness: Effects of Exogenous Thyrotropin-Releasing Hormone and Its Combination with Growth Hormone Secretagogues. *J Clin Endocrinol Metab* 1998; 83(2): 309–319.

59. Mesotten D, Van den Berghe G. Changes within the GH/IGF-I/IGFBP axis in critical illness. *Crit Care Clin* 2006; 22(1): 17–28, v.

60. Fliers E, Guldenaar SE, Wiersinga WM, Swaab DF. Decreased hypothalamic thyrotropin-releasing hormone gene expression in patients with nonthyroidal illness. *J Clin Endocrinol Metab* 1997; 82(12): 4032–4036.

61. Bacci V, Schussler GC, Kaplan TB. The relationship between serum triiodothyronine and thyrotropin during systemic illness. *J Clin Endocrinol Metab* 1982; 54(6): 1229–1235.

62. Hamblin PS, Dyer SA, Mohr VS et al. Relationship between thyrotropin and thyroxine changes during recovery from severe hypothyroxinemia of critical illness. *J Clin Endocrinol Metab* 1986; 62(4): 717–722.

63. Peeters RP, Wouters PJ, van Toor H, Kaptein E, Visser TJ, Van den Berghe G. Serum 3,3′,5′-triiodothyronine (rT3) and 3,5,3′-triiodothyronine/rT3 are prognostic markers in critically ill patients and are associated with postmortem tissue deiodinase activities. *J Clin Endocrinol Metab* 2005; 90(8): 4559–4565.

64. Van den Berghe G, de Zegher F, Lauwers P. Dopamine and the sick euthyroid syndrome in critical illness. *Clinical Endocrinology* 1994; 41(6): 731–737.

65. Faglia G, Ferrari C, Beck-Peccoz P, Spada A, Travaglini P, Ambrosi B. Reduced plasma thyrotropin response to thyrotropin releasing hormone after dexamethasone administration in normal subjects. Hormone And Metabolic Research Hormon-Und Stoffwechselforschung Hormones Et Metabolisme 1973; 5(4): 289–292.

66. van der Poll T, Romijn JA, Wiersinga WM, Sauerwein Hp. Tumor necrosis factor: a putative mediator of the sick euthyroid syndrome in man. *J Clin Endocrinol Metab* 1990; 71(6): 1567–1572.

67. Damas P, Reuter A, Gysen P, Demonty J, Lamy M, Franchimont P. Tumor necrosis factor and interleukin-1 serum levels during severe sepsis in humans. *Crit Care Med* 1989; 17(10): 975–978.

68. van der Poll T, Van Zee KJ, Endert E et al. Interleukin-1 receptor blockade does not affect endotoxin-induced changes in plasma thyroid hormone and thyrotropin concentrations in man. *J Clin Endocrinol Metab* 1995; 80(4): 1341–1346.

69. Boelen A, Platvoet-ter Schiphorst MC, Wiersinga WM. Immunoneutralization of interleukin-1, tumor necrosis factor, interleukin-6 or interferon does not prevent the LPS-induced sick euthyroid syndrome in mice. *J Endocrinol* 1997; 153(1): 115–122.

70. Boelen A, Platvoet-ter Schiphorst MC, Wiersinga WM. Association between serum interleukin-6 and serum 3,5,3′-triiodothyronine in nonthyroidal illness. *J Clin Endocrinol Metab* 1993; 77(6): 1695–1699.

71. Boelen A, Schiphorst MC, Wiersinga WM. Relationship between serum 3,5,3′-triiodothyronine and serum interleukin-8, interleukin-10 or interferon gamma in patients with nonthyroidal illness. *J Endocrinol Invest* 1996; 19(7): 480–483.

72. Fekete C, Gereben B, Doleschall M et al. Lipopolysaccharide induces type 2 iodothyronine deiodinase in the mediobasal hypothalamus: implications for the nonthyroidal illness syndrome. *Endocrinology* 2004; 145(4): 1649–1655.

73. Fekete C, Singru PS, Sarkar S, Rand WM, Lechan RM. Ascending brainstem pathways are not involved in lipopolysaccharide-induced suppression of thyrotropin-releasing hormone gene expression in the hypothalamic paraventricular nucleus. *Endocrinology* 2005; 146(3): 1357–1363.

74. Baur A, Bauer K, Jarry H, Kohrle J. Effects of proinflammatory cytokines on anterior pituitary 5′-deiodinase type I and type II. *J Endocrinol* 2000; 167(3): 505–515.

75. Zeold A, Doleschall M, Haffner MC et al. Characterization of the nuclear factor-kappa B responsiveness of the human dio2 gene. *Endocrinology* 2006; 147(9): 4419–4429.

76. Nadeau S, Rivest S. Effects of circulating tumor necrosis factor on the neuronal activity and expression of the genes encoding the tumor necrosis factor receptors (p55 and p75) in the rat brain: a view from the blood-brain barrier. *Neuroscience* 1999; 93(4): 1449–1464.

77. Boelen A, Kwakkel J, Wiersinga WM, Fliers E. Chronic local inflammation in mice results in decreased TRH and type 3 deiodinase mRNA expression in the hypothalamic paraventricular nucleus independently of diminished food intake. *J Endocrinol* 2006; 191(3): 707–714.

78. Alkemade A, Friesema EC, Unmehopa UA et al. Neuroanatomical pathways for thyroid hormone feedback in the human hypothalamus. *J Clin Endocrinol Metab* 2005; 90(7): 4322–4334.

79. Pizzagalli F, Hagenbuch B, Stieger B, Klenk U, Folkers G, Meier PJ. Identification of a novel human organic anion transporting polypeptide as a high affinity thyroxine transporter. *Mol Endocrinol* 2002; 16(10): 2283–2296.

80. Trajkovic M, Visser TJ, Mittag J et al. Abnormal thyroid hormone metabolism in mice lacking the monocarboxylate transporter 8. *J Clin Invest* 2007; 117(3): 627–635.

81. Sugiyama D, Kusuhara H, Taniguchi H et al. Functional characterization of rat brain-specific organic anion transporter (Oatp14) at the blood-brain barrier: high affinity transporter for thyroxine. *J Biol Chem* 2003; 278(44): 43489–43495.

82. Clerget-Froidevaux MS, Seugnet I, Demeneix BA. Thyroid status co-regulates thyroid hormone receptor and co-modulator genes specifically in the hypothalamus. *FEBS Lett* 2004; 569(1–3): 341–345.

83. Lechan RM, Fekete C. Role of melanocortin signaling in the regulation of the hypothalamic-pituitary-thyroid (HPT) axis. *Peptides* 2006; 27(2): 310–325.

84. Ahima RS, Saper CB, Flier JS, Elmquist JK. Leptin regulation of neuroendocrine systems. *Front Neuroendocrinol* 2000; 21(3): 263–307.

85. Sergeyev V, Broberger C, Hokfelt T. Effect of LPS administration on the expression of POMC, NPY, galanin, CART and MCH mRNAs in the rat hypothalamus. *Brain Res Mol Brain Res* 2001; 90(2): 93–100.

86. Fliers E, Unmehopa UA, Manniesing S, Vuijst CL, Wiersinga WM, Swaab DF. Decreased neuropeptide Y (NPY) expression in the infundibular nucleus of patients with nonthyroidal illness. *Peptides* 2001; 22(3): 459–465.

87. Van den Berghe G, de Zegher F, Bouillon R. Acute and Prolonged Critical Illness as Different Neuroendocrine Paradigms. *J Clin Endocrinol Metab* 1998; 83(6): 1827–1834.

88. Van den Berghe G. Novel insights into the neuroendocrinology of critical illness. *Eur J Endocrinol* 2000; 143(1): 1–13.

89. Van den Berghe G. Dynamic neuroendocrine responses to critical illness. *Front Neuroendocrinol* 2002; 23(4): 370–391.

90. Gardner DF, Kaplan MM, Stanley CA, Utiger RD. Effect of tri-iodothyronine replacement on the metabolic and pituitary responses to starvation. *N Engl J Med* 1979; 300(11): 579–584.

91. Utiger RD. Decreased extrathyroidal triiodothyronine production in nonthyroidal illness: benefit or harm? *Am J Med* 1980; 69(6): 807–810.

92. Van den Berghe G, Wouters P, Weekers F et al. Reactivation of Pituitary Hormone Release and Metabolic Improvement by Infusion of Growth Hormone-Releasing Peptide and Thyrotropin-Releasing Hormone in Patients with Protracted Critical Illness. *J Clin Endocrinol Metab* 1999; 84(4): 1311–1323.

93. Van den Berghe G, Baxter RC, Weekers F et al. The combined administration of GH-releasing peptide-2 (GHRP-2), TRH and GnRH to men with prolonged critical illness evokes superior endocrine and metabolic effects compared to treatment with GHRP-2 alone. *Clin Endocrinol (Oxf)* 2002; 56(5): 655–669.

94. Vaughan GM, Mason AD, Jr., McManus WF, Pruitt BA, Jr. Alterations of mental status and thyroid hormones after thermal injury. *J Clin Endocrinol Metab* 1985; 60(6): 1221–1225.

95. Becker RA, Vaughan GM, Ziegler MG et al. Hypermetabolic low triiodothyronine syndrome of burn injury. *Crit Care Med* 1982; 10(12): 870–875.

96. Bettendorf M, Schmidt KG, Grulich-Henn J, Ulmer HE, Heinrich UE. Tri-iodothyronine treatment in children after cardiac surgery: a double-blind, randomised, placebo-controlled study. *Lancet* 2000; 356(9229): 529–534.

97. Debaveye Y, Van den Berghe G. Is there still a place for dopamine in the modern intensive care unit? *Anesth Analg* 2004; 98(2): 461–468.

98. Van den Berghe G, de Zegher F, Vlasselaers D et al. Thyrotropin-releasing hormone in critical illness: from a dopamine-dependent test to a strategy for increasing low serum triiodothyronine, prolactin, and growth hormone concentrations. *Crit Care Med* 1996; 24(4): 590–595.

11 The Adrenal Response to Critical Illness

Mikael Alves,
Xavi Borrat, MD
and Djillali Annane, MD, PhD

INTRODUCTION

The integrity of the hypothalamic pituitary adrenal (HPA) axis and the noradrenergic system are essential to survive critical illness as stressed almost a century ago when bilateral hemorrhage of the adrenals were associated with

From: *Contemporary Endocrinology: Acute Cause to Consequence*
Edited by: G. Van den Berghe, DOI: 10.1007/978-1-60327-177-6_11,
© Humana Press, New York, NY

215

fatal outcome in meningococcemia. In the past two decades, it has become consensual that overwhelming systemic inflammation is the hallmark of most of critical illnesses and likely accounts for progression of organs failure and death. Whether excessive systemic inflammation during critical illness results from an inappropriate response of the HPA axis has been extensively investigated and remains unclear. This review will discuss the mechanisms of inadequate HPA response to critical illness and the benefit/risk of glucocorticoids during critical illness.

EVIDENCE OF IMPAIRED HYPOTHALAMIC PITUITARY ADRENAL AXIS DURING CRITICAL ILLNESS

The first demonstration of critical illness associated adrenal insufficiency was reported in patients with fulminate meningococcemia (1). Several decades later abnormal cortisol metabolism was observed in patients with severe abdominal infection and renal or liver failure (2). Then, in the early nineties, Koo and colleagues demonstrated that induction of peritonitis by cecal ligature and puncture in rats resulted in decreased corticosterone synthesis (3). In these experiments, as compared to sham-operated animals, septic animals had higher circulating levels of ACTH but similar levels of corticosterone and decreased adrenals concentration of corticosterone. Furthermore, administration of ACTH resulted in lower increment in cortisol in septic animals. In a similar model of polymicrobial

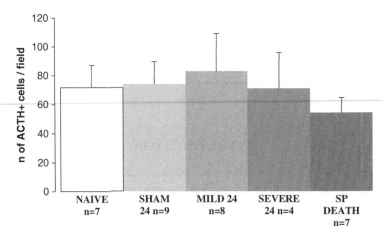

Fig. 1. Male Wistar rats were exposed to cecal ligature and puncture producing increasing severity of sepsis. Sham-operated animals remained sepsis free. ACTH synthesizing cells were counted after careful dissection of the pituitary gland and immunoassaying preparation. There was a slight increase in the number of ACTH positive cells in the mild septic group suggesting sepsis induced recruitment of cells. By contrast, in more severe sepsis there was a gradual decrease in the number of ACTH positive cells suggesting pituitary failure.

sepsis, adrenocortical cells sensitivity to ACTH decreased with the intensity of inflammation with subsequent abolition of circadian rhythm of corticosterone synthesis *(4)*. In another animal study, the number of ACTH synthesizing cells and the amount of ACTH release by these cells decreased with increasing severity of sepsis following peritonitis (Fig. 1, personal communication). Sepsis associated adrenal insufficiency was also documented in large animals *(5)*. Impaired HPA axis is not specific to sepsis and decreased adrenal responsiveness to corticotrophin may for example complicate trauma and hemorrhage in rats *(6)*. A number of observational clinical studies suggested that abnormal HPA axis may occur in patients with sepsis, burns, trauma, liver diseases, or many other acute illnesses *(7–11)*. In a recent study, the integrity of the HPA axis was investigated in patients with severe sepsis using the overnight metyrapone test *(12)*. Remarkably, when compared to healthy volunteers or non-septic critically ill patients, about 60% of patients with severe sepsis had abnormal response to metyrapone suggestive of secondary adrenal insufficiency in 80% of cases.

MECHANISMS OF IMPAIRED HYPOTHALAMIC-PITUITARY ADRENAL RESPONSE TO CRITICAL ILLNESS

Signalization to the Hypothalamic-Pituitary Axis

During systemic inflammation, the hypothalamic pituitary adrenal axis is activated both via neural routes and via blood-borne cytokines. Afferent fibres of noradrenergic and the vagus nerve sense the threat at the level of tissues with subsequent activation of neurons within the Locus Coeruleus that synapse on cholinergic inter-neurons in the parvocellular nuclei. Acetylcholine stimulates the release of corticotrophin releasing factor through muscarinic receptor and this effect is enhanced by nitric oxide or carbon monoxide and inhibited by hydrogen sulfide. Hence, in LPS challenged or septic animals, vagotomy enhanced the systemic inflammatory response, an effect fully prevented by electrical stimulation of the vagus nerve *(13)*. The blood-borne inflammatory mediators, via hypophysial portal capillaries, reached the hypothalamus and the brain areas lacking a blood-brain barrier (i.e., circum ventricular organs), or can cross the blood brain barrier via specific transport systems *(14)*. Glial cells can also produce a number of cytokines such Interleukin (IL)-1, IL-2 and IL-6 *(15)*, and in endotoxin challenged animals, IL-6 was expressed in the anterior pituitary *(16)* and in patients with sepsis, both TNF and IL-1β were expressed in the parvocellular and supraoptic nuclei *(17)*. Subsequent over-expression of the inducible NO synthase (iNOS) may prolong the synthesis of hypothalamic hormones *(18,19)*. The pituitary and pineal glands also expressed the anti-inflammatory cytokines IL-10, IL-13, and IL-1 receptor antagonist which may counterbalance the stimulatory effects of the pro-inflammatory mediators on the neurohormones *(20)*. Cytokines can also directly act on the anterior pituitary, particularly to stimulate ACTH synthesis and release *(21)*, and on the adrenal gland to stimulate cortisol synthesis. Hence, in critical illness, it is thought that the degree of activation of the HPA axis parallels the intensity of the systemic inflammatory response and may be mediated by IL-6 *(22)*. One may consider the ratios ACTH/IL-6 or cortisol/IL-6 in plasma as markers of the balance between systemic inflammation and the neuroendocrine response. Nevertheless, there is still no validated index of the appropriateness of HPA axis activation.

Critical Illness Associated Vascular Damage of the Hypothalamic Pituitary Adrenal Axis

The pituitary is characterized by a weak arterial supply particularly in the *pars distalis* and thus is exposed to ischemia and necrosis in case of sudden cardiovascular collapse. The hypothalamus may also be susceptible to vascular damage. For example, in a cohort of 330 septic shock, brain ischemia or hemorrhage were found in 7% and 10% of patients, respectively *(23)*. The adrenal glands are characterized by limited venous drainage and thus the increased arterial flow during stress results in prompt enlargement of the glands subsequently exposing them to hemorrhagic or necrotic damage. Cardiovascular or renal failure, positive blood cultures, coagulation disorders and anticoagulant are the main risk factors for adrenal vascular damage *(24)*.

Critical Illness Associated Inflammation of the Hypothalamic Pituitary Adrenal Axis

As mentioned above, brain expression of cytokines like IL-1 upregulates the inducible nitric oxide synthase (iNOS), particularly in the wall of vessels neighboring pituitary and hypothalamic cells. The subsequent accumulation of NO behaves as a neurotoxin. Then, NO was shown to cause neuronal apoptosis in critical illnesses like sepsis *(25)*. In endotoxin-challenged animals, a number of other mediators (e.g., substance P, superoxide radicals, carbon monoxide, prostaglandins) are upregulated and may further alter the synthesis of the hypothalamic-pituitary hormones *(26)*. Likewise, a number of pro-inflammatory mediators may interfere with cortisol synthesis by the adrenal cells. Tumour necrosis factor has a dual effect on adrenocortical cells function. Corticosterone production is inhibited by TNF at concentrations ranging from 0.1 to 100 ng/ml *(27)* and enhanced by higher concentrations (200 to 500 ng/ml) *(28)*. Interleukin-6 may enhance basal and post ACTH corticosterone release by adrenocortical cells in culture *(29)* whereas it is inhibited by IL-10 *(30)*. Exposure of rats' adrenocortical cells to serum from patients with septic shock resulted in inhibition of both basal and ACTH

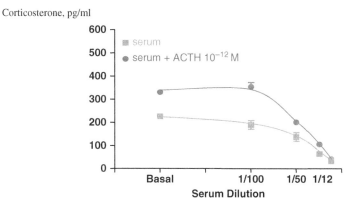

Fig. 2. Adrenocortical cells of rats were cultured and exposed to serum from a patient with septic shock. Serum from septic shock dramatically decreased in a concentration dependent manner corticosterone production by cells.

stimulated corticosterone production (Fig. 2, personal communication). Neutrophils derived corticostatins may compete with ACTH on their binding sites and thus block corticosterone synthesis. Finally, it has been suggested that some viruses may share identical amino-acid sequences with ACTH *(31)*. These viruses may compete with ACTH at the receptor levels. Alternately, the host producing viral antibodies may directly interact with ACTH and account for adrenal insufficiency.

Critical Illness Associated Tissue Resistance to Corticosteroids

Once produced, cortisol is release in the circulation and binds to cortisol binding globulin (CBG) and albumin with only about 10% of circulating unbound hormone. At tissues levels, elastase released from polymorphonuclear cells frees cortisol from its carrier allowing the free hormone to passively enter the cells or binds to membrane sites. In the cytosol, cortisol binds to a specific receptor to form a very active complex with subsequent down or upregulation of thousands of genes *(32)*. During critical illness, a rapid decrease in CBG and albumin levels occurs increasing in the proportion of unbound hormone which however may be less effectively delivered to target tissues *(33)*. Other mechanisms of tissue resistance to corticosteroids may include down regulation of the glucocorticoid receptor alpha or decrease in its affinity for cortisol. Cortisol may also be inactivated by over expression of the 11 beta hydroxysteroid dehydrogenase *(34)*. Exposure of peripheral polymorphonuclear cells to plasma from patients with unresolving acute respiratory distress syndrome demonstrated that systemic inflammation is associated with decreased ratio of glucocorticoid receptor alpha over nuclear factor kappa B suggesting acquired glucocorticoid resistance

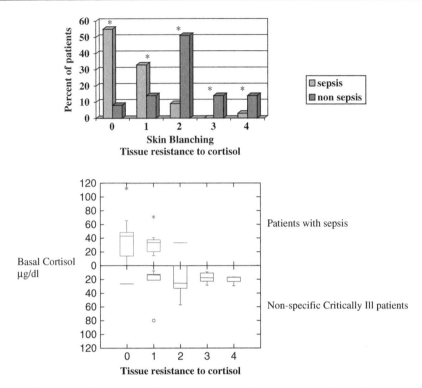

Fig. 3. *Top panel*: distribution of skin blanching 18 hours after topical administration of glucocorticoids. Score 0= no skin blanching – score 1= mottled areas of skin blanching – score 3= skin blanching limited to the area of application – score 4 =skin blanching beyond the area of application. There were significantly (p = 0.02) more patients with a score of 0, 1 or 2 among severe sepsis than among non septic critically ill patients. There was a significant (p<0.001) inverse relationship between basal cortisol levels and a low score of skin blanching (*bottom panel*).

syndrome *(33)*. Dermal application of a glucocorticoid in patients with septic shock failed to induce skin blanching in about three quarter of cases suggesting peripheral tissue resistance (Fig. 3, personal communication). In addition, serum cortisol levels inversely correlated with the intensity of skin blanching. The use of several drugs in the critically ill may further contribute to tissue resistance to corticosteroids or may accelerate their metabolism.

DIAGNOSIS OF IMPAIRED HYPOTHALAMIC PITUITARY ADRENAL AXIS DURING CRITICAL ILLNESS

Clinical symptoms of adrenal insufficiency like fever, abdominal pain, vomiting, hypotension, or altered consciousness are very common signs in the critically ill patients and thus are unhelpful for the recognition of impaired HPA axis. Similarly, hyponatremia and hyperkaliemia or changes in eosinophil count are non specific findings in the intensive care unit.

Although there is no consensus on how to diagnose adrenal insufficiency in critically ill patients, in practice, physicians should rely on the standard short corticotrophin test. The insulin tolerance test cannot be used for intensive care unit for several reasons. This test is cumbersome and requests trained physicians and nurses. Critical illness is almost always associated with insulin resistance lowering the reliability of the insulin tolerance test. Furthermore the on/off response type renders the test very dangerous, increasing the risk of profound hypoglycaemia particularly in the sedated patients. The overnight metyrapone test is also cumbersome and dangerous to be performed in critically ill patients. Nevertheless, it was used in one study and pending systematic cortisol replacement therapy at the end of the test, no serious complications were observed (12). This test relies on evaluation of increase in plasma concentrations of corticotrophin and 11B deoxycortisol after metyrapone induced fall in cortisol levels. It is unlikely that corticotrophin and 11 B deoxycortisol could be measured in a timely fashion for routine use in the ICU. The standard high dose corticotrophin remains the most practical test for the diagnosis of HPA axis impairment during critical illness. In critically ill patients with normal response to metyrapone test, i.e., presumably having normal adrenal function, the basal total cortisol level was never lower than 10 μg/dl and delta cortisol was never lower than 9 μg/dl (12). In this study, none of the patients with abnormal response to metyrapone had basal or stimulated cortisol levels higher than 44 μg/dl. Thus, during critical illness, a basal cortisol level lower than 10μg/dl or an increment in cortisol lower than 9 μg/dl are suggestive of impaired HPA axis. In patients with low albumin levels, total cortisol levels are less reliable (36) and because free cortisol levels could not be obtained in a timely fashion, the diagnosis of adrenal insufficiency in these patients remains problematic. However, the delta cortisol may not be affected by serum albumin levels, suggesting that using the increment in cortisol levels after ACTH remains a valuable diagnostic tool in these patients (37). Recently, it was shown that salivary concentrations of free cortisol may be reliably obtained in critically ill patients (38). Whether recognition of adrenal insufficiency in these patients may rely on determination of salivary cortisol concentrations remains to be investigated. Finally, computed tomography scan can help demonstrating damage to the adrenal glands (39).

CLINICAL CONSEQUENCES OF CRITICAL ILLNESS ASSOCIATED IMPAIRED HPA AXIS

In animals, removal of the adrenal cortex increased dramatically the death rate following endotoxin whereas animals with intact adrenal cortex and destruction of the medulla have similar risk of death than sham-operated animals (40). In critically ill patients a number of large observational studies have investigated the prevalence of adrenal insufficiency and have shown increased risk of death associated with presumed adrenal insufficiency *(7–11)*. Hospital mortality was close to 60% in patients with severe sepsis and adrenal insufficiency and only 22% in those with normal response to the overnight metyrapone test *(12)*. Critically ill patients with adrenal insufficiency are more likely hypotensive and require higher doses of vasopressor. They are also more likely to have mechanical ventilation weaning failure *(41)*.

TREATMENT WITH GLUCOCORTICOIDS DURING CRITICAL ILLNESS

Critical illness is thought to be characterized by uncontrolled systemic inflammation which may result from inadequate cortisol synthesis or acquired tissue resistance to cortisol. Glucocorticoids are potent immuno-modulatory drugs and act through genomic as well as non-genomic effects *(32)*. In addition, glucocorticoids have numerous cardiovascular and metabolic effects which may contribute to the restoration of homeostasis during critical illness.

Immuno-Modulatory Effects of Glucocorticoids Administration During Critical Illness

The molecular mechanisms have been extensively described elsewhere *(42)*. In conditions of excessive and deleterious systemic inflammation like acute respiratory distress syndrome or severe sepsis, glucocorticoids have been shown to attenuate inflammation without causing immune-suppression.

In patients with acute respiratory distress syndrome, moderate doses of glucocorticoids (1 mg/kg/day of methylprednisolone) were associated with enhanced glucocorticoid receptor-mediated functions leading to significant reductions in nuclear factor-kappa B DNA binding and transcription of tumour necrosis factor and interleukin-1B *(34)*. In five randomized controlled trials of prolonged treatment with moderate doses of glucocorticoids have shown a rapid and profound decrease in both lung and plasma concentrations of pro-inflammatory cytokines and a dramatic fall in neutrophils count in the bronchial-alveolar fluids *(43–47)*. The favorable effects of glucocorticoids on systemic and lung inflammation was associated with improved lung compliance and function and prevention of dissemination of inflammation to other organs. Thus, patients were weaned earlier from the ventilator, developed fewer organ failures and fewer super-infections and left earlier the intensive care unit.

In severe sepsis, moderate doses (around 200 mg per day) of hydrocortisone resulted in a significant attenuation of the systemic inflammatory response syndrome, a dramatic reduction in plasma levels of C-reactive proteins, of phospholipase A2 and of neutrophil elastase *(48)*. Several randomized controlled trials have shown that such dose of hydrocortisone induced a substantial decrease in circulating levels of most pro-inflammatory cytokines *(49,50)*. Ex vivo studies on polymorphonuclear cells demonstrated that hydrocortisone prevents the up-regulation of late pro-inflammatory mediators like the macrophage migrating inhibitory factor *(51)*. Of note, circulating levels of anti-inflammatory cytokines were either not affected by hydrocortisone therapy or even significantly reduced *(49)*. Finally, hydrocortisone therapy was not associated with significant alteration in HLA-DR expression on the monocytes surface *(49)*. Taken together these data suggested that moderate doses of hydrocortisone down regulate both early and late pro-inflammatory mediators without causing immune suppression. Subsequently, in severe sepsis, hydrocortisone therapy fastened organs failure resolution without increasing the risk of super-infection. The reduction in local or systemic inflammation was demonstrated in a number of severe infections like bacterial meningitis, pneumocystis pneumonia, typhoid fever, croup, or severe cases of H5N1 avian influenza.

Administration of moderate doses of glucocorticoids have been successful in restoring immune homeostasis in other critical illnesses. Moderate doses of glucocorticoids significantly reduced circulating TNF, IL-6, and IL-8 levels in patients after cardiac surgery with cardiopulmonary bypass *(52)*. Hydrocortisone therapy was found to produce similar favorable effects on inflammation and organ dysfunction in critically ill patients with acute liver diseases *(10,11)*, and in high risk surgical patients *(53)* .

Effects of Glucocorticoids Administration on Survival from Critical Illness

Most of physicians refrain to use short course of high dose glucocorticoids (e.g., 30 mg/kg of methylprednisolone) in patients with severe sepsis or acute respiratory failure as they have been proven to be ineffective *(54)*. By contrast, the benefit/risk of a prolonged treatment with moderate doses of glucocorticoids may be favorable in several critical illnesses such as severe sepsis or acute respiratory failure.

In 18 critically ill patients, as compared with standard treatment alone, 100 mg twice daily of hydrocortisone dramatically improved intensive care unit survival rate (90% vs. 12.5%) *(55)*. There were 14 randomized clinical trials of long course (one week or more) with moderate doses 200 to 300 mg of hydrocortisone per day, or 1 mg/kg/day of methylprednisolone) in patients with severe sepsis or acute respiratory failure, accounting for 1496 patients *(43–45,47,49,50,56–63)*. The pooled estimate from these studies showed a significant (p=0.01) reduction in mortality with glucocorticoids (Fig. 4, personal

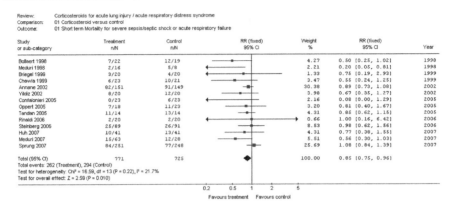

Fig. 4. Meta-analysis of 14 randomized controlled trials in patients with severe sepsis, septic shock, acute lung injury or acute respiratory distress syndrome.

communication). Indeed, there were 262/771 deaths in the glucocorticoids treated group and 294/725 deaths in the control group. The relative risk of dying was 0.85 (95% CI: 0.75 to 0.96) in favor of treatment with glucocorticoids. There was no heterogeneity across the studies (chi-square statistic = 16.59, p = 0.22, and I2 = 21.7%). In other conditions than severe sepsis or acute respiratory failure, randomized clinical trial are needed to determine the benefit/risk profile of glucocorticoids therapy at moderate doses.

Side Effects of Glucocorticoids Administration During Critical Illness

Although meta-analysis of randomized clinical trials did not show an increased risk of gastro-intestinal bleeding or of super-infection with glucocorticoids therapy given at moderate doses (*54*), these serious adverse events are common complications of glucocorticoids. Therefore, it is mandatory to carefully and systematically screen for super-infection in glucocorticoids – treated critically ill patients, all the more that this treatment will blunt the febrile response to infection. Similarly, these patients may benefit from systematic stress ulcer prophylaxis. Glucocorticoids therapy is almost always associated with increased blood glucose levels and intensive insulin therapy may be paramount in these patients to counteract the potential hyperglycaemia related morbidity.

CONCLUSION

In conclusion, the imbalance between the systemic inflammatory response and the hypothalamic pituitary adrenal axis is likely a determinant of critical illness pathophysiology and outcome. At this time, the short corticotrophin test remains the most accurate tool to identify critical illness related corticosteroids insufficiency. Patients with baseline cortisol levels of less than 10µg/dl or an increment after 250µg ACTH of less than 9 µg/dl are very likely adrenal insufficient. Cumulative evidence from randomized controlled trials suggests that patients with severe sepsis or acute respiratory failure benefit from prolonged treatment with moderate doses of glucocorticoids.

REFERENCES

1. Waterhouse R. Case of suprarenal apoplexy. *Lancet* 1911; 1: 577.
2. Melby JC et al. Comparative studies on adrenal cortical function and cortisol metabolism in healthy adults and in patients with shock due to infection. *J Clin Invest* 1958; 37: 1791–1798.
3. Koo DJ et al. Adrenal insufficiency during the late stage of polymicrobial sepsis. *Crit Care Med* 2001; 29: 618–622.
4. Carlson DE et al. Cecal ligation and puncture in rats interrupts the circadian rhythms of corticosterone and adrenocortical responsiveness to adrenocorticotrophic hormone. *Crit Care Med* 2006; 34: 1178–1184.
5. Burkitt JM et al. Relative adrenal insufficiency in dogs with sepsis. *J Vet Inter Med* 2007; 21: 226–231.
6. Wang P et al. Mechanism of adrenal insufficiency following trauma and severe hemorrhage: role of hepatic 11beta-hydroxysteroid dehydrogenase. *Arch Surg* 1999; 134: 394–401.
7. Annane D et al. A 3-level prognostic classification in septic shock based on cortisol levels and cortisol response to corticotropin. *JAMA* 2000; 283: 1038–1045.
8. Dimopoulo I et al. Hypothalamic-pituitary-adrenal axis dysfunction in critically ill patients with traumatic brain injury: incidence, pathophysiology, and relationship to vasopressor dependence and peripheral interleukin-6 levels. *Crit Care Med* 2004; 32: 404–408.
9. Lipiner-Friedman D et al. Adrenal function in sepsis: the retrospective Corticus cohort study. *Crit Care Med* 2006; 35: 1012–1018.
10. Marik PE et al. The hepatoadrenal syndrome: a common yet unrecognized clinical condition. *Crit Care Med* 2005; 33: 1254–1259.
11. Tsai MH et al. Adrenal insufficiency in patients with cirrhosis, severe sepsis and septic shock. *Hepatology* 2006; 43: 673–681.
12. Annane D et al. Diagnosis of adrenal insufficiency in severe sepsis and septic shock. *Am J Respir Crit Care Med* 2006; 174: 1319–1326.
13. Borovikova LV et al. Vagus nerve stimulation attenuates the systemic inflammatory response to endotoxin. *Nature* 2000; 405: 458–462.
14. Banks WA et al. Leptin enters the brain by a saturable system independent of insulin. *Peptides* 1996; 17: 305–311.
15. Koenig JI Presence of cytokines in the hypothalamic-pituitary axis. *Prog Neuroendocrinoimmunol* 1991; 4: 143–147.
16. Spangelo BL et al. Production of interleukin- 6 by anterior pituitary cells in vitro. *Endocrinology* 1990; 126: 582–586.
17. Sharshar T et al. The neuropathology of septic shock. *Brain Pathol.* 2004; 14: 21–33.
18. McCann SM et al. The mechanism of action of cytokines to control the release of hypothalamic and pituitary hormones in infection. *Ann NY Acad Sci* 2004; 917: 4–18.
19. Sharshar T et al. Apoptosis of neurons in cardiovascular autonomic centres triggered by inducible nitric oxide synthase after death from septic shock. *Lancet* 2003; 362: 1799–1805.

20. Wong ML et al. Interleukin (IL) 1b, IL-1 receptor antagonist, IL-10, IL-13 gene expression in the central nervous system and anterior pituitary during systemic inflammation: pathophysiological implications. *PNAS USA* 1997; 93: 227–232.
21. Rettori V et al. An interleukin-1α-like neuronal system in the preoptic-hypothalamic region and its induction by bacterial lipopolysaccharide in concentrations which alter pituitary hormone release. *Neuroimmunomodulation* 1994; 1: 251–258.
22. Gloddek J et al. The intrapituitary stimulatory effect of lipopolysaccharide on ACTH secretion is mediated by paracrine-acting IL-6. *Exp Clin Endocrinol Diabetes* 2001; 109: 410–415.
23. Annane et al. Norepinephrine plus dobutamine versus epinephrine alone for the management of septic shock. *Lancet* 2007; 370: 676–84.
24. Prigent H et al. Science review: mechanisms of impaired adrenal function in sepsis and molecular actions of glucocorticoids. *Crit Care* 2004; 8: 243–252.
25. Sharshar T et al. Apoptosis of neurons in cardiovascular autonomic centres triggered by inducible nitric oxide synthase after death from septic shock. *Lancet* 2003; 362: 1799.
26. Maxime V et al. Metabolism modulators in sepsis: The abnormal pituitary response. *Crit Care Med* 2007; 35: S596–601.
27. Jaattela M et al. Tumor necrosis factor as a potent inhibitor of adrenocorticotropin-induced cortisol production and steroidogenic P450 enzyme gene expression in cultured human fetal adrenal cells. *Endocrinology* 1991; 128: 623–629.
28. Swain MG et al. Tumor necrosis factor-alpha stimulates adrenal glucocorticoid secretion in cholestatic rats. *Am J Physiol* 1996; 270: G987–G991.
29. Salas MA et al. Interleukin-6 and ACTH act synergistically to stimulate the release of corticosterone from adrenal gland cells. *Clin Exp Immunol.* 1990; 79: 470–473.
30. Smith EM et al. IL-10 as a mediator in the HPA axis and brain. *J Neuroimmunol* 1999; 100: 140–148.
31. Wheatland R. Molecular mimicry of ACTH in SARS – implications for corticosteroids treatment and prophylaxis. *Med Hypotheses* 2004; 63: 855–862.
32. Barnes PJ. How corticosteroids control inflammation: Quintiles Prize Lecture 2005. *Br J Pharmacol.* 2006; 148: 245–254.
33. Beishuizen A et al. Patterns of corticosteroid-binding globulin and the free cortisol index during septic shock and multitrauma. *Intensive Care Med.* 2001; 27: 1584–91.
34. Meduri GU et al. Nuclear factor-kappaB- and glucocorticoid receptor alpha- mediated mechanisms in the regulation of systemic and pulmonary inflammation during sepsis and acute respiratory distress syndrome. Evidence for inflammation-induced target tissue resistance to glucocorticoids. *Neuroimmunomodulation* 2005; 12: 321–338.
35. Pretorius E et al. Cortisol resistance in conditions such as asthma and the involvement of 11beta-HSD-2: a hypothesis. *Horm Metab Res* 2006; 38: 368–376.
36. Hamrahian AH et al. Measurements of serum free cortisol in critically ill patients. *N Engl J Med* 2004; 350: 1629–1638.
37. Salgado DR. Adrenal function testing in patients with septic shock. *Crit Care* 2006; 10: R149.
38. Arafah BM et al. Measurement of Salivary Cortisol Concentration in the Assessment of Adrenal Function in Critically Ill Subjects: A Surrogate Marker of the Circulating Free Cortisol. *J Clin Endocrinol Metab* 2007; 92: 2965–71.
39. Chanques G et al. Enlarged adrenals during septic shock. *Intensive Care Med.* 2007; 33: 1671–2.
40. Witek-Janusek L et al. Role of the adrenal cortex and medulla in the young rats' glucoregulatory response to endotoxin. *Shock* 1995; 3: 434–439.

41. Huang CJ et al. Association between adrenal insufficiency and ventilator weaning. *Am J Respir Crit Care Med.* 2006; 173: 276–280.

42. Rhen T et al. Antiinflammatory action of glucocorticoids–new mechanisms for old drugs. *N Engl J Med.* 2005; 353: 1711–1723.

43. Meduri GU et al. Effect of prolonged methylprednisolone therapy in unresolving acute respiratory distress syndrome. A randomized controlled trial. *JAMA* 1998; 280: 159–65.

44. Confalonieri M et al. Hydrocortisone infusion for severe community-acquired pneumonia: a preliminary randomized study. *Am J Respir Crit Care Med* 2005; 171: 242–248.

45. Steinberg KP, et al. Efficacy and safety of corticosteroids for persistent acute respiratory distress syndrome. *N Engl J Med* 2006; 354: 1671–1684.

46. Annane D et al. Effect of low doses of corticosteroids in septic shock patients with or without early acute respiratory distress syndrome. *Crit Care Med* 2006; 34: 22–30.

47. Meduri GU et al. Methylprednisolone infusion in early severe ARDS: results of a randomized controlled trial. *Chest* 2007; 131: 954–963.

48. Briegel J et al. Low-dose hydrocortisone infusion attenuates the systemic inflammatory response syndrome. The Phospholipase A2 Study Group. *Clin Investig.* 1994; 72: 782–787.

49. Keh D et al. Immunologic and hemodynamic effects of "low-dose" hydrocortisone in septic shock: a double-blind, randomized, placebo-controlled, crossover study. *Am J Respir Crit Care Med.* 2003; 167: 512–520.

50. Oppert M et al. Low-dose hydrocortisone improves shock reversal and reduces cytokine levels in early hyperdynamic septic shock. *Crit Care Med.* 2005; 33: 2457–2464.

51. Maxime V et al. Corticoids normalize leukocyte production of macrophage migration inhibitory factor in septic shock. *J Infect Dis.* 2005; 191: 138–44.

52. Celik JB et al. Methylprednisolone prevents inflammatory reaction occurring during cardiopulmonary bypass: effects on TNF-alpha, IL-6, IL-8, IL-10. *Perfusion.* 2004; 19: 185–191.

53. Rivers EP et al. Adrenal insufficiency in high-risk surgical ICU patients. *Chest.* 2001; 119: 889–896.

54. Annane et al. Corticosteroids for severe sepsis and septic shock: a systematic review and meta-analysis. *BMJ.* 2004; 329: 480.

55. McKee JL et al. Cortisol replacement in severely stressed patients. *Lancet.* 1985; 1:484.

56. Bollaert PE et al. Reversal of late septic shock with supraphysiologic doses of hydrocortisone. *Crit Care Med.* 1998; 26: 645–650.

57. Chawla K et al. Hydrocortisone reverses refractory septic shock. *Crit Care Med* 1999; 27: A33.

58. Annane et al. Effect of treatment with low doses of hydrocortisone and fludrocortisone on mortality in patients with septic shock. *JAMA.* 2002; 288: 862–871.

59. Yildiz O et al. Physiological-dose steroid therapy in sepsis. *Crit Care* 2002; 6: 251–259.

60. Tandan SM et al. Low dose steroids and adrenocortical insufficiency in septic shock: a double-blind randomised controlled trial from India. *Am J Respir Crit Care Med* 2005; A24.

61. Rinaldi S et al. Low-dose hydrocortisone during severe sepsis: effects on microalbuminuria. *Crit Care Med* 2005; 34: 2334–2339.

62. Huh JW et al. Effect of low doses of hydrocortisone in patient with septic shock and relative adrenal insufficiency: 3 days versus 7 days treatment. *Crit Care Med* 2007; 34: A101.

63. Sprung CL et al. The CORTICUS randomized, double-blind, placebo-controlled study of hydrocortisone therapy in patients with septic shock. *N Engl J Med* 2008; 34: 61–9.

12 Catecholamines and Vasopressin During Critical Illness

Pierre Asfar, MD, PhD, Peter Radermacher, MD, PhD, and Enrico Calzia, MD, PhD

From: *Contemporary Endocrinology: Acute Cause to Consequence*
Edited by: G. Van den Berghe, DOI: 10.1007/978-1-60327-177-6_12,
© Humana Press, New York, NY

INTRODUCTION

Treatment of systemic hypotension aims at maintaining an adequate oxygen delivery to the tissue by increasing the circulating volume as the first approach, and by applying vasoactive drugs if fluid therapy alone is not sufficient to restore an adequate cardiovascular function. With respect to their main pharmacodynamic profiles, vasoactive drugs are commonly subdivided into inotropes, mainly including catecholamines like epinephrine, dopamine, and dobutamine, and vasopressors like phenylephrine and vasopressin (1). The subdivision into these categories, however, does not completely hold true as many of these drugs, especially catecholamines often reveal properties of both classes.

In this chapter, we will present the current rationale of vasoactive drug therapy during shock and discuss their interactions with metabolism and immune system. We will particularly focus on the septic shock as this condition represents not only the most frequent type of shock (2), but also the most common cause of death in intensive care unit.

CLINICAL PHARMACOLOGY AND PRACTICAL USE
OF CATECHOLAMINES

As just mentioned, the traditional subdivision of catecholamines into inotropes, that is, mainly acting on β receptors, and vasopressors, that is, mainly acting on α receptors, should be regarded cautiously since, to a substantial degree, most of them act on both receptor types. Exceptions are dopexamine and isoproterenol as pure β-adrenergic agonists, and phenylephrine, which is the only pure α-agonist.

Dobutamine has a weak affinity for α and β_2 and a stronger affinity for β_1-adrenergic receptors. Therefore it is used to combine its inotropic (β_1) and vasodilating (β_2) effects; the latter property can decrease the systemic resistance, and may therefore be advantageous in septic shock where dobutamine and norepinephrine can be combined in order to counterbalance an excessive vasoconstriction (1).

Norepinephrine, in contrast, is a strong, non-specific α-agonist with an inotropic effect related to its affinity to β_1-receptors. This β_1-related effect of norepinephrine is particularly important as it maintains or even increases cardiac output, thus compensating, at least partially, for the increased afterload induced by the strong α–mediated vasoconstriction.

Epinephrine exerts the strongest agonistic action on both α- and β-receptors. The use of epinephrine is generally limited to shock states resistant to dobutamine or norepinephrine treatment while it is not recommended by international guidelines *(3–4)*. Nevertheless some authors are still debating on the use of epinephrine as the first drug in septic shock *(5)*.

Dopamine, the natural agonist for dopaminergic receptors, also has pharmacologically important and dose-dependent effects on the adrenoreceptors. At low doses the β-adrenergic related inotropic action predominates, while, at higher dosages, the effects of this drug are mainly dominated by the α–mediated vasoconstriction.

Despite of these fairly well understood specific mechanisms of receptor interaction, however, the pharmacological actions of catecholamines in the clinical settings are not always fully predictable. During septic shock, for example, norepinephrine kinetics and dynamics are unpredictable *(5)*, and even the dopamine plasma concentration measured in healthy subjects *(7)* during fixed infusion rate, differed from the theoretically predicted one. In addition, the underlying disease may change receptor properties in terms of densities and binding affinity, and desensitization may be the reason behind the well known inter- and intrasubject variability of catecholamine-effects *(8,9,10)*. For these reasons, vasoactive drug therapy of septic shock still remains largerly based on empiric experience. Prospective randomized trials comparing the different drugs are not available until yet, and even a Cochrane Database *(11)* concluded that there is no evidence until yet supporting any difference between specific catecholamines in terms of effectivness or safety. On the other hand, useful suggestions for a practical approach to catecholamine therapy may be derived from the literature. For example, according to the data presented in a review article, norepinephrine seems to be more potent than dopamine for reversing hypotension *(12)*. Furthermore, in a recent multiple centers observational study the use of dopamine, but not that of norepinephrine or dobutamine, was an independent risk factor for intensive care unit mortality in patients with septic shock *(13)*. Another observational study supports the benefit of norepinephrine on survival in septic shock compared to other catecholamines *(14)*. Currently, a trial comparing norepinephrine plus dobutamine versus epinheprine *(15)* is still ongoing, and, as already mentioned before, there is an emerging discussion around the use of epinephrine as first line drug *(5)*, although it is not recommended for that scope by any guideline until yet. In contrast, the practical approach for using catecholamines in septic shock summarized by the Surviving Sepsis Campaign *(16)* should be considered as the most actual recommendation.

The question whether vasoactive drugs should be titrated targeting at a specific arterial pressure threshold *(17,18)* in septic shock also still remains an open issue. In fact, beneficial effects of increased blood pressure were observed in experimental study but not confirmed by human studies until yet, and recommendations like that of titrating norepinephrine to increase mean arterial pressure not above 65-70 mmHg *(19)* are still not sufficiently supported by scientific data. At least in cardiac surgery patients with vasodilatory shock, for example, increasing mean arterial pressure by norepinephrine from 60 to 90 mm Hg does not seem to affect intestinal mucosal perfusion and gastric or splanchnic oxygen demand/supply ratio. On the other hand, in a recent investigation conducted on rats Dubniks et al. *(21)* nicely demonstrated that maintaining perfusion pressure by noradrenaline under conditions of increased vascular permeability induces a potentially deleterious loss of plasma volume. However, the increased vascular permeability-model used for this study only partially mimicks properties of septic shock, thus limiting the practical conclusions from the investigation *(21,22)*. In contrast, Sennoun et al. *(23)* presented experimental data obtained in a rat model of septic shock, showing that norepinephrine combined with volume resuscitation allowed maintaining aortic and mesenteric blood flow and results in better tissue oxygenation than fluid resuscitation alone. Early use of norepinephrine was even more advantageous in terms of mesenteric perfusion, lactate levels, and infused volume when compered to delayed therapy.

In a more generic sense an agreement on the endpoints of therapy of septic shock is still lacking; for example, the observed correlation between high lactate levels and increased mortality in septic shock *(24)* seems to suggest the usefulness of this variable as a therapeutic guide, but lactate metabolism in septic patients is rather complex to quantify and an increase may be due to other factors than tissue hypoxia *(5,25,26,27)*. In particular, catecholamines, and especially epinephrine, may induce an increase in lactate production derived from direct stimulation of glycolysis without impairment of the oxygen availability to the cell *(5,28,29)*. In addition, even the strategy of targeting at a supranormal oxygen delivery *per se*, previously considered as one of the main goals of therapy in septic shock patients, has been abandoned, since different studies *(16,30)* clearly demonstrated its ineffectivness.

In summary, the best strategy for vasoactive support in septic patients is still a matter of debate; an individualized therapy which also considers the particular condition of the patient is likely to prove as the right approach in clinical practice, but it will probably even remain the most difficult to achieve.

CATECHOLAMINES AND REGIONAL PERFUSION

Albeit of crucial importance, the specific impact of catecholamines and other vasoactive drugs on the perfusion of different organs, epecially the kidney and the splanchnic organs, in critical care patients is still not fully explained *(31–32)*. In fact, observations in healthy subjects cannot be easily translated to pathological conditions, and the perfusion of liver and splanchnic region are difficult to study in the clinical context. Furthermore, since a general consensus regarding the methods to assess splanchnic blood flow and metabolism in critically ill patients is still lacking, some authors refuse definitive conclusions regarding different effects of norepinephrine and dopamine on this region *(31)*. An agreement only exists around the fact that adequate fluid resuscitation is a prerequisite for any successful vasoactive therapy *(3-4)*.

Dopamine

Theoretically, lower doses of dopamine which should act on both the β_2 and the dopaminergic receptors are expected to increase splanchnic perfusion. In contrast, higher doses should rather be deleterious due to the increasing α-effect *(1)*. However, there is no clear clinical evidence supporting these theories. In fact, both low and high dose have been considered responsible for mixed results ranging from increased *(33–34)* to constant and decreased splanchnic blood flow *(35)*. Nevertheless, at least when compared to epinephrine in septic shock, dopamine seems to maintain a better balance between oxygen demand and supply as suggested by the lower gradient between mixed venous and hepatic vein oxygen saturation *(36)*.

In contrast to splanchnic blood flow, the effects of dopamine on renal perfusion are much better understood. As expected, a combined afferent and efferent arteriolar dilation induced by low doses of dopamine increases renal blood flow, however, without augmenting glomerular filtration rate due to the simultaneous decrease in intraglomerular pressure. In contrast, at higher concentrations dopamine causes a marked renal vasoconstriction. Dopamine not only has effects on renal hemodynamics, it further participates in renal sodium regulation by reducing the proximal reabsorption and, at least under physiological conditions, by contributing to natriuresis as appropriate response to modest volume expansion. Nevertheless, the concept of using low dose infusions for protecting the kidney against hypoperfusion *(37)* has been abandoned, since no clinical study could yet demonstrate any benefit of low dose dopamine infusions for preventing or treating acute renal failure *(38,39,40,41,42,43)* despite an increase in urine output. In particular, the randomized clinical trial conducted by the clinical trials group of the Australian and New Zealand intensive care societies *(44)* provided convincing evidence that the so-called low-dose dopamine therapy does not protect shock patients from renal failure.

Norepinephrine

Similar as for dopamine, the net effect of norepinephrine on splanchnic hemodynamics remains ambiguous. In fact, clinical studies demonstrated increased *(45)*, unchanged *(46–47)*, or variable effects on splanchnic blood flow *(46)*.

Furthermore, the comparison of norepinephrine and other catecholamines is often confused by the frequent addition of dobutamine. Especially in the case of human septic shock, however, the combined use of dobutamine and norepinephrine resulted in an increased splanchnic perfusion when compared to norepinephrine alone (48); this observation led to the widely accepted recommendation for combining these two drugs (3–4). Two further clinical studies revealed potential benefits of norepinephrine when compared to other catecholamines with regard to splanchnic perfusion. In fact, De Backer and colleagues (36) found a higher fractional splanchnic blood flow in septic patients with norepinephrine than with epinephrine, and Guerin et al. (32) showed that norepinephrine was superior to dopamine for maintaining fractional splanchnic blood flow and hepato-splanchnic energy balance in a comparable group of patients.

The effect of norepinephrine on renal hemodynamic is complex inasmuch it directly increases afferent arteriolar tone and enhances the efferent arteriolar resistance through a mediation by renin and angiotensin II. As a net effect, it should decrease renal blood flow without affecting the intraglomerular pressure and thus the filtration rate. Clinical studies, however, do not fully confirm these theoretical considerations. In fact, several studies reported an improvement in renal blood flow under norepinephrine, especially when the drug was used to restore arterial blood pressure during vasodilatory shock (49). Clearly, the question of the dependency of renal perfusion on systemic pressure is of crucial importance but still remains unsolved. Only one experimental study performed by Bellomo et al. (50), which analyzed the effect of norepinephrine infusion in dogs, allowed concluding that during endotoxemia norepinephrine effectively improves renal blood flow and that this effect it is not related to an increased perfusion pressure.

Several clinical studies suggest the efficacy and safety of norepinephrine for supporting renal function (51,52,53,54) in septic shock. Interestingly, the only randomized controlled study comparing norepinephrine and dopamine with regard to renal effects during septic shock suggests that the former is superior not only in reversing hypotension but also for increasing urine output (55). In a recent review the same authors identified norepinephrine as an independent predictor of survival during septic shock (14). Interestingly, in an experimental study Langenberg et al. (56) observed that in septic shock acute kidney injury developed concomitantly with increased renal blood flow, while recovery of renal function was rather associated with relative vasoconstriction and decrease in renal perfusion. These data challenge the common view that renal failure in septic shock is related to renal hypoperfusion, and therefore raise intriguing questions on the adequate hemodynamic therapy to prevent this complication in patients with sepsis (57).

Epinephrine

Epinephrine is at least as efficient as norepinephrine and even superior to dopamine in restoring hypotension; nevertheless its potentially deleterious effects on regional perfusion limit the utility of this drug to a rescue therapy in severe shock states, once other vasoactive drugs have failed *(36)*. The impairment on PCO_2 gap, splanchnic blood flow, difference between mixed and hepatic venous hemoglobin oxygen saturation, glucose release, and lactate production *(58)* under epinephrine clearly show the negative effects exerted by this drug on the splanchnic region *(36,59–60)*. Interestingly, an alternative point of view is offered by Levy *(5)* who argues against the traditional negative consideration of epinephrine during septic shock.

Unfotunately, there are no human studies on the renal effects of epinephrine until yet. The ongoing debate on the detailed role of epinephrine in septic shock has led to the large randomized trial comparing norepinephrine plus dobutamine versus epinephrine *(15)*. As long as more convincing data are available, however, the use of epinephrine during shock still remains a second line approach, mainly as a rescue therapy.

Dobutamine

Dobutamine has been tested in septic shock both as a unique agent as well as in combination with norepinephrine. Albeit the assumption that dobutamine may increase splanchnic blood flow as a consequence of a systemic increase of cardiac index is widely accepted *(61,62,63)*, its presumed selective beneficial effect on splanchnic hemodynamic has not been demonstrated yet *(61)*.

Dobutamine was proved to exert a beneficial effect on splanchnic perfusion when combined to norepinephrine; to this respect, dobutamine was even superior to epinephrine alone *(48)*. Therefore, dobutamine is recommended as the first line drug in septic shock when combined to norepinephrine.

Metabolic Effects of Catecholamines

An adequate perfusion and oxygen delivery to the different tissues do not guarantee a sufficient metabolic function, especially during and after a shock state. In fact, depending on the underlying disease and the therapeutic actions, metabolic effects may potentially influence the outcome. For example, during septic shock a hypermetabolic condition associated with insulin resistance, hyperlactatemia, and increased oxygen demand is a common finding, which are concomitant with impaired macro- and micorvascular organ perfusion and mitochondrial dysfunction *(64–65)*. In this context, interactions between vasoactive therapy and metabolism must be considered in order to avoid any further deterioration of the derangements already present. The complex interactions between glucose metabolism and catecholamines have been extensively reviewed in a recent article by Barth et al. *(66)*.

Epinephrine, for example, is known to induce prominent metabolic effects. Among these are hyperglycemia (induced by increasing both gluconeogenesis and glycogenolysis and by decreasing insulin release mainly through a β_2 mediated action), increased oxygen demand, and enhanced plasma lactate concentration *(5,67)*. Albeit these metabolic changes are part of the physiological response to stress, in the long term clinical setting of septic shock they can be detrimental because the drug-induced increase in gluconeogenesis may particularly impair the hepatic balance between oxygen supply and demand. Furthermore, since on the one hand plasma lactate concentration correlates with mortality *(24)*, and, on the other hand, epinephrine has been shown to increase lactate both in healthy subject and in septic patients *(64)*, it has been postulated that this drug could lead, through an excessive vasoconstriction, to a low perfusion-induced cellular hypoxia. These metabolic effects together with the epinephrine-induced reduction in splanchnic perfusion *(59)* represent the main arguments against the use of this drug as first line agent in septic shock *(3–4,68)*. Nevertheless, it is still unclear whether the hyperlactatemic and hyperglycemic metabolic response caused by epinephrine is associated with a mere calorigenic effect or reflects a condition of metabolic stress *(66)*.

In this context, a recent study by Levy et al. *(69)* assumes particular importance: in endotoxin-challenged rats, the authors elegantly showed that the hyperlactatemia during epinephrine infusion was not accompanied by a complementary increase in the lactate/pyruvate-ratio. The authors also confirmed their experimental observations in a clinical study providing evidence that during septic shock epinephrine increases lactate production mainly as the result of enhanced aerobic glycolysis associated with increased activity of Na-K-ATPase *(29)*. Although Levy et al. did not directly demonstrate the link between epinephrine and Na-K- ATPase stimulation in humans, they underscored the need to change the unique traditional interpretation of increased lactate production as a marker of cellular hypoxia.

With respect to norepinephrine-induced metabolic effects investigations permitting definitive conclusions are still lacking, but no evidence supports sustained negative effects until yet. In healthy volunteers, no substantial metabolic alterations were described except for a slightly increased glycaemia without any persisting effects on glucose production and a small increase in lactate concentration *(70)*,. During septic shock, De Backer et al. *(36)* reported higher glycaemia under norepinephrine when compared to dopamine, but did not find adverse metabolic effects.

With regard to the metabolic effect of dopamine, two studies underscored its supposed negative role on liver metabolism: Jakob et al. *(34)* demonstrated a decreased splanchnic oxygen consumption despite a increased splanchnic blood flow induced by dopamine infusion in septic patients. Guerin et al. finally *(32)*, compared dopamine and norepinephrine but did not find any difference in splanchnic blood flow despite a higher cardiac index and a similar mean arterial pressure in the dopamine group. The result of this hemodynamic difference was a lower splanchnic fractional flow associated with lower hepatic lactate uptake and higher hepatic venous lactate/pyruvate ratio; these results suggest a detrimental dopamine-related effect on hepatic energy balance. This hypothesis, however, had not been confirmed by De Backer *(36)*, who reported a similar metabolic profile during dopamine or norepinephrine infusion.

Dobutamine, as a weak agonist of β_2-receptors, and β_2-receptor, is known to stimulate gluconeogenesis. Surprisingly, dobutamine infusion caused a slight decrease in glucose production in both healthy subjects *(70)* and in patient with septic shock *(61)* or recovering from cardiac surgery *(71)*. This unexpected effect on carbohydrate metabolism led to the hypothesis that dobutamine may not have pronounced β_2-activity, and thus metabolic effects in vivo *(70)*.

Some authors argued that theoretically, due to the absence of major adverse metabolic properties of both norepinephrine and dobutamine, the combined administration of these two drugs may be safe with regard to splanchnic perfusion, in particular when compared to epinephrine *(59,70,72–73)*. This hypothesis, however, has not been tested experimentally until yet. Finally, despite the fairly scarce data available, the use of pure α-agonists, for example, phenylephrine, cannot be recommended: in two independent clinical studies replacing norepinephrine by phenylephrine, titrated to achieve comparable systemic hemodynamics, resulted in marked metabolic depression *(74,75)*.

IMMUNE MODULATION BY CATECHOLAMINES

An increasing body of evidence supports the role of adrenergic agents in the modulation of immune and inflammatory response in critically ill patients and experimental models. Almost all inflammatory cells express α and β adrenoreceptors on their surface *(76,77)* while D_1 and D_2 receptors are known to be present on lymphocytes and natural killer cells *(78)*. Immunomodulatory actions of catecholamines are predominantly mediated by β_2-receptors; although α_2-adrenoreceptors may also induce the production of a variety of pro-inflammatory cytokines *(79)*. Apart from these observations, however, the definitive and unique role of catecholamines in the complex network of inflammatory response, which presumably ranges from modulating T-helper cells migration and maturation *(80,81,82)*, and controlling cytokines expression *(83,84)* to directly promote apoptosis in immune cells *(85)* remains to be fully elucidated. Furthermore, some authors suggested that catecholamines may play an anti-inflammatory action by down-regulating the pro-inflammatory cytokine response. In this context, the interleukine-6 response of splanchnic reticuloendothelial tissues (86) seems to be mediated by ephinephrine, but not by norepinephrine, while the ephinephrine-induced increase in interleukine-10 may inhibit TNFα production (87). Another investigation suggests that dopamine may be responsible for a functional suppression of neutrophilis caused by the attenuation of the chemoattractant effect of interleukine (88). In addition to these direct effects on the immune system, dopamine interferes with the response to inflammation through its action on neuroendocrine system. Dopamine infusion suppresses the release of most of anterior pituitary dependent hormones and stimulates the synthesis of adrenal glucocorticoids (89). The concomitant inhibition of growth hormone pulsatile secretion (90), thyroid-stimulating hormone (91) and particularly prolactin, which enhances monocyte and B and T-cells response, may aggravate immune dysfunction and susceptibility to infection. In contrast, dopexamine had minimal effects on pituitary function in high-risk surgical patients (92) but still modulated cellular immune functions during experimental systemic inflammation (93). Interestingly, in a very recent experimental investigation in endotoxin-treated rats, Hofstetter et al. (94) demonstrated that norepinephrine, as well as vasopressin, counteracted the anti-inflammatory response induced by inhaled isoflurane, which consisted in an attenuated release of the cytokines TNFalpha and IL-1beta. Whether or not these catecholamine-induced alterations of immunological functions may somehow influence survival in sepsis and septic shock still remain to be defined.

In summary, catecholamines remain the cornerstone in the therapy of circulatory failure. However, clinicians must not only focus their attention on the hemodynamic effects, but also use a more rationale approach considering the metabolic, endocrinological, and immunological consequences of catecholamines administration. Looking at alternative strategies to catecholamines in the treatment of shock, evidences of beneficial effects on hemodynamic endpoints of vasopressin during septic shock are accumulating and will be discussed in the next chapters.

VASOPRESSIN AND ITS ANALOGOUS IN SHOCK THERAPY

Vasopressin is a natural hormone produced in magnocellular neurons of hypothalamus and released from the posterior hypophysis. Its secretion is stimulated in response to increases in plasma osmolality and decreases in systemic blood pressure.

Vasopressin and its analogue terlipressin exert their effects via vascular V1a receptors and renal tubular V2 receptors. V1a receptor stimulation leads to arterial vasoconstriction and V2 stimulation increases renal free water reabsorption.

Terlipressin has a higher vascular affinity for vascular receptors than vasopressin as assessed by a higher V1a/V2 receptor ratio compared to vasopressin (2.2 versus 1, respectively) *(95)*.

Abolished responsiveness of vascular smooth muscle to catecholamines stimulation is one of the mechanisms leading to hypotension during endotoxic shock *(96)*. The vasoconstrictor response to other agents such as angiotensin and vasopressin is similarly abolished *(97,98)* despite an increased plasmatic level of vasopressin as shown in sepsis or hypodynamic models of septic shock in baboons and dogs *(99,100)*. The decreased vascular responsiveness during sepsis is mediated by pro-inflammatory cytokines which exert a down regulation of V1 receptors *(101)*.

Conversely, Landry et al. reported a vasopressin deficiency and hypersensitivity *(102,103)* in human septic shock. In fact, these authors demonstrated that for a same level of mean arterial pressure in septic shock and in cardiogenic shock the vasopressin blood levels were dramatically lower in the former state. In addition, low dose vasopressin administration in vasodilatory septic *(102)* and in post-cardiopulmonary bypass shock showed a beneficial hemodynamic effect in humans *(104)*. Sharshar et al. *(105)* precisely characterized the circulating levels of vasopressin during the different phases of septic shock, concluding that the vasopressin concentration is almost always increased during the early phase of sepsis (first 6 hours), whereas it declines afterward (after 36 hours from the onset of shock). The cause for vasopressin deficiency is still controversial, but because the infusion of vasopressin can reach the expected plasma concentration, it seems unlikely that an increased clearance of this hormone is responsible for the low plasma level during sepsis. An exhaustion of neurohypophysis stores seems to be a more logical conclusion *(106)* as Sharshar et al. even speculated that this fall in vasopressin production may contribute to the development of hypotension. Jochberger et al. *(107)* argued against this latter hypothesis, because they failed to demonstrate any correlation between vasopressin levels and the presence of shock in a mixed critically ill population. These authors concluded that peripheral hyposensibility rather than deficiency would contribute to hypotension. The detailed mechanisms of vasopressin hypersensitivity in septic shock were reviewed most recently by Barret et al. and include changes in vasopressin receptor response, dysautonomic failure, interaction with other vasoconstrictors, and interaction with corticosteroids *(108)*.

HEMODYNAMIC EFFECTS OF VASOPRESSIN IN SEPTIC SHOCK: EXPERIMENTAL STUDIES

In hypodynamic endotoxic shock models, vasopressin infusion induces a decrease in cardiac output *(100,109,110)* and myocardial ischemia *(111)*. Moreover, a recent study in endotoxic rabbits *(112)* reported a detrimental effect of vasopressin on left ventricular systolic function (assessed by systolic aortic blood flow and maximal aortic acceleration). The investigators argued that the myocardial dysfunction was independent of the vasopressininduced increase in cardiac afterload but rather caused by an impairment of coronary perfusion or a direct effect on cardiac myocytes. However, the hypothesis of impairment coronary perfusion by vasopressin was not confirmed by Kang et al. in endotoxin-induced rabbit shock model *(113)* Using a pressure-conductance catheter technique to assess heart function as derived from left ventricular pressure-volume loops, we did not find any further impairment of myocardial systolic contractility nor diastolic relaxation related to vasopressin during resuscitated, long-term hyperdynamic norepinephrine-resuscitated fecal peritonitis-induced porcine septic shock (unpublished data).

In hyperdynamic endotoxic models, the hemodynamic effects of V1 agonists were dependent on the infusion rate of vasopressin or terlipressin. In a study where the infusion rate of V1 agonist was targeted to increase mean arterial pressure above physiological values (+ 20 mm Hg above baseline values) cardiac output decreased as well as oxygen consumption *(114,115)*. However, the use of low doses of V1 agonists in hyperdynamic endotoxic animals increased mean arterial pressure without detrimental effect on cardiac output *(116,117)*, and in a dose response study in endotoxemic pigs, Malay et al. demonstrated detrimental effects on blood flow in various organs athigher vasopressin infusion ratesonly *(117)*. Similarly, Albert et al. reported in endotoxic rabbits that mean arterial pressure increased proportionally with incremental boluses of vasopressin whereas aortic blood flow remained stable at least for the lowest doses *(118)*. Albeit using low dose terlipressin, our group reported a decrease in cardiac output associated to a hyperlactatemia *(119)* that was not originating from splanchnic circulation in long term hyperdynamic endotoxic shock in pigs. Compared to repeated high doses bolus administration (1mg) continuous infusion of low doses of terlipressin avoided a decrease in cardiac index and limited the raise of blood lactates in a live bacteria model of septic shock in pigs *(120)*.

In addition, low dose of V1 agonists were reported to improve survival in fluid resuscitated endotoxic rats *(116)* and in live bacteria septic shock in sheep *(121)* as well as in dogs *(122)*.

V1 AGONISTS IN SEPTIC SHOCK: CLINICAL STUDIES IN ADULT PATIENTS

In all published studies, V1 agonists increased mean arterial pressure and reduced noradrenaline requirements *(102,103,123–136)*. The effect of V1 agonists on cardiac output was more variable. Cardiac output decreased in ten studies *(123,125,126,130,131,133–136)* remained stable in two *(127,132)* and even increased in one *(129)*. Dünser et al. *(129)* prospectively randomized study, 48 patients with catecholamine resistant vasodilatory shock to receive either a combined infusion of vasopressin and norepinephrine or norepinephrine alone. Vasopressin-treated patients presented with significantly lower heart rate, norepinephrine requirements, and a lower incidence of new-onset tachyarrhythmias than noepinephrine patients. Mean arterial pressure, cardiac index, stroke volume, and stroke volume were significantly higher in patients treated with the association of vasopressin and norepinephrine. It must be noted that in this study 18 patients in each group (vasopressin versus norepinephrine) were treated with milrinone to overcome excess peripheral vasconstriction.

In all of the studies, vasopressin and terlipressin were able to reduce the need for other vasopressors, and, in some cases, a complete weaning from norepinephrine was possible. The ability to increase or restore sensitivity to catecholamines remains the major rationale for supporting the use of vasopressin as a rescue therapy when conventional catecholamines have failed.

During the European Congress of Intensive Care Medicine held in Barcelona in Spain in 2006, Russell et al. reported the results of a multicenter randomized controlled trial of vasopressin and septic shock trial (VASST). Eight hundred and two patients were included and were stratified according to the initial dose of norepinephrine in order to determine severity groups (less and more severe). The overall mortality rate was the same in both groups. Surprisingly, the subgroup analysis showed a significant lower mortality in the less severe patients with septic shock, whereas the mortality rate was similar in the most severe patients. At first glance, these unexpected results argue against the concept of vasopressin as a rescue therapy of the hemodynamic failure during septic shock but rather in favor of an early administration. Nevertheless, these primary results should be interpreted with caution until the complete publication of this controlled study.

Interestingly very little safety data is available in the literature. Except for some case reports related to skin ischemia injuries, only Dünser et al. reported their experience of side effects of vasopressin in 63 critically ill patients with catecholamine-resistant vasodilatory shock. In this retrospective study, new ischemic skin lesions occurred in 19 of 63 patients (30%). Body mass index, pre-existent peripheral arterial occlusive disease, presence of septic shock, and norepinephrine requirements were significantly higher in patients with ischemic skin lesions. These patients required significantly more units of fresh frozen plasma and thrombocyte concentrates than patients without ischemic skin lesions. Pre-existent peripheral arterial occlusive disease and presence of septic shock were independently associated with the occurrence of ischemic skin lesions during vasopressin therapy *(137)*. These results were prospectively confirmed by the VASST study reported by Russell et al. in Barcelona in 2006: while the rate of serious adverse event was similar in both groups (vasopressin versus noepinephrine), the authors reported a higher rate of digital ischemia with vaso-pressin (p = 0.06).

EFFECTS OF V1 AGONISTS ON SPLANCHNIC CIRCULATION: EXPERIMENTAL STUDIES

V1a agonists are proposed in the treatment of vasodilatory shock states and especially in septic shock (138). However, V1a agonists may induce macro- and microcirculatory disturbances in some vascular beds due to excessive vaso-constriction which is not counterbalanced by positive inotropic effect. Since splanchnic circulation is thought to play a central role during septic shock, assessment of efficiency, and side effects of a potent vasoconstrictor such as V1a agonist on this circulation is mandatory.

Schmid et al. have assessed the effect of incremental vasopressin doses on mesenteric, renal and iliac blood flows in anesthetized dogs (139). Vasopressin decreased blood flow in all these three vascular. However, mesenteric and renal blood flows expressed as percentage of cardiac output significantly increased whereas it decreased in the ileac vascular bed suggesting a redistribution of blood flow towards the splanchnic organs. In an ex vivo study in rabbit, vaso-pressin had vasoconstrictor effect on renal artery but not on mesenteric artery, and this vasoconstriction was inhibited by nitric oxide (140). Hence, depending on the species and experimental model, V1 agonist's effects on regional hemo-dynamics are potentially different.

V1 agonists are thought to potentially jeopardize splanchnic hemodynamics due to their potent vasoconstrictor effects such as reported by Lazlo et al. There are various models of gastric injuries in rats (141), in which infusing V1 receptor antagonist reduced the gastric mucosal damage (142). Recently, our group reported in non fluid-resuscitated endotoxic rats that infusion of terli-pressin exhibited dramatically decreased splanchnic blood flow. Conversely, in fluid challenged endotoxic animals splanchnic blood flow as well as ileal micro-circulation assessed by laser Doppler technique was well-maintained (116). The role of fluid challenge, hence, seems crucial for the hemodynamic response. Indeed, whenever the experimental design led to a hypodynamic state, infus-ing a V1 agonist induced detrimental macro- or micro-circulatory effects in the splanchnic area (110,143). Conversely, when animals were in hyperdy-namic state, different studies in various species did not report harmful effects on splanchnic hemodynamics (110,119,121). Beside the role of fluid chal-lenge, the infusion rate and timing of vasopressin infusion is important as well.

Malay et al. reported the effects of incremental doses on global and regional circulation in fluid-resuscitated endotoxic pig model *(117)*. In this study, low doses of vasopressin, such as typically used in the clinical management of septic shock, raised arterial pressure without detrimental effect on mesenteric, renal, iliac and carotid blood flows. However, moderately higher doses of vasopressin induced ischemia in the mesenteric and renal circulations. Bennet et al. compared temporal changes of cardiovascular responses of vasopressin versus norepinephrine on blood pressure and renal, mesenteric and hindquarter blood flow during continuous infusion of endotoxin in conscious rats. The authors showed that vasopressin exhibited a better and earlier pressor response in the renal and hindquarter vascular beds but not in the mesenteric vascular bed *(144)*.

Interestingly, a study by Westphal et al. nicely illustrated the importance of the dose of V1 agonist. The authors analysed the ilear villous microcirculation with videomicroscopy, using high dose vasopressin in a rat model peritonitis-induced septic shock (0.006 UI/min/340 g of body weight approximately 1.23 UI/min for a human of 70 kg). As expected, vasopressine markedly increased mean arterial pressure, but also reduced blood flow of continuously perfused terminal arterioles. During shock, plasma of vasopressin concentration decreased below baseline, and infusion of vasopressin induced supra-physiologic concentration of the hormone, which in turn probably led to an excessive vasoconstriction *(145)*.

Knotzer et al. *(146)* report the effects of an incremental infusion vasopressin in endotoxic pigs. The results of the present investigation certainly have to be interpreted within the limits of this experimental model, but also in the light of another recent publication of the same group reporting the effects of incremental doses of vasopressin in normal, that is, healthy non-endotoxic pigs *(147)*. The main result of these two studies was that incremental vasopressin threatened splanchnic circulation by decreasing jejunal mucosal microvascluar $(\mu)PO_2$ in non-endotoxic pigs, while it had no further detrimental effect on mucosal oxygenation beyond that of endotoxin per se in endotoxic animals. Interestingly, infusing vasopressin in non-endotoxic animals decreased cardiac output and systemic oxygen delivery due to an excessive vasoconstriction, which in turn limited oxygen availability in jejunal mucosa. Conversely, during endotoxemia, vasopressin did not induce further decrease in cardiac output despite an effective vasoconstriction as mirrored by the level of mean arterial pressure.

Thus, as the reader may notice, it is rather difficult to draw a definitive conclusion on the effects of V1 agonists on splanchnic hemodynamics: most experimental studies assessing the effects of V1 agonist at low doses in hyperdynamic septic models did not demonstrate a detrimental effect.

EFFECTS OF V1 AGONISTS ON RENAL: EXPERIMENTAL STUDIES

The net effect of vasopressin on renal function is complex and differs widely between physiologic and pathologic conditions. In physiologic conditions, vasopressin induces water reabsorption by acting on V2 receptors in response to hyperosmolarity and with a different degree to hypotension. The simultaneous V1 receptor–mediated renal vascular response increases the efferent arteriolar tone with less or no effect on the afferent one. As a result, the glomerular pressure is increased while the total renal flow is slightly decreased (148). In endotoxemic rabbits, vasopressin induced an increase in mean arterial pressure associated with an increase in renal blood flow (113,118,143).

At the same time, a short negative feedback loop seems to be activated by vasopressin, which enhances local prostaglandin production through the V1 receptor. Prostaglandins, in particular PGE_2 (130), may minimize the antidiuretic and the vascular response to vasopressin, maintaining renal perfusion.

EFFECTS OF V1 AGONISTS ON REGIONAL CIRCULATIONS DURING SEPTIC SHOCK: CLINICAL STUDIES

Very few studies report the effects of V1 agonist on splanchnic circulation in patients with septic shock. Among the studies related to the systemic effects of V1 agonist none of them reported clinical detrimental renal or splanchnic side effect (102,123–125,127–130,136). However, the simple clinical assessment may not be sufficient to affirm the absence of harm of V1 agonist on splanchnic circulation.

In a prospective controlled study in 16 patients with septic shock refractory to catecholamines, Tsuneyoshi et al. (124) reported a significant increase in urinary output in 10 patients with vasopressin associated with a decreased arterial lactate concentration in surviving patients. In a double blinded study comparing the effects of a four-hour continuous infusion of vasopressin with those of norepinephrine in 24 patients with septic shock, Patel et al. (127) reported a significantly increased diuresis affiliated with a significant improve increatinine clearance during vasopressin. Interestingly, gastric-arterial PCO_2 gradient remained unaltered in both groups. These beneficial effects on creatinine clearance as well as neutral effects on gastric-arterial PCO_2 gradient were confirmed by Lauzer et al. (136). In the above-mentioned randomised controlled study, Dünser et al., comparing the combination of vasopressin (4UI/h) with norepinephrine versus norepinephrine alone, also assessed parameters of visceral organ perfusion and function. In this study, gastric-arterial PCO_2 gradient rose after one hour of norepinephrine infusion and remained stable until the end of the study with norepinephrine alone whereas the combination of vasopressin and nore-pinephrine induced a progressive raise of gastric-arterial PCO_2 gradient reaching the same values at 48 hours of the study. However, patients treated with vasopressin and norepinephrine exhibited a significant increase in plas-matic bilirubin concentrations suggesting an impaired liver blood flow or a direct effect on hepatic function mediated by vasopressin. In a short-term study in 12 patients with septic shock Klinzing et al. *(131)* reported that a switch from norepinephrine (0.18 to 1.1 µg/kg/min) to high dose of vasopressin (0.06 to 1.8 UI/min) significantly increased gastric-arterial PCO_2 gradient from 18 ± 27 to 37 ± 27 mm Hg. However tonometric variations do not always mirror splanchnic blood flow changes *(149)*. Indeed in the same study, splanchnic blood flow was invasively assessed with continuous indocyanin green dye infusion and hepatic venous catheterization. Vasopressin significantly decreased cardiac index from 3.8 ±1.3 to 3.0 ± 1.1 l/min/m^2 and oxygen consumption, while fractional splanchnic blood flow (expressed as per cent of cardiac output) increased significantly from 11 ± 8 to 26 ± 17%. The potential detrimental effects of V1 agonist on gastric-mucosal PCO_2 gradient were not confirmed by Morelli et al. *(134)* who reported the effects of a bolus of 1 mg of terlipressin in 15 patients with septic shock treated with a combination of norepinephrine and dobutamine to induce a high cardiac output. Terlipressin increased mean arterial pressure and mean pulmonary artery pressure but lowered cardiac output, oxygen delivery, and consumption as well as arterial lactate concentrations. Nevertheless, it did not alter the gastric-arterial PCO_2 gradient and even increased gastric mucosal perfusion assessed with laser Doppler flowmetry. Given these controversial data, the hemodynamic effects of low doses of V1 agonists on splanchnic circulation in patients with septic shock are still not fully understood and justify further studies.

The net effect of vasopressin on renal function is complex and widely differs between physiologic and pathologic conditions. In physiologic conditions, vaso-pressin induces water reabsorption via its actionon V2 receptors in response to hyperosmolarity and to hypotension. The simultaneous V1 receptor–mediated renal vascular response increases the efferent arteriolar tone with less or no effect on the afferent one. As a result, the glomerular pressure is increased while the total renal flow is slightly decreased. At the same time, a short neg-ative feedback loop seems to be activated by vasopressin, enhancing the local prostaglandin production through the V1 receptor.

Different clinical studies performed in septic shock patients and either comparing norepinephrine and vasopressin, or replacing norepinephrine by vaso-pressin, showed increased or unchanged urine output during vasopressin infu-sion *(124,124,127,128,134–136)*, which was often associated with an increased creatinine clearance *(127,134–136)*. The exact mechanism of this diuretic effect is poorly understood. While there is no evidence that vasopressin doses higher than 0.04 U/min may increase urine output, a beneficial effect on renal function has been observed even at low doses of vasopressin (0.02 U/min). Despite these encouraging data, researchers *(150)* advocate a cautious approach, and further investigations are warranted before low-dose vasopressin can be considered a "renoprotective" therapy.

CONCLUSION

During hyperdynamic septic shock, data on the effects of low doses of V1 agonists on global hemodynamics are accumulating. However, to date, there is no definitive data confirming the superiority of V1 agonists in terms of mortality and morbidity. Given the potentially deleterious intrinsic metabolic and immune-modulating effects of catecholamines, however, it could be argued that decreasing the infusion rate of norepinephrine (or other catecholamines are a relevant target for patients with septic shock. Nevertheless, in view of our current knowledge today, the use of V1 agonist cannot only be recommended for day-to-day routine protocols as has to be restrained to clinical investigations until the complete publication of the large multicenter randomized trial (VASST) comparing vasopressin and norepinephrine in patients with septic shock.

REFERENCES

1. Kevin TT, Corley BVM. Inotropes and vasopressors in adults and foals. *Vet Clin Equine* 2004; 20: 77–106.
2. Landry DW, Oliver JA. The pathogenesis of vasodilatory shock. *N Engl J Med* 2001; 345: 588–595.
3. Dellinger RP, Carlet JM, Masur H, et al. Surviving sepsis campaign guidelines for management of severe sepsis and septic shock. *Intensive Care Med* 2004; 30: 536–555.
4. Beale RJ, Hollenberg SM, Vincent JL, et al. Vasopressor and inotropic support in septic shock: an evidence-based review. *Crit Care Med* 2004; 32: S455–S465.
5. Levy B. Bench-to-bedside review: Is there a place for epinephrine in septic shock?. *Crit Care*. 2005; 9: 561–565
6. Beloeil H, Mazoit X, Benhemou D, et al. Norepinephrine kinetics and dynamics in septic shock and trauma patients. *Br J Anaesth* 2005; 95: 782–788.
7. MacGregor DA, Smith TE, Prielipp RC, et al. Pharmacokinetics of dopamine in healthy male subjects. *Anesthesiology* 2000; 92: 338–346.
8. MacGregor DA, Prielipp RC, Butterworth JF, et al. Relative efficacy and potency of beta-adrenoceptor agonists for generating cAMP in human lymphocytes. *Chest* 1996; 109: 194–200.
9. Silverman HJ, Penaranda R, Orens JB, et al. Impaired beta-adrenergic receptor stimulation of cyclic adenosine monophosphate in human septic shock: association with myocardial hyporesponsiveness to catecholamines. *Crit Care Med* 1993; 21: 31–39.

10. Reinelt H, Radermacher P, Fischer G, et al. Dobutamine and dopexamine and the splanchnic metabolic response in septic shock. *Clin Intensive Care* 1997; 8: 38–41.

11. Mullner M, Urbanek B, Havel C, et al. Vasopressors for shock. *Cochrane Database Syst Rev* . 2004;(3):CD003709.

12. Beale RJ, Hollenberg SM, Vincent JL, et al. Vasopressor and inotropic support in septic shock: an evidence-based review. *Crit Care Med* 2004; 32: S455–465.

13. Sakr Y, Reinhart K, Vincent JL, et al. Does dopamine administration in shock influence outcome? Results of the Sepsis Occurence in Acutely Ill Patients (SOAP) Study. *Crit Care Med* 2006; 34: 589–597.

14. Martin C, Viviand X, Leone M, et al. Effect of norepinephrine on the outcome of septic shock. *Crit Care Med* 2000; 28: 2758–2765.

15. Annane D, Vignon P, Renault A, et al. Norepinephrine plus dobutamine versus epinephrine alone for management of septic shock: a randomised trial. *Lancet* 2007; 370: 676–684.

16. Dellinger RP, Carlet JM, Masur H, et al. Surviving sepsis campaign guidelines for management of severe sepsis and septic shock. *Intensive Care Med* 2004; 30: 536–555.

17. Bourgoin A, Leone M, Delmas A, et al. Increasing mean arterial pressure in patients with septic shock: effects on oxygen variables and renal function. *Crit Care Med* 2005; 33: 780–786.

18. De Backer D, Vincent JL. Norepinephrine administration in septic shock: how much is enough? *Crit Care Med* 2002; 30: 1398–1399.

19. Le Doux D, Astiz ME, Carpati CM, et al. Effects of perfusion pressure on tissue perfusion in septic shock. *Crit Care Med* 2000; 28: 2729–2732.

20. Nygren A, Thoren A, Ricksten SE. Norepinephrine and intestinal mucosal perfusion in vasodilatory shock after cardiac surgery. Shock 2007 epub ahead of print 10.1097/shk.0b013e318063e71f

21. Dubniks K, Persson J, Grände PO. Effect of blood pressure on plasma volume loss in the rat under increased permeability. *Intensive Care Med* 2007 epub ahead of print 10.1007/s00134-007-0756-2

22. Asfar P, Radermacher P, Marx G. Time out for vasopressors in increased microvascular permeability? *Intensive Care Med* 2007 epub ahead of print 10.1007/s00134-007-0757-1

23. Sennoun N, Montemont C, Gibot S, Lacolley P, Levy B. Comparative effects of early versus delayed use of norepinephrine in resuscitated endotoxic shock. *Crit Care Med* 2007; 35: 1736–1740

24. Bakker J, Coffernils M, Leon M, et al. Blood lactate levels are superior to oxygen derived variables in predicting outcome in human septic shock. *Chest* 1991; 99: 956–962. B.

25. Leverve X. Lactate in the intensive care unit : pyromaniac, sentinel or fireman ? *Crit Care* 2005; 9: 622–623.

26. Valenza F, Aletti G, Fossali T, et al. Lactate as a marker of energy failure in critically ill patients: hypothesis. *Crit Care* 2005; 9: 588–593.

27. Howard J, Luchette F, Mc Carter F et al. Lactate is an unreliable indicator of tissue hypoxia in injury or sepsis. Lancet 1999; 354: 505–508.

28. Träger K, Radermacher P, De Backer D, et al. Metabolic effects of vasoactive agents. *Curr Opin in Anaesth* 2001; 14: 157–163.

29. Levy B, Gibot S, Franck P, et al. Relation between muscle Na + K + ATPase activity and raised lactate concentrations in septic shock: a prospective study. *Lancet* 2005; 365: 871–875.

30. Gattinoni L, Brazzi L, Pelosi P, et al. A trial of goal-oriented hemodynamic therapy in critically ill patients. *N Engl J Med* 1995; 333: 1025–1032.

31. Asfar P, De Backer D, Meier-Hellmann A, et al. Clinical review: influence of vasoactive and other therapies on intestinal and hepatic circulations in patients with septic shock. *Crit Care* 2004; 8: 170–179.

32. Guerin JP, Levraut J, Samat-Long C, et al. Effects of dopamine and norepinephrine on systemic and hepatosplanchnic hemodynamics, oxygen exchange, and energy balance in vasoplegic septic patients. *Shock* 2005; 23: 18–24.

33. Meier-Hellmann A, Bredle DL, Specht M, et al. The effects of low-dose dopamine on splanchnic blood flow and oxygen uptake in patients with septic shock. *Intensive Care Med* 1997; 23: 31–37.

34. Jakob SM, Ruokonen E, Takala J. Effects of dopamine on systemic and regional blood flow and metabolism in septic and cardiac surgery patients. *Shock* 2002; 18: 8–13.

35. Gelman S, Mushlin P. Catecholamine-induced changes in the splanchnic circulation affecting systemic hemodynamics. *Anesthesiology* 2004; 100: 434–439.

36. De Backer D, Creteur J, Silva E, et al. Effects of dopamine, norepinephrine, and epinephrine on the splanchnic circulation in septic shock: which is best? *Crit Care Med* 2003; 31: 1659–1667.

37. Denton MD, Chertow GM, Brady HR. "Renal dose" of dopamine for the treatment of acute renal failure : scientific rationale, experimental studies and clinical trias. *Kidney Int* 1996; 49: 4.

38. Friedrich JO, Adhikari N, Herridge MS, et al. Meta-analysis: low-dose dopamine increases urine output but does not prevent renal dysfunction or death. *Ann Intern Med* 2005; 142: 510–524.

39. Lassingg A, Donner E, Grubhofer G, et al. Lack of renoprotective effects of dopamine and furosemide during cardiac surgery. *J Am Soc Nephrol* 2000; 11: 97.

40. Marik PE, Iglesias J. Low dose dopamine does not prevent acute renal failure in patients with septic shock and oliguria. NORASEPT II Study investigators. *Am J Med* 1999; 107: 387.

41. Hoogenberg K, Smit AJ, Girbes ARJ: Effects of low-dose dopamine on renal and systemic hemodynamics during incremental norepinephrine infusion in healthy volunteers. *Crit Care Med* 1998; 26: 260–265.

42. Girbes ARJ, Lieverse AG, Smit AJ, et al. Lack of specific hemodynamic effects of different doses of dopamine after infrarenal aortic surgery. *Br J Anaesth* 1996; 77: 153–157.

43. Girbes ARJ, Patten MT, McCloskey BV, et al. The renal and neurohumoral effects of the addition of low-dose dopamine in septic critically ill patients. *Intensive Care Med* 2000; 26: 1685–1689.

44. Australian and New Zeeland Intensive Care Society (ANZICS) Clinical Trials Group. Low-dose dopamine in patients with early renal dysfunction: a placebo controlled randomised trial. *Lancet* 2000; 356: 2139–2143

45. Meier-Hellmann A, Specht M, Hannemann L, et al. Splanchnic blood flow is greater in septic shock treated with norepinephrine than in severe sepsis. *Intensive Care Med* 1996; 22: 1354–1359.

46. Ruokonen E, Takala J, Kari A. Regional blood flow and oxygen transport in septic shock. *Crit Care Med* 1993; 21: 1296–1303.

47. Ruokonen E, Takala J, Uusaro A. Effect of vasoactive treatment on the relationship between mixed venous and regional oxygen saturation. *Crit Care Med* 1991; 19: 1365–1369.

48. Duranteau J, Sitbon P, Teboul JL. Effects of epinephrine, norepinephrine, or the combination of norepinephrine and dobutamine on gastric mucosa in septic shock. *Crit Care Med* 1999; 28: 893–900.

49. Bellomo R, Giantomasso DD. Noradrenaline and the kidney: friends or foes? *Crit Care* 2001; 5: 294–298.

50. Bellomo R, Kellum JA, Wisniewski SR, et al. Effects of norepinephrine on the renal vasculature in normal and endotoxemic dogs. *Am J Respir Crit Care Med* 1999; 159: 1186–1192.

51. Hesselvik JF, Brodin B. Low dose norepinephrine in patients with septic shock and oliguria: effects on afterload, urine flow, and oxygen transport. *Crit Care Med* 1989; 17: 179–180.

52. Meadows D, Edwards JD, Wilkins RG, et al. Reversal of intractable septic shock with norepinephrine therapy. *Crit Care Med* 1988; 16: 663–666.

53. Martin C, Eon B, Saux P, Aknin P, et al. Renal effects of norepinephrine used to treat septic shock patients. *Crit Care Med* 1990; 18: 282–285.

54. Desjars P, Pinaud M, Bugnon D, et al. Norepinephrine therapy has no deleterious renal effects in human septic shock. *Crit Care Med* 1990; 18: 1048–1049.

55. Martin C, Papazian L, Perrin G, et al. Norepinephrine or dopamine for the treatment of hyperdynamic septic shock? *Chest* 1993; 103: 1826–1831.

56. Langenberg C, Wan L, Egi M, et al. Renal blood flow and function during recovery from experimental septic acute kidney injury. *Intensive Care Med* 2007; 33: 1614–1618

57. Matejovic M, Radermacher P, Joannidis M. Acute kidney injury in sepsis: Is renal blood flow more than just an innocent bystander? *Intensive Care Med* 2007; 33: 1498–1500

58. Totaro RJ, Raper RF. Epinephrine-induced lactic acidosis following cardiopulmonary bypass. *Crit Care Med* 1997; 25: 1693–1699.

59. Meier-Hellmann A, Reinhart K, Bredle DL, et al. Epinephrine impairs splanchnic perfusion in septic shock. *Crit Care Med* 1997; 25: 399–404.

60. Levy B, Bollaert PE, Charpentier C, et al. Comparison of norepinephrine and dobutamine to epinephrine for hemodynamics, lactate metabolism, and gastric tonometric variables in septic shock: a prospective randomized study. *Intensive Care Med* 1997; 23: 282–287.

61. Reinelt H, Radermacher P, Fischer G, et al. Effects of a dobutamine-induced increase in splanchnic blood flow on hepatic metabolic activity in patients with septic shock. *Anesthesiology* 1997; 86: 818–824.

62. Ruokonen E, Uusaro A, Alhava E, et al. The effect of dobutamine infusion on splanchnic blood flow and oxygen transport in patients with acute pancreatitis. *Intensive Care Med* 1997; 23: 732–737.

63. Creteur J, De Backer D, Vincent JL. A dobutamine test can disclose hepatosplanchnic hypoperfusion in septic patients. *Am J Respir Crit Care Med* 1999; 160: 839–845.

64. Träger K, DeBacker D, Radermacher P. Metabolic alterations in sepsis and vasoactive drug-related metabolic effects. *Curr Opin Crit Care* 2003; 9: 271–278.

65. Brealey D, Brand M, Hargreaves I et al. Association between mitochondrial dysfunction and severity and outcome of septic shock. *Lancet* 2002; 360: 219–23.

66. Barth E, Albuszies G, Baumgart K, et al. Glucose metabolism and catecholamines. *Crit Care Med* 2007; 35: S508–S518

67. Ensinger H, Träger K. Metabolic effect of vasoactive drugs. In: Vincent JL, editor. Yearbook of intensive care and emergency medicine. New York Springer Verlag; 2002. p. 499–509.

68. Wilson J, Woods I, Fawcett J, et al. Reducing the risk of major elective surgery: randomised controlled trial of preoperative optimisation of oxygen delivery. *BMJ* 1999; 318: 1099–1103.

69. Levy B, Mansart A, Bollaert PE, et al. Effects of epinephrine and norepinephrine on hemo-dynamics, oxidative metabolism, and organ energetics in endotoxemic rats. *Intensive Care Med* 2003; 29: 292–300.

70. Ensinger H, Geisser W, Brinkmann A, et al. Metabolic effects of norepinephrine and dobutamine in healthy volunteers. *Shock* 2002;18(6): 495–500. B.

71. Ensinger H, Rantala A, Vogt J, et al. Effect of dobutamine on splanchnic carbohydrate metabolism and amino acid balance after cardiac surgery. *Anesthesiology* 1999; 91: 1587–1595.

72. Marik PE, Mohedin M. The contrasting effects of dopamine and norepinephrineon systemic and splanchnic oxygen utilization in hyperdynamic sepsis. *J Am Med Assoc* 1994; 272: 1354–1357.

73. Levy B, Nace L, Bollaert PE, et al. Comparison of systemic and regional effects of dobutamine and dopexamine in norepinephrine-treated septic shock. *Intensive Care Med* 1999; 25: 942–948.

74. Reinelt H, Radermacher P, Kiefer P, Fischer G, Wachter U, Vogt J, Georgieff M. Impact of exogenous beta-adrenergic receptor stimulation on hepatosplanchnic oxygen kinetics and metabolic activity in septic shock.*Crit Care Med*. 1999; 27: 325–331

75. Morelli A, lange M, Ertner C, Dünser M, Rehberg S, Bachetoni A, D'Allesadnro M, Van AKen H, Guarracino F, Pietropaoli P, Traber DL, Westphal M. Short-term effects of phenylephrine on systemic and regional hemodynamics in patients with septic shock: a crossover study. *Shock* 2007 epub ahead of print 10.1097/shk.0b013e31815810ff

76. Khan MM, Sansoni P, Silverman ED, et al. Beta-adrenergic receptors on human suppressor, helper, and cytolytic lymphocytes. *Biochem Pharmacol* 1986; 35: 1137–1142.

77. Landmann R. Beta-adrenergic receptors in human leukocyte subpopulations. *Eur J Clin Invest* 1992; 22(Suppl 1): 30–36.

78. Santambrogio L, Lipartiti M, Bruni A, et al. Dopamine receptors on human T- and B-lymphocytes. *J Neuroimmunol* 1993; 45: 113–119.

79. Bergquist J, Ohlsson B, Tarkowski A. Nuclear factor kappa B is involved in the catecholaminergic suppression of immunocompetent cells. *Ann NY Acad Sci* 2000; 917: 281–289.

80. Maestroni GJ. Dendritic cell migration controlled by alpha 1b-adrenergic receptors. *J Immunol*. 2000; 165: 6743–6747.

81. Maestroni GJ. Short exposure of maturing, bone marrow-derived dendritic cells to norepinephrine: impact on kinetics of cytokine production and development. *J Neuroimmunol*. 2002; 129: 106–114.

82. Sanders VM, Baker RA, Ramer-Quinn DS, et al. Differential expression of the beta2-adrenergic receptor by Th1 and Th2 clones: implications for cytokine production and B cell help. *J Immunol*. 1997; 158: 4200–4210.

83. Pastores SM, Hasko G, Vizi ES, et al. Cytokine production and its manipulation by vasoactive drugs. *New Horiz* 1996; 4: 252–264.

84. Guirao X, Kumar A, Katz J, et al. Catecholamines increase monocyte TNF receptors and inhibit TNF through beta 2-adrenoreceptor activation. *Am J Physiol* 1997; 273: E1203–E1208.

85. Oberbeck R. Therapeutic implications of immune-endocrine interactions in the critically ill patients. *Curr Drug Targets Immune Endocr Metabol Disord* 2004; 4: 129–139.

86. Bergmann M, Gornikiewicz A, Tamandl D, et al. Continuous therapeutic epinephrine but not norepinephrine prolongs splanchnic IL-6 production in porcine endotoxic shock. *Shock* 2003; 20: 575–581.

87. van der Poll T, Coyle SM, Barbosa K, et al. Epinephrine inhibits tumor necrosis factor-alpha and potentiates interleukin 10 production during human endotoxemia. *J Clin Invest* 1996, 97: 713–719.

88. Sookhai S, Wang JH, Winter D, et al. Dopamine attenuates the chemoattractant effect of interleukin- 8: a novel role in the systemic inflammatory response syndrome. *Shock* 2000, 14: 295–299.

89. Van den Berghe G, de Zegher F. Anterior pituitary function during critical illness and dopamine treatment. *Crit Care Med* 1996; 24: 1580–1590.

90. Van den Berghe G, de Zegher F, Lauwers P, et al. Growth hormone secretion in critical illness: effect of dopamine. *J Clin Endocrinol Metab* 1994; 79: 1141–1146.

91. Van den Berghe G, de Zegher F, Lauwers P. Dopamine and the sick euthyroid syndrome in critical illness. *Clin Endocrinol (Oxf)* 1994; 41: 731–737.

92. Schilling T, Grundling M, Strang CM, et al. Effects of dopexamine, dobutamine or dopamine on prolactin and thyreotropin serum concentrations in high-risk surgical patients. *Intensive Care Med* 2004; 30: 1127–1133.

93. Oberbeck R. Dopexamine and cellular immune functions during systemic inflammation. *Immunobiology* 2004; 208: 429–438.

94. Hofstetter C, Boost KA, Hoegl S,et al. Norepinephrine and vasopressin counteract anti-inflammatory effects of isoflurane in endotoxemic rats. *Int J Mol Med* 2007; 20: 597–604

95. Bernadich C, Bandi JC, Melin P, et al. Effects of F-180, a new selective vasoconstrictor peptide, compared with terlipressin and vasopressin on systemic and splanchnic hemodynamics in a rat model of portal hypertension. *Hepatology* 1998; 27: 351–356.

96. Chernow B, Roth BL. Pharmacologic manipulation of the peripheral vasculature in shock: clinical and experimental approaches. Circ Shock 1986; 18: 141–155.

97. Schaller MD, Waeber B, Nussberger J, et al. Angiotensin II, vasopressin, and sympathetic activity in conscious rats with endotoxemia. *Am J Physiol* 1985; 249: H1086–1092.

98. Hollenberg SM, Tangora JJ, Piotrowski MJ, et al. Impaired microvascular vasoconstrictive responses to vasopressin in septic rats. *Crit Care Med* 1997; 25: 869–873.

99. Wilson MF, Brackett DJ. Release of vasoactive hormones and circulatory changes in shock. *Circ Shock* 1983; 11: 225–234.

100. Cronenwett JL, Baver-Neff BS, Grekin RJ, et al. The role of endorphins and vasopressin in canine endotoxin shock. *J Surg Res* 1986; 41: 609–619.

101. Bucher M, Hobbhahn J, Taeger K, et al. Cytokine-mediated downregulation of vasopressin V(1A) receptors during acute endotoxemia in rats. *Am J Physiol Regul Integr Comp Physiol* 2002; 282: R979–984.

102. Landry DW, Levin HR, Gallant EM, et al. Vasopressin deficiency contributes to the vasodilation of septic shock. *Circulation* 1997; 95: 1122–1125.

103. Landry DW, Levin HR, Gallant EM, et al. Vasopressin pressor hypersensitivity in vasodilatory septic shock. *Crit Care Med* 1997; 25: 1279–1282.

104. Argenziano M, Choudhri AF, Oz MC, et al. A prospective randomized trial of arginine vasopressin in the treatment of vasodilatory shock after left ventricular assist device placement. *Circulation* 1997; 96: S286–S290.

105. Sharshar T, Blanchard A, Paillard M, et al. Circulating vasopressin levels in septic shock. *Crit Care Med* 2003; 31: 1752–1758.

106. Sharshar T, Carlier R, Blanchard A, et al. Depletion of neurohypophyseal content of vasopressin in septic shock. *Crit Care Med* 2002; 30: 497–500.

107. Jochberger S, Mayr VD, Luckner G, et al. Serum vasopressin concentrations in critically ill patients. *Crit Care Med* 2006; 34: 293–299.
108. Barrett LK, Singer M, Clapp LH. Vasopressin: mechanisms of action on the vasculature in health and in septic shock. *Crit Care Med* 2007; 35: 33–40.
109. Wilson MF, Brackett DJ, Archer LT, et al. Mechanisms of impaired cardiac function by vasopressin. *Ann Surg* 1980; 191: 494–500.
110. Martikainen TJ, Tenhunen JJ, Uusaro A, et al. The effects of vasopressin on systemic and splanchnic hemodynamics and metabolism in endotoxin shock. *Anesth Analg* 2003; 97: 1756–1763.
111. Avontuur JA, Bruining HA, Ince C. Inhibition of nitric oxide synthesis causes myocardial ischemia in endotoxemic rats. *Circ Res* 1995; 76: 418–425.
112. Faivre V, Kaskos H, Callebert J, et al. Cardiac and renal effects of levosimendan, arginine vasopressin, and norepinephrine in lipopolysaccharide-treated rabbits. *Anesthesiology* 2005; 103: 514–521.
113. Kang CH, Kim WG. The effect of vasopressin on organ blood flow in an endotoxin-induced rabbit shock model. *J Invest Surg* 2006; 19: 361–369.
114. Westphal M, Stubbe H, Sielenkamper AW, et al. Terlipressin dose response in healthy and endotoxemic sheep: impact on cardiopulmonary performance and global oxygen transport. *Intensive Care Med* 2003; 29: 301–308.
115. Westphal M, Stubbe H, Sielenkamper AW, et al. Effects of titrated arginine vasopressin on hemodynamic variables and oxygen transport in healthy and endotoxemic sheep. *Crit Care Med* 2003; 31: 1502–1508.
116. Asfar P, Pierrot M, Veal N, et al. Low-dose terlipressin improves systemic and splanchnic hemodynamics in fluid-challenged endotoxic rats. *Crit Care Med* 2003; 31: 215–220.
117. Malay MB, Ashton JL, Dahl K, et al. Heterogeneity of the vasoconstrictor effect of vasopressin in septic shock. *Crit Care Med* 2004; 32: 1327–1331.
118. Albert M, Losser MR, Hayon D, et al. Systemic and renal macro- and microcirculatory responses to arginine vasopressin in endotoxic rabbits. *Crit Care Med* 2004; 32: 1891–1898.
119. Asfar P, Hauser B, Ivanyi Z, et al. Low-dose terlipressin during long-term hyperdynamic porcine endotoxemia: effects on hepatosplanchnic perfusion, oxygen exchange, and metabolism. *Crit Care Med* 2005; 33: 373–380.
120. Lange M, Morelli A, Ertmer C, et al. Continuous Versus Bolus Infusion of Terlipressin in Ovine Endotoxemia. Shock 2007 epub ahead of print 10.1097/shk.0b013e318050c78d
121. Sun Q, Dimopoulos G, Nguyen DN, et al. Low-dose vasopressin in the treatment of septic shock in sheep. *Am J Respir Crit Care Med* 2003; 168: 481–486.
122. Minneci PC, Deans KJ, Banks SM, et al. Differing effects of epinephrine, norepinephrine, and vasopressin on survival in a canine model of septic shock. *Am J Physiol Heart Circ Physiol* 2004; 287: H2545–2554.
123. Malay MB, Ashton RC, Jr., Landry DW, et al. Low-dose vasopressin in the treatment of vasodilatory septic shock. *J Trauma* 1999; 47: 699–703.
124. Tsuneyoshi I, Yamada H, Kakihana Y, et al. Hemodynamic and metabolic effects of low-dose vasopressin infusions in vasodilatory septic shock. *Crit Care Med* 2001; 29: 487–493.
125. Holmes CL, Walley KR, Chittock DR, et al. The effects of vasopressin on hemodynamics and renal function in severe septic shock: a case series. *Intensive Care Med* 2001; 27: 1416–1421.

126. Dünser MW, Mayr AJ, Ulmer H, et al. The effects of vasopressin on systemic hemodynamics in catecholamine-resistant septic and postcardiotomy shock: a retrospective analysis. *Anesth Analg* 2001; 93: 7–13.

127. Patel BM, Chittock DR, Russell JA, et al. Beneficial effects of short-term vasopressin infusion during severe septic shock. *Anesthesiology* 2002; 96: 576–582.

128. O'Brien A, Clapp L, Singer M. Terlipressin for norepinephrine-resistant septic shock. *Lancet* 2002; 359: 1209–1210.

129. Dünser MW, Mayr AJ, Ulmer H, et al. Arginine vasopressin in advanced vasodilatory shock: a prospective, randomized, controlled study. *Circulation* 2003;107: 2313–2319.

130. Leone M, Albanese J, Delmas A, et al. Terlipressin in catecholamine-resistant septic shock patients. *Shock* 2004;22: 314–319.

131. Klinzing S, Simon M, Reinhart K, et al. High-dose vasopressin is not superior to norepinephrine in septic shock. *Crit Care Med* 2003;31: 2646–2650.

132. van Haren FM, Rozendaal FW, van der Hoeven JG. The effect of vasopressin on gastric perfusion in catecholamine-dependent patients in septic shock. *Chest* 2003;124: 2256–2260.

133. Luckner G, Dünser MW, Jochberger S, et al. Arginine vasopressin in 316 patients with advanced vasodilatory shock. *Crit Care Med* 2005;33: 2659–2666.

134. Morelli A, Rocco M, Conti G, et al. Effects of terlipressin on systemic and regional haemodynamics in catecholamine-treated hyperkinetic septic shock. *Intensive Care Med* 2004;30: 597–604.

135. Albanese J, Leone M, Delmas A, et al. Terlipressin or norepinephrine in hyperdynamic septic shock: a prospective, randomized study. *Crit Care Med* 2005;33: 1897–1902.

136. Lauzier F, Levy B, Lamarre P, et al. Vasopressin or norepinephrine in early hyperdynamic septic shock: a randomized clinical trial. *Intensive Care Med* 2006;32: 1782–1789.

137. Dunser MW, Mayr AJ, Tur A, et al. Ischemic skin lesions as a complication of continuous vasopressin infusion in catecholamine-resistant vasodilatory shock: incidence and risk factors. *Crit Care Med* 2003;31: 1394–1398.

138. Landry DW, Oliver JA. The pathogenesis of vasodilatory shock. *N Engl J Med* 2001;345: 588–595.

139. Schmid PG, Abboud FM, Wendling MG, et al. Regional vascular effects of vasopressin: plasma levels and circulatory responses. *Am J Physiol* 1974;227: 998–1004.

140. Garcia-Villalon AL, Garcia JL, Fernandez N, et al. Regional differences in the arterial response to vasopressin: role of endothelial nitric oxide. *Br J Pharmacol* 1996;118: 1848–1854.

141. Laszlo F, Karacsony G, Pavo I, et al. Aggressive role of vasopressin in development of different gastric lesions in rats. *Eur J Pharmacol* 1994;258: 15–22.

142. Laszlo F, Whittle BJ. Constitutive nitric oxide modulates the injurious actions of vasopressin on rat intestinal microcirculation in acute endotoxaemia. *Eur J Pharmacol* 1994;260: 265–268.

143. Guzman JA, Rosado AE, Kruse JA. Vasopressin vs norepinephrine in endotoxic shock: systemic, renal, and splanchnic hemodynamic and oxygen transport effects. *J Appl Physiol* 2003;95: 803–809.

144. Bennett T, Mahajan RP, March JE, et al. Regional and temporal changes in cardiovascular responses to norepinephrine and vasopressin during continuous infusion of lipopolysaccharide in conscious rats. *Br J Anaesth* 2004;93: 400–407.

145. Westphal M, Freise H, Kehrel BE, et al. Arginine vasopressin compromises gut mucosal microcirculation in septic rats. *Crit Care Med* 2004;32: 194–200.

146. Knotzer H, Maier S, Dünser MW, et al. Arginine vasopressin does not alter mucosal tissue oxygen tension and oxygen supply in an acute endotoxemic pig model. *Intensive Care Med* 2006;32: 170–174.

147. Knotzer H, Pajk W, Maier S, et al. Arginine vasopressin reduces intestinal oxygen supply and mucosal tissue oxygen tension. *Am J Physiol Heart Circ Physiol* 2005;289: H168–173.

148. Boffa JJ, Arendshorst WJ. Maintenance of renal vascular reactivity contributes to acute renal failure during endotoxemic shock. *J Am Soc Nephrol* 2005;16: 117–124.

149. Creteur J, De Backer D, Vincent JL. Does gastric tonometry monitor splanchnic perfusion? *Crit Care Med* 1999;27: 2480–2484.

150. Holmes CL. Is low-dose vasopressin the new reno-protective agent? *Crit Care* Med 2004;32: 1972–1974.

13 The Diabetes of Injury: Novel Insights and Clinical Implications

Ilse Vanhorebeek, PhD *and Greet Van den Berghe,* MD, PhD

CONTENTS

From: *Contemporary Endocrinology: Acute Cause to Consequence*
Edited by: G. Van den Berghe, DOI: 10.1007/978-1-60327-177-6_13,
© Humana Press, New York, NY

INTRODUCTION

Whereas blood glucose levels normally are tightly regulated within the narrow range of 60–140 mg/dl, they usually rise during critical illness, irrespective of whether the patient had diabetes or not before the insult. This dysregulation of glucose homeostasis during critical illness has been labeled 'stress diabetes' or 'diabetes of injury' *(1,2)*. For a long time, it has been considered to be an adaptive and beneficial stress response. Indeed, according to a classic dogma moderate hyperglycemia in critically ill patients is beneficial for organs that largely rely on glucose for their energy supply but do not require insulin for glucose uptake, such as the brain and blood cells. Also, the development of hyperglycemia was regarded as a buffer against occasional hypoglycemia and consequent brain injury with tight glucose management. However, above the threshold of 220 mg/dl hyperglycemia-induced osmotic diuresis and fluid shifts occur. Furthermore, knowledge from the diabetes literature indicates that uncontrolled and pronounced hyperglycemia predisposes to infectious complications *(2,3)*. Hence, until recently, the state of the art tolerated blood glucose levels up to 220 mg/dl in fed critically ill patients with only excessive hyperglycemia exceeding this value being treated *(4)*. Nowadays though, this approach has lost its foundations. Several studies already clearly identified the development of (even moderate) hyperglycemia as an important risk factor in terms of mortality and morbidity of critically ill patients suffering from a wide variety of underlying diseases *(5–16)*. Of crucial importance, however, was the demonstration by a landmark study that normalization of blood glucose levels with intensive insulin therapy during critical illness reduced mortality and morbidity of the patients in a surgical intensive care unit (ICU) *(17)*. This study has had a major impact worldwide. We here give an overview of the findings of that study and others performed or initiated after it, discuss some questions that have been raised with regard to efficacy and safety of the therapy in light of the available evidence, highlight the practical implications of how to safely implement intensive insulin therapy, and delineate the insights obtained so far into the mechanisms by which this therapy establishes its clinical benefits.

INTENSIVE INSULIN THERAPY TO THE TARGET OF NORMOGLYCEMIA IN CRITICAL ILLNESS: THE LEUVEN STUDIES

Associations between hyperglycemia and adverse outcome do not necessarily reflect a causal relationship, as the degree of hyperglycemia may be a marker of more severe illness. To demonstrate causality interference with a treatment that prevents hyperglycemia and assessment of its impact are needed. The first study on this topic included mechanically ventilated adult patients admitted to the ICU predominantly after extensive, complicated surgery or trauma, or after medical complications of major surgical procedures ($n = 1548$) *(17)*. Patients assigned to the conventional approach received insulin only if glucose concentrations exceeded 215 mg/dl with the aim of keeping concentrations between 180 and 200 mg/dl, resulting in mean morning blood glucose levels of 153 mg/dl (hyperglycemia). Insulin was administered to the patients in the intensive insulin therapy group to maintain blood glucose levels between 80 and 110 mg/dl, which resulted in mean blood glucose levels of 103 mg/dl (normoglycemia). When admission levels were not taken into account, mean blood glucose levels were 158 mg/dl in the conventional and 98 mg/dl in the intensive inulin therapy group.

In the intention-to-treat patient population tight blood glucose control with insulin lowered ICU mortality from 8.0% to 4.6% (absolute risk reduction, ARR of 3.4%) and in-hospital mortality from 10.9% to 7.2% (ARR of 3.7%) (Fig. 1). The benefit was much larger in the target population of patients who required intensive care for at least 5 days, with a reduction of ICU mortality from 20.2% to 10.6% (ARR of 9.6%) and of in-hospital mortality from 26.3% to 16.8% (ARR of 9.5%) (Fig. 1). The choice of the target population as patients in the ICU for at least 5 days was made arbitrarily, based on another study with a similar target population *(18)*. In retrospect, it appeared that the impact of the intervention increased with the duration of its application and that a substantial benefit was present with at least 3 days of intensive insulin therapy. Besides saving lives, intensive insulin therapy substantially prevented several critical illness-associated complications. The incidence of critical illness polyneuropathy as well as the development of blood stream infections and acute renal failure

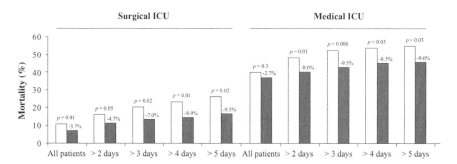

Fig. 1. Impact of intensive insulin therapy on in-hospital mortality of surgical and medical ICU patients in relation to duration of treatment *(17,22)*. *Open bars* represent the conventionally treated patients, *grey bars* represent the patients who received intensive insulin therapy.

requiring dialysis or hemofiltration were reduced. Fewer patients acquired liver dysfunction with hyperbilirubinemia. The need for red blood cell transfusions decreased. In addition, patients were less dependent on prolonged mechanical ventilation and intensive care. About 63% of the patients were included in the study after complicated cardiac surgery. Improvement of long-term outcome with intensive insulin therapy given for at least a third day in ICU was demonstrated for this subgroup in a follow-up study (19). Indeed, the survival benefit was maintained up to 4 years after randomization. Risk for hospital readmission and dependency on medical care were similar in both groups. Short-term glycemic control with insulin during intensive care did not induce a substantial burden for the patients, their relatives or society, but the perceived quality of social and family life appeared to be moderately compromised. In patients with isolated brain injury, intensive insulin therapy protected the central and peripheral nervous system from secondary insults and improved long-term rehabilitation (20). Finally, a *post-hoc* analysis on healthcare resource utilization illustrated the economic advantages of intensive insulin therapy, with substantial cost savings compared with conventional insulin therapy (21).

After the first study in the Leuven surgical ICU, a second large randomized, controlled trial on strict blood glucose control with intensive insulin therapy was started in the Leuven medical ICU (22). The medical study was powered to demonstrate or exclude an absolute reduction of 7% in the risk of death of long-stay patients needing at least a third day of intensive care. The power calculation was based on the outcome results of the surgical study, that had indicated that the impact of intensive insulin therapy was dependent on the duration of its application and substantial benefit was present from three days of treatment onwards (Fig. 1). Inclusion of 1200 patients was necessary in order to obtain the required 700 long-stay patients, as expected long stay cannot be identified upon admission. The same insulin-titration protocol was used as in the surgical study, resulting in mean morning blood glucose levels of 105 mg/dl in the intensive insulin therapy group versus 160 mg/dl for the conventional glucose management.

In-hospital mortality of the intention-to-treat population of 1200 patients was reduced from 40.0% to 37.3% (ARR of 2.7%) (Fig. 1). Statistically, this difference was not significant, which is not surprising as the study was not powered for this endpoint, but after correction for well-known upon-admission risk factors (malignancy, diabetes, kidney failure, upon-admission APACHE II, TISS-28, CRP, creatinine, ALT) the difference did reach statistical significance (odds ratio for intensive insulin 0.77, 95% confidence interval 0.60–0.99, $p = 0.04$). In the target group of long-stay patients tight glycemic control with insulin significantly reduced in-hospital mortality from 52.5% to 43.0% (ARR of 9.5%) (Fig. 1). Intensive insulin therapy significantly reduced morbidity in the intention-to-treat group of patients. New development of kidney injury occurred less frequently, the therapy allowed earlier weaning from mechanical ventilation and earlier discharge from the ICU and from the hospital. The positive effect on morbidity was even more striking in the target group. These long-stay patients were discharged from the hospital alive on average 10 days earlier than those who received conventional insulin therapy and fewer of them developed hyper-bilirubinemia. The incidence of critical illness polyneuropathy and/or myopathy was also reduced *(23)*. In contrast to the surgical patients, there was no difference in bacteremia or prolonged antibiotic therapy requirement for medical ICU patients, but the number of patients with hyperinflammation was lower *(22)*.

When the surgical and medical patient populations were mixed in a pooled data set of the two Leuven studies hospital mortality was reduced from 23.6% to 20.4% (ARR of 3.2%, $p = 0.04$) for all patients according to intention-to-treat analysis and from 37.9% to 30.1% (ARR of 7.8%, $p = 0.002$) in the patients who remained in the ICU for at least 3 days *(24)*. New development of kidney injury during ICU stay and critical illness polyneuropathy were reduced to almost half.

OTHER STUDIES ON INTENSIVE INSULIN THERAPY IN CRITICAL ILLNESS

The clinical benefits of intensive insulin therapy were largely confirmed in an observational study that assessed the impact of implementing a tight glucose management protocol in 'real life' intensive care for a heterogeneous medical/surgical patient population (n = 1600) *(25)*. Intravenous insulin was administered only if glucose levels exceeded 200 mg/dl on 2 successive measurements and aimed to lower glycemia below 140 mg/dl. Mean glucose levels of 131 mg/dl were reached. Hence, blood glucose control was somewhat less strict than in the Leuven studies. Comparison with historical controls as a reference, who had mean glucose levels of 152 mg/dl, showed that the implementation of the glucose control protocol resulted in a hospital mortality reduction from 20.9% to 14.8% (ARR of 6.1%), decreased length of ICU stay, lower incidence of newly developed renal failure, and reduced need for red blood cell transfusion. No effect was seen on the occurrence of severe infections, but this complication was not frequently present in the baseline period. An extended study in the same hospital ($n = 5365$) demonstrated a mortality reduction from 19.5% to 14.8% (ARR 4.7%) *(26)*. Implementation of the glucose management protocol substantially saved money *(27)*.

A small ($n = 61$) prospective, randomized, controlled study in a predominantly general surgical patient population, targeted glucose levels between 80 and 120 mg/dl with intensive insulin therapy. This resulted in mean daily glucose levels of 125 mg/dl versus 179 mg/dl in the standard glycemic control group and lower incidence of total nosocomial infections *(28)*.

Intravenous insulin infusion was used to eliminate hyperglycemia in an observational study of diabetic cardiac surgery patients. In-hospital mortality was significantly lower, deep sternal wound infections developed less frequently, and length of hospital stay was shortened *(29)*.

In a surgical trauma, ICU mean blood glucose levels decreased from 141 mg/dl to 125 mg/dl after implementation of a glucose control protocol. This coincided with fewer intraabdominal abscesses and fewer postinjury ventilator days *(30)*.

Patients with severe sepsis and septic shock were studied in a prospective, randomized, multi-center trial volume substitution and insulin therapy in severe sepsis (VISEP) *(31)*. Two treatment strategies were assessed simultaneously: type of fluid resuscitation and intensive insulin therapy. The insulin arm of the study was stopped prematurely because the rate of hypoglycemia in the intensive treatment group (12.1%) was considered unacceptably high. At this moment 488 patients were included and 90-day mortality was 29.5% in the intensive versus 32.8% in the conventional insulin treatment arm (ARR of 3.3%, not significant) *(32)*.

The prospective, randomized, controlled, multi-center GLUCONTROL trial was designed to investigate whether tight glycemic control to 80–110 mg/dl with insulin improves survival in a mixed population of critically ill patients *(33)*. However, the targeted glycemic control was not reached (unintended protocol violation) and the risk of hypoglycemia was considered high. Therefore, the steering and safety committee of this trial decided to stop enrollment of patients after a first interim analysis ($n = 855$).

It is striking that the available randomized studies all found a uniform 3–4% reduction in the risk of death in the intention-to-treat patient populations *(17,22,24,32)*. To assign this difference as statistically significant the study needs to be adequately powered and anticipated baseline risk of death needs to be taken into account. For instance, critically ill patients in medical ICUs often have a higher baseline severity of illness and higher intrinsic risk of death than surgical ICU patients. Hence, a higher number of medical ICU patients would need to be included compared to surgical ICU patients to demonstrate a similar absolute risk reduction. The relative reduction in the risk of death was higher in the surgical than in the medical Leuven ICU study, but a similar (although not statistically significant, as anticipated by powering for the target group of long-stay patients) absolute mortality risk reduction was found. This consistency in the absolute rather than relative risk reduction is in line with prevention of a certain number of avoidable deaths with intensive insulin therapy by preventing additional pathology during intensive care, rather than that the therapy is curing a disease.

The multi-center trial, called NICE-SUGAR (Normoglycemia in Intensive Care Evaluation and Survival Using Glucose Algorithm Regulation) is currently including patients from a mixed medical/surgical population *(34)*. It is the only clinical trial that is currently ongoing that is designed with sufficient statistical power (>5000 patients to be incluced) to assess the impact of strict blood glucose control with intensive insulin therapy on survival.

WHAT SHOULD BE THE TARGET OF GLUCOSE CONTROL WITH INTENSIVE INSULIN THERAPY?

In the clinical studies on intensive insulin therapy, it is impossible to completely distinguish the impact of insulin infusion from that of blood glucose control as both are done concomitantly. Therefore, a four-arm design study was set up in a rabbit model of prolonged critical illness *(35)*. Two normoinsulinemic and two hyperinsulinemic groups were each controlled to either normal or elevated glucose levels. The study revealed that glycemic control mediated the survival benefit of intensive insulin therapy, independent of insulin. Indeed, mortality was 41.4% in hyperglycemic versus 11.1% in normoglycemic rabbits, whereas insulin levels did not contribute to the survival benefit.

The clinical data are in agreement with this experimental observation. In the Leuven surgical study, the risk of death appeared to be linearly correlated with the degree of hyperglycemia, with no clear cut-off level below which there was no further benefit *(36)*. Conventionally treated patients who developed severe hyperglycemia (150–200 mg/dl) carried the highest risk of death, this risk was intermediate for patients who received conventional insulin therapy and who developed only moderate hyperglycemia (110–150 mg/dl), whereas the lowest risk was present in the patients whose blood glucose levels were controlled to strict normoglycemia below 110 mg/dl with intensive insulin therapy. This relation of risk of death with strata of glucose control was confirmed in the mixed medical/surgical patient population, with most benefit gained when glycemia was controlled below 110 mg/dl *(24)*. Patients with diabetes appeared to behave differently though, with an inverse pattern for the 3 strata of glucose control, although no significant differences were noted among these 3 levels.

Glycemic control also accounted for most effects of intensive insulin therapy on morbidity of critical illness *(17,24,36)*. Tight glycemic control below 110 mg/dl appeared to be of crucial importance for the prevention of bacteremia, anemia, and acute renal failure *(24,36)* and for reducing the risk of critical illness polyneuropathy, for which a positive linear correlation was observed with glycemia *(20)*.

The superior clinical benefit with glucose control below 110 mg/dl underscores the importance of achieving the normoglycemic target range. Seventy percent of the patients allocated to intensive insulin therapy in the Leuven studies *(17,22,24)* actually achieved a mean daily blood glucose level below 110 mg/dl. At the time of interim analysis of the GLUCONTROL study, median (interquartile range) levels of glucose were 147 (127–163) mg/dl in the conventional and 118 (109–131) mg/dl in the intensive insulin group (Preiser JC, data presented at the 19th European Symposium on Intensive Care Medicine, Barcelona, Spain, September 2006). This means that tight glycemic control was achieved in only approximately 25% of the patients on intensive insulin therapy.

FEAR FOR HYPOGLYCEMIA: DOES IT OUTWEIGH THE CLINICAL BENEFITS OF INTENSIVE INSULIN THERAPY?

Severe (<30 mg/dl) or prolonged hypoglycemia can cause convulsions, coma, and irreversible brain damage as well as cardiac arrhythmias. The risk of hypoglycemia is a concern when intensive insulin therapy is administered to critically ill patients, as early hypoglycemic symptoms are not easily recognized in ICU patients *(4)*. Indeed, the patients themselves may be unable to recognize or communicate hypoglycemic symptoms, but also, clinical symptoms may be masked by concomitant diseases and by inherent intensive care treatments such as sedation, analgesia, and mechanical ventilation.

The risk of hypoglycemia (glucose $\leq$ 40 mg/dl) increased with intensive insulin therapy from 0.8 to 5.1% in the surgical *(17)* and from 3.1 to 18.7% in the medical ICU study *(22)*. Patients with sepsis appeared to be particularly susceptible, with an overall incidence of hypoglycemia of 11.4% (2.9% for conventional and 19.6% for intensive insulin therapy) versus 3.9% for patients without sepsis (1.2% for conventional and 6.8% for intensive insulin therapy) *(37)*. These brief hypoglycemic episodes did not cause early deaths. Only minor immediate and transient morbidity was seen in a minority of patients and no late neurological sequellae occurred among hospital survivors *(24)*. Hence, the biochemical hypoglycemia was not associated with obvious clinical problems. However, it cannot be completely excluded that the occurrence of hypoglycemia counteracted some of the survival benefit of intensive insulin therapy. Indeed, the risk of hypoglycemia coincided with a higher risk of death (OR of 3.2 in the surgical *(17)* and OR of 2.9 in the medical ICU study *(22)*, when corrected for randomization, APACHE II score, history of diabetes, history of malignancy, and common diagnostic subgroups), equally in both conventional and intensive insulin groups. It is interesting, however, that a higher mortality was observed with spontaneous hypoglycemia than with hypoglycemic events during insulin infusion. In a recent nested-case control study, where case and control subjects were matched for baseline risk factors and time in ICU before development of hypoglycemia, no causal link was found between the hypoglycemic event and death *(38)*. These observations support the view that hypoglycemia in ICU patients who receive intensive insulin therapy may merely identify patients at high risk of dying rather than representing a risk on its own *(39)*. Moreover, higher severity of illness, with a higher incidence of liver and kidney failure, makes patients more susceptible to the development of hypoglycemia. As most benefit was gained with the tightest blood glucose control, the risk of hypoglycemia should be weighed against improved outcome. Nevertheless, the utmost care has to be taken to avoid hypoglycemia.

The incidence of hypoglycemia was comparable for the Leuven studies (11%) and GLUCONTROL (10%), but the achievement of tight glucose control was dramatically different *(17,22,24,33)*. Importantly, if optimal blood glucose control, that is, to normoglycemia, is not achieved and hypoglycemia is frequent, the therapy is not likely to bring about benefit and thus only exposes patients to risks. If hypoglycemia does develop, it should be corrected promptly but with the caution not to overcorrect, as recent animal experiments suggest that neuronal death can be triggered by glucose reperfusion and activation of neuronal NADPH oxidase *(40)*.

DO ALL PATIENTS BENEFIT FROM INTENSIVE INSULIN THERAPY?

A novel intervention can only be advocated for patients who are likely to benefit from the therapy. Therefore, the databases of the 2 Leuven studies were pooled to look at large diagnostic subgroups of mixed medical/surgical patients *(17,22,24,37)*. Intensive insulin therapy reduced mortality and morbidity of patients with cardiovascular, respiratory, gastrointestinal/hepatic disease or surgery, of patients with active malignancy and of those with sepsis upon ICU admission *(24,37)*. All these subgroups had a quite comparable absolute reduction in the risk of death. Morbidity of patients with a prior history of diabetes tended to be reduced with administration of intensive insulin therapy. However, they showed no survival benefit and the risk of death in relation to strata of glucose control was rather the inverse (although not significantly different) as for the other groups (vide supra). Hence, while awaiting further studies, it may be advisable to lower glucose levels less aggressively and set the treatment goal for patients with diabetes to the glucose levels obtained prior to the acute insult. Interestingly, patients with diabetes who were on insulin treatment prior to critical illness had a tendency for an increased risk of death (odds ratio 1.39, 95% confidence interval 0.96–2.01, $p = 0.08$), whereas those who had previously been treated with medication other than insulin had a lower risk of death (odds ratio 0.61, 95% confidence interval 0.40–0.93, $p = 0.02$), as revealed by multivariate logistic regression analysis that corrected for other upon admission risk factors such as severity of illness and cancer, and for intensive insulin therapy in ICU (odds ratio 0.78, 95% confidence interval 0.63–0.96, $p = 0.02$). The exact reason for this statistical association remains to be investigated.

In both Leuven studies, the survival benefit obtained with intensive insulin therapy was more pronounced when the patients received this therapy for at least a few days (17,22) and a striking parallelism was observed between both studies for this time effect (Fig. 1). An apparent difference in both studies was that in the medical study a higher, but not statistically significant, number of intensive insulin-treated short-stay patients died (56/209) than in the conventional group (42/224), which was of concern to the practicing clinician. It would suggest possible harm by brief treatment, whereas it is virtually impossible to predict which patient will require more than 3 days of intensive care. However, selection bias likely explains this observation: a *post hoc* exploratory mortality analysis revealed that for 36 short-stay patients intensive care had been limited or withdrawn within 72 hours after ICU admission for reasons of futility, imbalanced among the conventional ($n = 10$) and intensive ($n = 26$) insulin therapy groups. The apparent mortality difference disappeared after correction for the well-known upon-admission risk factors that are the major reasons for therapy restriction. Importantly, when the datasets from the surgical and the medical study were pooled, statistical power was sufficient to show that brief insulin treatment for less than 3 days did not cause harm (24).

COULD HIGH-DOSE INSULIN ADMINISTRATION HARM THE CRITICALLY ILL PATIENT?

Not only hyperglycemia, but also the dose of insulin administered to the critically ill patients was associated with a high risk of death (17,24,36,41). This further indicates that it was the blood glucose control and/or other metabolic effects of insulin that accompany tight blood glucose control, and not the insulin dose administered per se, that contributed to the improved survival with intensive insulin therapy. The association between high insulin dose and mortality can be explained by more severe insulin resistance in the sicker patients, who have a high risk of death. Alternatively, it could point to a true deleterious effect of hyperinsulinemia. In patients who received intensive insulin therapy circulating levels of insulin were, however, only transiently higher in spite of the large difference in insulin dose administered compared with conventionally treated patients (42). More study is needed to address this important question, as potential harm to some patients cannot be definitively excluded with the available evidence.

PRACTICAL CONSIDERATIONS WHEN IMPLEMENTING TIGHT GLYCEMIC CONTROL

Implementation of strict blood glucose control in the routine clinical setting of certain ICUs may prove to be a challenge. A strong leader in the team has to drive the change in practice. The best way to achieve blood glucose control during intensive care is by continuous insulin infusion. The use of oral anti-diabetic agents in patients with previously diagnosed diabetes should be discontinued. Obviously, clear guidelines are needed as well as adequate education and training of the medical and nursing staff, the latter being the ones who should titrate the insulin infusions. Inevitably, frequent blood glucose determinations are necessary and will increase the working load for the nurses. In the research setting of the two Leuven studies the nursing staff was unaltered compared to before the onset of the study, with 1 nurse taking care of 2 patients *(17,22)*.

Avoiding hypoglycemia is a special concern and specific preventive mesures include the concomitant administration of insulin and carbohydrates and close monitoring of blood glucose levels, also after stable glucose levels are obtained. Obviously, the insulin dose should be adequately reduced during interruption of enteral feeding. The development of an accurate and reliable continuous blood glucose sensor, and preferably a closed-loop system for computer-assisted blood glucose control, will likely help to avoid hypoglycemia and to reduce the nursing workload. Hence, availability of such a device is likely to facilitate implementation of tight blood glucose control in ICU.

Evidently, one needs to be able to rely on the accuracy of the blood glucose determinations. As routine central hospital laboratories deliver glucose values too slowly for use in a glucose regulation protocol, bed-side point-of-care methods are used instead. Importantly, differences between systems and methods of detection, the use of plasma versus whole blood and patient variables (extremes of haematocrit, pH, oxygenation, medications, and temperature) can influence the glucose readings and result in different absolute values *(43,44)*. This might have implications for comparing the appropriate glucose targets and algorithms for glucose control in relation to the glycemic control of the Leuven studies. Both Leuven studies used whole arterial blood and determined glucose with an ABL blood gas analyzer (shown to be accurate, rapid, and user-friendly *(45)*) and by HemoCue. The absence of an arterial line may make tight blood glucose control very difficult as capillary blood glucose values, obtained by finger stick *(46–48)* or measurements in fluid obtained from subcutaneous sites *(49,50)* do not appear to be reliable in the ICU setting.

When all these considerations are taken into account and the conditions ful-filled, successful implementation of strict blood glucose control with intensive insulin therapy is feasible, as has already been shown *(25)*.

HOW DOES INTENSIVE INSULIN THERAPY IMPROVE OUTCOME FROM CRITICAL ILLNESS?

Development of Stress Hyperglycemia and Mechanism by Which Intensive Insulin Therapy Achieves Blood Glucose Control

Glucose production by the liver is enhanced in critical illness by an upregu-lation of both gluconeogenesis and glycogenolysis, despite high blood glucose levels and augmented insulin secretion. The mechanism is not completely clear, but increased levels of glucagon, cortisol, growth hormone, catecholamines, and cytokines all play a role *(51–56)*. Several of their effects indeed counteract the normal actions of insulin. Impaired glucose uptake also contributes to the development of hyperglycemia. Critically ill patients are immobilized, which means that the important excercise-stimulated glucose uptake in skeletal muscle is likely abolished. Insulin-stimulated glucose uptake by glucose transporter-4 (GLUT-4) is compromized *(57,58)*. Whole body glucose uptake is increased, however, but mainly takes place in tissues that are not dependent on insulin for glucose uptake, such as the nervous system and the blood cells *(2,59)*. The com-bined picture of higher levels of insulin, elevated hepatic glucose production, and impaired peripheral glucose uptake reflects the development of peripheral insulin resistance during critical illness.

Data from the studies performed by our group suggest that mainly stim-ulation of glucose uptake by skeletal muscle explains how intensive insulin therapy lowers circulating glucose levels in critically ill patients, rather than an effect of insulin on hepatic glucose handling *(60,61)*. This is illustrated by improved responsiveness of the insulin-regulated genes GLUT-4 (controlling insulin-stimulated glucose uptake) and hexokinase-II (rate-limiting enzyme in intracellular insulin-stimulated glucose metabolism) in skeletal muscle, in con-trast to the lack of an effect of intensive insulin therapy on insulin-regulated genes in the liver, including glucokinase (rate-limiting enzyme for insulin-mediated glucose uptake and glycogen synthesis in liver), phosphoenolpyruvate carboxykinase (rate-limiting for gluconeogenesis), and insulin-like growth fac-tor binding protein-1. These findings were corroborated by a recent study that showed that the metabolic insulin signal was increased in post-mortem skeletal muscle biopsies from patients who received intensive insulin therapy, as illus-trated by an increase in the assocation between insulin-receptor-substrate-1 and phosphoinositide-3-kinase and increased phosphorylation of Akt, whereas no effect was seen in liver *(42)*.

Does Parenteral Nutrition Take Part in the Effect of Intensive Insulin Therapy?

Criticism has been raised with regard to the feeding regimen that was followed in the Leuven studies. Official guidelines were followed though *(17,22,62)*, with enteral feeding attempted as soon as possible after hemodynamic stabilization of the patients, but early administration of parenteral feeding to compensate for the deficit when the caloric target could not be reached. It was suggested that the patients in this way were at risk of overfeeding and that intensive insulin therapy would merely serve to offset risk associated with 'excessive' parenteral glucose. Analysis of the pooled dataset of the two Leuven studies *(24)* argues against such criticism, by showing a mortality benefit independent of strata of glucose control. Indeed, intensive insulin therapy lowered mortality both in the lowest and the highest tertile of parenteral glucose load in the intention-to-treat population and in all tertiles of parenteral feeding for patients treated in intensive care for at least 3 days. Moreover, the most pronounced benefit was present for patients who received the smallest amount of parenteral feeding. Although the Leuven feeding regimen is different from the approach adopted in many centers, where parenteral nutrition is started only late after admission to the ICU with prolonged failure of enteral nutrition, it looks like the fear for complications of overfeeding may be exaggerated and needs to be reassessed in the era of tight glycemic control *(63)*.

Intensive Insulin Therapy Protects Against Glucose Toxicity in Critical Illness

As indicated above, preventing hyperglycemia is crucial to obtain the clinical benefits of intensive insulin therapy. It is striking that by avoiding even a moderate degree of hyperglycemia only during the relatively short period the patients needed intensive care, this strategy prevented the most feared complications of critical illness. Downregulation of glucose transporters is the normal response of cells to protect themselves from deleterious effects of moderate hyperglycemia *(64)*. In patients with diabetes, the time frame in which chronic hyperglycemia causes severe complications is several orders of magnitude longer than the time it took to prevent life-threatening complications in critical illness. This indicates that hyperglycemia would be more acutely toxic in critically ill patients than in healthy individuals or diabetic patients. Upregulation of insulin-independent glucose uptake mediated by the facilitative glucose transporters GLUT-1, GLUT-2, or GLUT-3 may play a role. Several factors induced in critical illness, including cytokines, angiotensin II, endothelin-1, vascular endothelial growth factor, transforming growth factor-β? but also the development of hypoxia have been shown to increase the expression and membrane localization of GLUT-1 and GLUT-3 in different cell types *(65–69)*, which may overrule the normal downregulatory protective response against hyperglycemia. Furthermore, GLUT-2 and GLUT-3 allow glucose to enter cells directly proportional to the extracellular glucose level over the range of glycemia present in critical illness *(70)*. Hence, cellular glucose overload may develop in hepatocytes, endothelial, epithelial and immune cells, renal tubules, the central and peripheral nervous system, pancreatic β-cells, and gastrointestinal mucosa. In contrast, cells and tissues that predominantly rely on insulin-dependent glucose transport via GLUT-4, such as skeletal muscle, may be relatively protected against hyperglycemia-induced cellular glucose overload and toxicity.

Mitochondrial dysfunction and the associated bioenergetic failure have been regarded as factors contributing to multiple organ failure, the most common cause of death in sepsis and prolonged critical illness, and have indeed been related to lethal outcome in patients and in a resuscitated long-term rat model of sepsis *(71,72)*. Intensive insulin therapy protected hepatocytic mitochondria from severe ultrastructural and functional damage *(73)*, whereas no effect was seen in skeletal muscle. These data are consistent with the concept that insulin therapy prevented hyperglycemia-induced mitochondrial damage to hepatocytes. Together with a similar protection of other cellular systems with passive glucose uptake this could theoretically explain some of the beneficial effects of intensive insulin therapy in severe illness.

All major components of innate immunity are compromised by high glucose levels *(74)*, including polymorphonuclear neutrophil function and intracellular bactericidal and opsonic activity *(75–78)*. This may play a role in the increased susceptibility of critically ill patients to develop severe infections *(3,79)*. Importantly, intensive insulin therapy largely prevented severe nosocomial infections and lethal sepsis in critically ill patients *(17,37)*. Glucose control with insulin beneficially affected innate immunity in an animal model of prolonged critical illness, by preservation of phagocytosis and oxidative burst function of monocytes *(80)*.

Several decades ago, the infusion of glucose together with insulin and potassium (GIK) emerged as a metabolic cocktail to reduce early mortality and morbidity of patients with acute myocardial infarction and yielded promising results. However, no clinical benefits were found in two recent large, randomized trials on GIK therapy in patients with acute myocardial infarction (CREATE-ECLA) and patients with diabetes and myocardial infarction (DIGAMI-2) *(81,82)*. GIK infusion for 24 hours after acute stroke also failed to reduce mortality *(83,84)*. Importantly, neither study performed or succeeded in tight blood glucose control, which may explain the disappointing results.

Intensive Insulin Therapy also Exerts Non-glycemic Effects

The serum lipid profile of critically ill patients is severely disturbed: triglyceride levels are elevated (due to an increase in very-low-density lipoprotein), whereas levels of high-density lipoprotein (HDL)- and low-density lipoprotein (LDL)-cholesterol are low *(85–87)*. Intensive insulin therapy prevented the rise in serum triglycerides during full nutritional support and substantially increased circulating HDL and LDL and the level of cholesterol associated with these lipoproteins *(60)*. Serum triglycerides and free fatty acids were also decreased when burned children were treated with insulin *(88)*. Triglycerides have an important role in energy provision, lipoproteins in transportation of lipid components and endotoxin scavenging *(89–91)*. Hence, a contribution of the (partial) correction of the lipid profile to improved outcome may be expected. This has indeed been confirmed in multivariate logistic regression analysis, where the effect on dyslipidemia surprisingly even surpassed the effect of glycemic control *(60)*.

Insulin has well-recognized anabolic properties, including stimulation of muscle protein synthesis and attenuation of protein breakdown *(92–94)*. Therefore, the administration of insulin has been put forward as an intervention to attenuate the hypercatabolic state of prolonged critical illness *(95,96)*. Such an anabolic effect was not obvious from clinical observation in the surgical ICU trial *(17)*, but a higher protein content was measured in post-mortem skeletal muscle biopsies of patients who received intensive insulin therapy *(73)* and in a rabbit model of prolonged critical illness weight loss was prevented *(80)*. Altered regulation at the level of the somatotropic axis appeared not to be involved *(97)*.

Anti-inflammatory properties of insulin are illustrated by lowered serum C-reactive protein (CRP) and mannose-binding lectin levels with intensive insulin therapy *(98)*. This effect was independent of infection prevention. In a rabbit model a similar attenuation of the CRP response was seen *(80)*. Insulin therapy had no major effect on an extensive series of pro- and anti-inflammatory cytokines in surgical critically ill patients *(99)*. This is in contrast with a study of burned children, where the administration of insulin resulted in lower levels of pro-inflammatory cytokines and proteins and stimulation of the anti-inflammatory cascade, but only late after the insult *(88)*. Similar results were obtained from studies on endotoxemic rats and pigs and thermally injured rats *(100–102)*. These anti-inflammatory effects of insulin therapy may have been direct, but prevention of hyperglycemia may have been crucial as well.

It has also been shown that insulin is able to improve myocardial function and protect the myocardium during acute myocardial infarction, open heart surgery, endotoxic shock, and other critical conditions *(103,104)*. This may be due to direct anti-apoptotic properties of insulin independent of glucose uptake and involving insulin signalling *(103,105,106)*, but avoiding hyperglycemia is crucial as well (vide supra) *(103)*. Intensive insulin therapy protected the endothelium, which related to its prevention of organ failure and death *(99)*. Lower levels of adhesion molecules indicated that endothelial activation was reduced. Inhibition of excessive iNOS-induced NO release is likely involved. Levels of asymmetric dimethylarginine, an arginine derivative and endogenous inhibitor of nitric oxide synthase activity, were also reduced *(107)*. This was associated with a better outcome, most likely mediated by reducing the inhibition of the constitutively expressed endothelial nitric oxide synthase *(108)*, contributing to preservation of organ blood flow.

Finally, the cortisol response to critical illness was attenuated by intensive insulin therapy, which statistically related to improved outcome *(109)*. Altered cortisol-binding activity was not involved.

CONCLUSION

More and more evidence argues against the concept that the diabetes of injury is an adaptive, beneficial response in the modern ICU era. Maintenance of normoglycemia with intensive insulin therapy has been shown to improve survival and reduce morbidity of critically ill patients. Demonstration of these clinical benefits appears to depend on the quality of blood glucose control (target of sustained normoglycemia has to be reached in a large enough fraction of patients, with avoidance of overlapping glucose levels with the control group, and prevention of excessive hypoglycemia) and the statistical power of the studies. Higher reductions in the absolute risk of death and in morbidity are seen when the therapy is continued for at least a few days. Substantial progress has been made in the understanding of the mechanisms underlying the clinical benefits of intensive insulin therapy. Much more is to be learnt about the exact pathways involved, as well as the relative contribution of preventing glucose toxicity and direct non-glycemic effects of insulin.

Acknowledgment   The work was supported by research grants from the Katholieke Universiteit Leuven (GOA2007/14) and the Fund for Scientific Research (FWO), Flanders, Belgium (G.0533.06). I. Vanhorebeek is a Postdoctoral Fellow of the FWO, Flanders, Belgium.

REFERENCES

1. Thorell A, Nygren J, Ljungqvist O. Insulin resistance: a marker of surgical stress. *Curr Opin Clin Nutr Metab Care* 1999; 2:69–78.
2. McCowen KC, Malhotra A, Bistrian BR. Stress-induced hyperglycaemia. *Crit Care Clin* 2001; 17:107–124.

3. Pozzilli P, Leslie RD. Infections and diabetes: mechanisms and prospects for prevention. *Diabet Med* 1994; 11:935–941.

4. Boord JB, Graber AL, Christman JW, et al. Practical management of diabetes in critically ill patients. *Am J Respir Crit Care Med* 2001; 164:1763–1767.

5. Krinsley JS. Association between hyperglycemia and increased hospital mortality in a heterogeneous population of critically ill patients. *Mayo Clin Proc* 2003; 78:1471–1478.

6. Yendamuri S, Fulda GJ, Tinkoff GH. Admission hyperglycemia as a prognostic indicator in trauma. *J Trauma* 2003; 55:33–38.

7. Laird AM, Miller PR, Kilgo PD, et al. Relationship of early hyperglycemia to mortality in trauma patients. *J Trauma* 2004; 56:1058–1062.

8. Rovlias A, Kotsou S. The influence of hyperglycemia on neurological outcome in patients with severe head injury. *Neurosurgery* 2000; 46:335–342.

9. Jeremitsky E, Omert LA, Dunham M, et al. The impact of hyperglycemia on patients with severe brain injury. *J Trauma* 2005; 58:47–50.

10. Capes SE, Hunt D, Malmberg K, et al. Stress hyperglycemia and prognosis of stroke in nondiabetic and diabetic patients: a systematic overview. *Stroke* 2001; 32:2426–2432.

11. Capes SE, Hunt D, Malmberg K, et al. Stress hyperglycaemia and increased risk of death after myocardial infarction in patients with and without diabetes: a systematic overview. *Lancet* 2000; 355:773–778.

12. Bolton CF. Sepsis and the systemic inflammatory response syndrome: neuromuscular manifestations. *Crit Care Med* 1996; 24:1408–16.

13. Faustino EV, Apkon M. Persistent hyperglycemia in critically ill children. *J Pediatr* 2005; 146:30–34.

14. Vriesendorp TM, Morélis QJ, DeVries JH, et al. Early post-operative glucose levels are an independent risk factor for infection after peripheral vascular surgery. A retrospective study. *Eur J Vasc Endovasc Surg* 2004; 28:520–525.

15. Garg R, Bhutani H, Alyea E, Pendergrass M. Hyperglycemia and length of stay in patients hospitalized for bone marrow transplantation. *Diabet Care* 2007; 30:993–994.

16. Ganji MR, Charkchian M, Hakemi M, et al. Association of hyperglycemia on allograft function in the early period after renal transplantation. *Trans Proc* 2007; 39:852–854.

17. Van den Berghe G, Wouters P, Weekers F, et al. Intensive insulin therapy in critically ill patients. *N Engl J Med* 2001; 345:1359–1367.

18. Takala J, Ruokonen E, Webster NR, et al. Increased mortality associated with growth hormone treatment in critically ill adults. *N Engl J Med* 1999; 341:785–792.

19. Ingels C, Debaveye Y, Milants I, et al. Strict blood glucose control with insulin during intensive care after cardiac surgery: impact on 4-years survival, dependency on medical care and quality of life. *Eur Heart J* 2006; 27:2716–2724.

20. Van den Berghe G, Schoonheydt K, Becx P, et al. Insulin therapy protects the central and peripheral nervous system of intensive care patients. *Neurology* 2005; 64:1348–1353.

21. Van den Berghe G, Wouters PJ, Kesteloot K, et al. Analysis of healthcare resource utilization with intensive insulin therapy in critically ill patients. *Crit Care Med* 2006; 34: 612–616.

22. Van den Berghe G, Wilmer A, Hermans G, et al. Intensive insulin therapy in medical intensive care patients. *N Engl J Med* 2006; 354:449–461.

23. Hermans G, Wilmer A, Meersseman W, et al. Impact of intensive insulin therapy on neuromuscular complications and ventilator-dependency in MICU. *Am J Respir Crit Care Med* 2007; 175:480–489.

24. Van den Berghe G, Wilmer A, Milants I, et al. Intensive insulin therapy in mixed medical/surgical ICU: benefit versus harm. *Diabet* 2006; 55:3151–3159.

25. Krinsley JS. Effect of an intensive glucose management protocol on the mortality of criti-
     cally ill adult patients. *Mayo Clin Proc* 2004; 79:992–1000.
26. Krinsley JS. Glycemic control, diabetic status, and mortality in a heterogenous population
     of critically ill patients before and during the era of intensive glycemic management: six
     and one-half years experience at a university-affiliated community hospital. *Semin Thorac
     Cardiovasc Surg* 2006; 18:317–325.
27. Krinsley JS, Jones RL. Cost analysis of intensive glycemic control in critically ill adult
     patients. *Chest* 2006; 129:644–650.
28. Grey NJ, Perdrizet GA. Reduction of nosocomial infections in the surgical intensive-care
     unit by strict glycemic control. *Endocr Pract* 2004; 10:46–52.
29. Furnary AP, Wu Y. Clinical effects of hyperglycemia in the cardiac surgery population: the
     Portland Diabetic Project. *Endocr Pract* 2006; 12:22–26.
30. Reed CC, Stewart RM, Sherman M, et al. Intensive insulin protocol improves glucose con-
     trol and is associated with a reduction in intensive care unit mortality. *J Am Coll Surg* 2007;
     204:1048–1055.
31. Brunkhorst FM, Kuhnt E, Engel C, et al. Intensive insulin therapy in patient with severe
     sepsis and septic shock is associated with an increased rate of hypoglycemia – results from
     a randomized multicenter study (VISEP) (abstract). *Infection* 2005; 33(Suppl1):19.
32. http://webanae.med.uni-jena.de/WebObjects/DSGPortal.woa/WebServerResources/sepnet/
     visep.html
33. National Institutes of Health: Glucontrol study: comparing the effects of two glucose
     control regimens by insulin in intensive care unit patients (article online). Available
     from http://www.clinicaltrials.gov/ct/show/NCT00107601 and http://www.glucontrol.org/.
     Accessed August 31, 2007.
34. National Institutes of Health: Normoglycemia in intensive care evaluation and survival
     using glucose algorithm regulation (NICE-SUGAR study) (article online). Available from
     http://www.clinicaltrials.gov/ct/show/NCT00220987 Accessed August 31, 2007.
35. Ellger B, Debaveye Y, Vanhorebeek I, et al. Survival benefits of intensive insulin therapy in
     critical illness. Impact of normoglycemia versus glycemia-independent actions of insulin.
     Diabetes 2006; 55:1096–1105.
36. Van den Berghe G, Wouters PJ, Bouillon R, et al. Outcome benefit of intensive insulin
     therapy in the critically ill: insulin dose versus glycemic control. *Crit Care Med* 2003;
     31:359–366.
37. Van Cromphaut S, Wilmer A, Van den Berghe G. Intensive insulin therapy for patients with
     sepsis in the ICU? *New Engl J Med* 2007; 6:1179–1181.
38. Vriesendorp TM, DeVries JH, van Santen S, et al. Evaluation of short-term consequences
     of hypoglycemia in an intensive care unit. *Crit Care Med* 2006; 34:26714–2718.
39. Mackenzie I, Ingle S, Zaidi S, et al. Hypoglycemia? So what! *Intensive Care Med* 2006;
     32:620–621.
40. Suh SW, Gum ET, Hamby AM, et al. Hypoglycemic neuronal death is triggered by glucose
     reperfusion and activation of neuronal NADPH oxidase. *J Clin Invest* 2007; 117: 910–918.
41. Finney SJ, Zekveld C, Elia A, et al. Glucose control and mortality in critically ill patients.
     JAMA 2003; 290:2041–2047.
42. Langouche L, Vander Perre S, Wouters PJ, et al. Effect of intensive insulin therapy on
     insulin sensitivity in the critically ill. *J Clin Endocrinol Metab* 2007; 92:3890–3897.
43. Dungan K, Chapman J, Braithwaite SS, et al. Glucose measurement:confounding issues in
     setting targets for inpatient management. *Diabet Care* 2007; 30:403–409.

44. Louie RF, Tang Z, Sutton DV, et al. Point-of-Care glucose testing. Effects of critical care variables, influence of reference instruments and a modular glucose meter design. *Arch Pathol Lab Med* 2000; 124:257–266.

45. Corstjens AM, Ligtenberg JJM, van der Horst ICC, et al. Accuracy and feasibility of point-of-care and continuous blood glucose analysis in critically ill ICU patients. *Crit Care* 2006; 10:R135.

46. Lacara T, Domagtoy C, Lickliter D, et al. Comparison of point-of-care and laboratory glucose analysis in critically ill patients. *Am J Crit Care* 2007; 16:336–347.

47. Kanji S, Buffie J, Hutton B, et al. Reliability of point-of-care testing for glucose measurement in critically ill adults. *Crit Care Med* 2005; 33:2778–2785.

48. Atkin SH, Dasmahapatra A, Jaker MA, et al. Fingerstick glucose determination in shock. *Ann Intern Med* 1991; 114:1020–1024.

49. Vlasselaers D, Schaup L, van den Heuvel I, et al. Monitoring blood glucose with microdialysis of interstitial fluid in critically ill children. *Clin Chem* 2007; 53:536–537.

50. Klonoff DC. Subcutaneous continuous glucose monitoring in severe burn patients. *Crit Care Med* 2007; 35:1445–1446.

51. Hill M, McCallum R. Altered transcriptional regulation of phosphoenolpyruvate carboxykinase in rats following endotoxin treatment. *J Clin Invest* 1991; 88:811–816.

52. Khani S, Tayek JA. Cortisol increases gluconeogenesis in humans: its role in the metabolic syndrome. *Clin Sci* (Lond) 2001; 101:739–747.

53. Watt MJ, Howlett KF, Febbraio MA, et al. Adrenalin increases skeletal muscle glycogenolysis, pyruvate dehydrogenase activation and carbohydrate oxidation during moderate exercise in humans. *J Physiol* 2001; 534:269–278.

54. Flores EA, Istfan N, Pomposelli JJ, et al. Effect of interleukin-1 and tumor necrosis factor/cachectin on glucose turnover in the rat. *Metabolism* 1990; 39:738–743.

55. Sakurai Y, Zhang XJ, Wolfe RR. TNF directly stimulates glucose uptake and leucine oxidation and inhibits FFA flux in conscious dogs. *Am J Physiol* 1996; 270: E864–E872.

56. Lang CH, Dobrescu C, Bagby GJ. Tumor necrosis factor impairs insulin action on peripheral glucose disposal and hepatic glucose output. *Endocrinology* 1992; 130:43–52.

57. Wolfe RR, Durkot MJ, Allsop JR, et al. Glucose metabolism in severely burned patients. *Metabolism* 1979; 28:1031–1039.

58. Wolfe RR, Herndon DN, Jahoor F, et al. Effect of severe burn injury on substrate cycling by glucose and fatty acids. *N Engl J Med* 1987; 317:403–408.

59. Mizock BA. Alterations in carbohydrate metabolism during stress: a review of the literature. *Am J Med* 1995; 98:75–84.

60. Mesotten D, Swinnen JV, Vanderhoydonc F, et al. Contribution of circulating lipids to the improved outcome of critical illness by glycemic control with intensive insulin therapy. *J Clin Endocrinol Metab* 2004; 89:219–226.

61. Mesotten D, Delhanty PJ, Vanderhoydonc F, et al. Regulation of insulin-like growth factor binding protein-1 during protracted critical illness. *J Clin Endocrinol Metab* 2002; 87:5516–5523.

62. Jolliet P, Pichard C, Biolog G, et al. Enteral nutrition in intensive care patients: a practical approach. *Intensive Care Med* 1998; 24:848–859.

63. Heidegger C-P, Romand J-A, Treggiari MM, Pichard C. Is it now time to promote mixed enteral and parenteral nutrition for the critically ill patient? *Intensive Care Med* 2007; 33:963–969.

64. Klip A, Tsakiridis T, Marette A, Ortiz PA. Regulation of expression of glucose transporters by glucose: a review of studies in vivo and in cell cultures. *FASEB J* 1994; 8:43–53.

65. Pekala P, Marlow M, Heuvelman D, Connolly D. Regulation of hexose transport in aortic endothelial cells by vascular permeability factor and tumor necrosis factor alfa, but not by insulin. *J Biol Chem* 1990; 265:18051–18054.

66. Shikhman AR, Brinson DC, Valbracht J, Lotz MK. Cytokine regulation of facilitated glucose transport in human articular chondrocytes. *J Immunol* 2001; 167:7001–7008.

67. Quinn LA, McCumbee WD. Regulation of glucose transport by angiotensin II and glucose in cultured vascular smooth muscle cells. *J Cell Physiol* 1998; 177:94–102.

68. Clerici C, Matthay MA. Hypoxia regulates gene expression of alveolar epithelial transport proteins. *J Appl Physiol* 2000; 88:1890–1896.

69. Sanchez-Alvarez R, Tabernero A, Medina JM. Endothelin-1 stimulates the translocation and upregulation of both glucose transporter and hexokinase in astrocytes: relationship with gap junctional communication. *J Neurochem* 2004; 89:703–714.

70. Tirone TA, Brunicardi C. Overview of glucose regulation. *World J Surg* 2001; 25:461–467.

71. Brealey D, Brand M, Hargreaves I, et al. Association between mitochondrial dysfunction and severity and outcome of septic shock. *Lancet* 2002; 360:219–223.

72. Brealey D, Karyampudi S, Jacques TS, et al. Mitochondrial dysfunction in a long-term rodent model of sepsis and organ failure. *Am J Physiol Regul Integr Comp Physiol* 2004; 286:R491–497.

73. Vanhorebeek I, De Vos R, Mesotten D, et al. Strict blood glucose control with insulin in critically ill patients protects hepatocytic mitochondrial ultrastructure and function. *Lancet* 2005; 365:53–59.

74. Turina M, Fry DE, Polk HC Jr. Acute hyperglycemia and the innate immune system: clinical, cellular, and molecular aspects. *Crit Care Med* 2005; 33:1624–1633.

75. Rassias AJ, Marrin CA, Arruda J, et al. Insulin infusion improves neutrophil function in diabetic cardiac surgery patients. *Anesth Analg* 1999; 88:1011–1016.

76. Nielson CP, Hindson DA. Inhibition of polymorphonuclear leukocyte respiratory burst by elevated glucose concentrations in vitro. *Diabetes* 1989; 38:1031–1035.

77. Perner A, Nielsen SE, Rask-Madsen J. High glucose impairs superoxide production from isolated blood neutrophils. *Intensive Care Med* 2003; 29:642–645.

78. Rayfield EJ, Ault MJ, Keusch GT, et al. Infection and diabetes: the case for glucose control. *Am J Med* 1982; 72:439–450.

79. Furnary AP, Zerr KJ, Grunkemeier GL, Starr A. Continuous intravenous insulin infusion reduces the incidence of deep sternal wound infection in diabetic patients after cardiac surgical procedures. *Ann Thor Surg* 1999; 67:352–360.

80. Weekers F, Giuletti A-P, Michalaki M, et al. Endocrine and immune effects of stress hyperglycemia in a rabbit model of prolonged critical illness. *Endocrinology* 2003; 144:5329–5338.

81. The CREATE-ECLA Trial Group Investigators. Effect of glucose-insulin-potassium infusion on mortality in patients with acute ST-segment elevation myocardial infarction. The CREATE-ECLA randomized controlled trial. *JAMA* 2005; 293:437–446.

82. Malmberg K, Ryden L, Wedel H, et al. Intense metabolic control by means of insulin in patients with diabetes mellitus and acute myocardial infarction (DIGAMI-2): effects on mortality and morbidity. *Eur Heart J* 2005; 26:650–661.

83. Scott JF, Robinson GM, French JM, et al. Glucose potassium insulin infusions in the treatment of acute stroke patients with mild to moderate hyperglycemia. The Glucose Insulin in Stroke Trial (GIST). *Stroke* 1999; 30:793–799.

84. Gray CS, Hildreth AJ, Sandercock PA, et al. Glucose-insulin-potassium infusions in the management of post-stroke hyperglycaemia: the UK Glucose Insulin in Stroke Trial (UK-GIST). *Lancet Neurol* 2007; 6:397–406.

85. Lanza-Jacoby S, Wong SH, Tabares A, et al. Disturbances in the composition of plasma lipoproteins during gram-negative sepsis in the rat. *Biochim Biophys Acta* 1992; 1124: 233–240.

86. Khovidhunkit W, Memon RA, Feingold KR, Grunfeld C. Infection and inflammation-induced proatherogenic changes of lipoproteins. *J Infect Dis* 2000; 181:S462–S472.

87. Carpentier YA, Scruel O. Changes in the concentration and composition of plasma lipoproteins during the acute phase response. *Curr Opin Clin Nutr Metab Care* 2002; 5:153–158.

88. Jeschke MG, Klein D, Herndon DN. Insulin treatment improves the systemic inflammatory reaction to severe trauma. *Ann Surg* 2004; 239:553–560.

89. Tulenko TN, Sumner AE. The physiology of lipoproteins. *J Nucl Cardiol* 2002; 9:638–649.

90. Harris HW, Grunfeld C, Feingold KR, Rapp JH. Human very low density lipoproteins and chylomicrons can protect against endotoxin-induced death in mice. *J Clin Invest* 1990; 86:696–702.

91. Harris HW, Grunfeld C, Feingold KR, et al. Chylomicrons alter the fate of endotoxin, decreasing tumor necrosis factor release and preventing death. *J Clin Invest* 1993; 91: 1028–1034.

92. Gore DC, Wolf SE, Sanford AP, et al. Extremity hyperinsulinemia stimulates muscle protein synthesis in severely injured patients. *Am J Physiol Endocrinol Metab* 2004; 286:E529–E534.

93. Agus MSD, Javid PJ, Ryan DP, Jaksic T. Intravenous insulin decreases protein breakdown in infants on extracorporeal membrane oxygenation. *J Pediatr Surg* 2004; 39:839–844.

94. Zhang XJ, Chinkes DL, Irtun O, Wolfe RR. Anabolic action of insulin on skin wound protein is augmented by exogenous amino acids. *Am J Physiol Endocrinol Metab* 2002; 282:E1308–E1315.

95. Vanhorebeek I, Van den Berghe G. Hormonal and metabolic strategies to attenuate catabolism in critically ill patients. *Curr Opin Pharmacol* 2004; 4:621–628.

96. Vanhorebeek I, Langouche L, Van den Berghe G. Endocrine aspects of acute and prolonged critical illness. *Nat Clin Pract Endocrinol Metab* 2006; 2:20–31.

97. Mesotten D, Wouters PJ, Peeters RP, et al. Regulation of the somatotropic axis by intensive insulin therapy during protracted critical illness. *J Clin Endocrinol Metab* 2004; 89: 3105–3113.

98. Hansen TK, Thiel S, Wouters PJ, et al. Intensive insulin therapy exerts anti-inflammatory effects in critically ill patients, as indicated by circulating mannose-binding lectin and C-reactive protein levels. *J Clin Endocrinol Metab* 2003; 88:1082–1088.

99. Langouche L, Vanhorebeek I, Vlasselaers D, et al. Intensive insulin therapy protects the endothelium of critically ill patients. *J Clin Invest* 2005; 115:2277–2286.

100. Jeschke MG, Klein D, Bolder U, Einspanier R. Insulin attenuates the systemic inflammatory response in endotoxemic rats. *Endocrinology* 2004; 145:4084–4093.

101. Brix-Christensen V, Andersen SK, Andersen R, et al. Acute hyperinsulinemia restrains endotoxin-induced systemic inflammatory response: an experimental study in a porcine model. *Anesthesiology* 2004; 100:861–870.

102. Klein D, Schubert T, Horch RE, et al. Insulin treatment improves hepatic morphology and function through modulation of hepatic signals after severe trauma. *Ann Surg* 2004; 240:340–349.

103. Das UN. Insulin: an endogenous cardioprotector. *Curr Opin Crit Care* 2003; 9:375–383.

104. Jonassen A, Aasum E, Riemersma R, et al. Glucose-insulin-potassium reduces infarct size when administered during reperfusion. *Cardiovasc Drugs Ther* 2000; 14:615–623.
105. Gao F, Gao E, Yue T, et al. Nitric oxide mediates the antiapoptotic effect of insulin in myocardial ischemia-reperfusion: the role of PI3-kinase, Akt and eNOS phosphorylation. *Circulation* 2002; 105:1497–1502.
106. Jonassen A, Sack M, Mjos O, Yellon D. Myocardial protection by insulin at reperfusion requires early administration and is mediated via Akt and p70s6 kinase cell-survival signalling. *Circ Res* 2001; 89:1191–1198.
107. Siroen MPC, van Leeuwen PAM, Nijveldt RJ, et al. Modulation of asymmetric dimethylarginine in critically ill patients receiving intensive insulin treatment: a possible explanation of reduced morbidity and mortality? *Crit Care Med* 2005; 33:504–510.
108. Nijveldt RJ, Teerlink T, van Leeuwen PA. The asymmetric dimethylarginine (ADMA)-multiple organ failure hypothesis. *Clin Nutr* 2003; 22:99–104.
109. Vanhorebeek I, Peeters RP, Vander Perre S, Jans I, Wouters PJ, Skogstrand K, Hansen TK, Bouillon R, Van den Berghe G. Cortisol response to critical illness: effect of intensive insulin therapy. *J Clin Endocrinol Metab* 2006; 91:3803–3813.

14 Disorders of Body Water Homeostasis

Suzanne Myers Adler, MD
and Joseph G. Verbalis, MD

CONTENTS

INTRODUCTION
OVERVIEW OF NORMAL WATER METABOLISM
HYPONATREMIA
HYPERNATREMIA
SUMMARY
REFERENCES

INTRODUCTION

Disorders of sodium and water homeostasis are among the most commonly encountered disturbances in the acute care setting, because many disease states cause defects in the complex mechanisms that control the intake and output of water and solute. Since body water is the primary determinant of extracellular fluid osmolality, disorders of body water balance can be categorized into hypoosmolar and hyperosmolar disorders, depending upon the presence of an excess or a deficiency of body water relative to body solute. The main constituent of plasma osmolality is sodium; consequently, hypoosmolar and hyperosmolar disease states are generally characterized by hyponatremia and hypernatremia, respectively. Both of these disturbances, as well as their overly rapid correction, can cause considerable morbidity and mortality *(1–4)*. After a brief review of normal water metabolism, this article focuses on the diagnosis and treatment of hyponatremia and hypernatremia in the acute care setting.

From: *Contemporary Endocrinology: Acute Cause to Consequence*
Edited by: G. Van den Berghe, DOI: 10.1007/978-1-60327-177-6_14,
© Humana Press, New York, NY

OVERVIEW OF NORMAL WATER METABOLISM

Whereas sodium metabolism is predominately regulated by the renin-angiotensin-aldosterone system (RAAS), water metabolism is controlled primarily by arginine vasopressin (AVP). AVP is a nine-amino acid peptide produced by cell bodies of magnocellular neurons located in the hypothalamic supraoptic and paraventricular nuclei and secreted into the bloodstream from axon terminals located in the posterior pituitary. The primary inputs to these hypothalamic neurons are via hypothalamic osmoreceptors and brainstem cardiovascular centers (5). Osmoreceptors located in the anterior hypothalamus stimulate AVP secretion in response to increased plasma osmolality and inhibit AVP secretion when plasma hypoosmolality is detected. Baroreceptors located in the carotid arteries and aortic arch also stimulate AVP secretion in response to decreases in mean arterial pressure or blood volume. AVP controls water permeability at the level of the nephron by binding to AVP V_2 receptors, causing aquaporin-2 (AQP2) water channel insertion into the luminal surface of collecting duct cells, thereby stimulating free water reabsorption and hence antidiuresis (6). Chronically, AVP also increases the synthesis of AQP2 in principal cells of the collecting duct, resulting in enhanced water permeability and maximal antidiuresis (7).

Many different neurotransmitters and hormones can stimulate AVP release, including acetylcholine, histamine, dopamine, prostaglandins, bradykinin, neuropeptide Y and angiotensin II. Many others inhibit AVP release, including nitric oxide, atrial natriuretic peptide, and opioids (8–10). Norepinephrine not only stimulates AVP release via α1-adrenoreceptors but also inhibits AVP release via α2-adrenoreceptors and β-adrenoreceptors (11,12). Since AVP secretion is influenced by so many different factors, any one of which may predominate in a given clinical circumstance, dysregulated AVP secretion is often the cause of impaired water homeostasis in acute illness.

HYPONATREMIA

Hyponatremia is a common electrolyte abnormality that varies greatly in its clinical presentation. It has been estimated that approximately 1% of hyponatremic patients have acute symptomatic hyponatremia, 4% have acute asymptomatic hyponatremia, 15–20% have chronic symptomatic hyponatremia, and 75–80% have chronic asymptomatic hyponatremia (13). The incidence of hyponatremia (serum [Na^+] ≤134 mmol/L) in an intensive care unit was prospectively found to be approximately 30% (14). The in-hospital mortality for critical care patients with hyponatremia approaches 40%, and hyponatremia has been shown to be an independent predictor of mortality in the intensive care unit *(15)*.

Hyponatremia is generally categorized based on serum tonicity as isotonic, hypotonic, or hypertonic. Although most instances of hyponatremia in acute illness are associated with hypotonicity, isotonic and hypertonic hyponatremia are also well-documented and are briefly discussed first.

Isotonic Hyponatremia

Isotonic hyponatremia is usually synonymous with so-called *pseudo-hyponatremia*, and must be distinguished from true hypoosmolality. Plasma osmolality may be measured directly in the laboratory by osmometry, or calculated based on the following formula:

$$\text{Posm (mOsm/kg } H_2O) = 2 \times \text{serum } [Na^+](\text{mmol/L})$$
$$+ \text{ glucose (mg/dL)}/18 + \text{BUN(mg/dL)}/2.8$$

Normal serum is typically comprised of 93% water and 7% non-aqueous factors, including lipids and proteins *(16)*. Although the non-aqueous components do not affect serum tonicity, in states of marked hyperproteinemia or hyperlipidemia (typically elevated chylomicrons or triglycerides), the non-aqueous proportion of serum is relatively increased with respect to the aqueous portion, thereby artifactually decreasing the concentration of Na^+/L of serum although the concentration of Na^+/L of serum water is unchanged. Because isotonic hyponatremia does not cause movement of water between the intracellular fluid (ICF) and extracellular fluid (ECF) compartments, it is not a meaningful cause of disturbed body fluid homeostasis in the acute care setting, but it must be distinguished from more pathological disorders.

Hypertonic Hyponatremia

Hypertonic hyponatremia has also been termed *translocational hyponatremia*, since the presence of osmotically active particles in the plasma induces an osmotic movement of water from the ICF to the ECF, and thereby decreases serum $[Na^+]$ even though serum osmolality remains elevated. Solutes such as glucose, mannitol, sorbitol, or radiocontrast agents all exert this effect. The generally accepted calculation to correct serum $[Na^+]$ for hyperglycemia is a decrease in serum $[Na^+]$ of 1.6 mmol/L for every 100 mg/dL increase in glucose concentration. However, some investigators have found a serum $[Na^+]$ correction factor of 2.4 mmol/L to be more accurate, especially at higher plasma glucose concentrations (e.g., > 400 mg/dL) *(17)*.

Hypotonic Hyponatremia

Of most relevance in the acute care setting is hypotonic hyponatremia, a condition indicative of an excess of water relative to solute in the ECF. Hypotonic hyponatremia can occur either as a result of solute *depletion*, a primary decrease in total body solute (often with secondary water retention), or solute *dilution*, a primary increase in total body water (often with secondary solute depletion) (Table 1) *(2,19)*. Hypotonic or hypoosmolar hyponatremia is generally subdivided according to the clinical ECF volume status. A recent retrospective analysis found the relative distributions of hypotonic hyponatremia in the intensive care setting to be 24% hypervolemic, 26% hypovolemic, and 50% euvolemic *(15)*.

HYPOVOLEMIC HYPOOSMOLAR HYPONATREMIA

Simultaneous water and sodium loss results in ECF volume depletion, with secondary AVP secretion and decreased free water excretion. Retention of water from ingested or infused fluids can then lead to the development of hyponatremia. Primary solute depletion can occur via renal or extrarenal sodium losses, each of which can have multiple etiologies.

Extrarenal solute losses. Vomiting, diarrhea, hemorrhage, excessive sweating, and dehydration all cause extrarenal losses of sodium and potassium, and the fluid loss that accompanies the solute losses is a potent stimulant to AVP secretion. Hyponatremia in hypovolemic shock secondary to volume loss (from hemorrhage or gastrointestinal free water losses), or distributive shock (secondary to sepsis where there is a relative hypovolemia from vasodilatation), is characterized by a urine sodium concentration (U_{Na}) generally less than 20 mmol/L, reflecting appropriate nephron function to maximize sodium reabsorption and hence conserve body solute and ECF volume.

Renal solute losses. Diuretics, mineralcorticoid deficiency, and nephropathies are all important etiologies of renal sodium loss that can lead to the development of hypovolemic hyponatremia. In patients on diuretics, hypokalemia from kaliuresis can worsen hyponatremia by causing a net movement of sodium intracellularly. Thiazides are more commonly associated with severe hyponatremia than are loop diuretics such as furosemide *(18)*. Renal solute loss is characterized by high urine sodium excretion, typically U_{Na} greater than 20 mmol/L, despite degrees of volume depletion that would normally activate mechanisms causing renal sodium conservation.

Patients with mineralcorticoid deficiency from primary adrenal insufficiency, or Addison's disease, can present in the acute care setting with either new-onset adrenal insufficiency or following a period of inadequate steroid replacement, and are typically profoundly volume depleted. Aldosterone secreted from the

Table 1
Pathogenesis Of Hypoosmolar Disorders

SOLUTE DEPLETION (PRIMARY DECREASES IN TOTAL BODY SOLUTE + SECONDARY WATER RETENTION)*:

1. RENAL SOLUTE LOSS
   Diuretic use
   Solute diuresis (glucose, mannitol)
   Salt wasting nephropathy
   Mineralocorticoid deficiency

2. NON-RENAL SOLUTE LOSS
   Gastrointestinal (diarrhea, vomiting, pancreatitis, bowel obstruction)
   Cutaneous (sweating, burns)
   Blood loss

SOLUTE DILUTION (PRIMARY INCREASES IN TOTAL BODY WATER SECONDARY SOLUTE DEPLETION)*:

1. IMPAIRED RENAL FREE WATER EXCRETION

   A. INCREASED PROXIMAL NEPHRON REABSORPTION
      Congestive heart failure
      Cirrhosis
      Nephrotic syndrome
      Hypothyroidism

   B. IMPAIRED DISTAL NEPHRON DILUTION
      Syndrome of Inappropriate antidiuretic hormone secretion (SIADH)
      Glucocorticoid deficiency

2. EXCESS WATER INTAKE
   Primary polydipsia

---

* Virtually all disorders of solute depletion are accompanied by some degree of secondary retention of water by the kidneys in response to the resulting intravascular hypovolemia; this mechanism can lead to hypoosmolality even when the solute depletion occurs via hypotonic or isotonic body fluid losses. Disorders of water retention can cause hypoosmolality in the absence of any solute losses, but often some secondary solute losses occur in response to the resulting intravascular hypervolemia and this can then further aggravate the dilutional hypoosmolality.

adrenal zona glomerulosa acts at the distal collecting duct to stimulate sodium reabsorption and hydrogen ion and potassium secretion. Conversely, aldosterone deficiency leads to excessive urinary sodium loss, intravascular volume depletion, and decreased glomerular filtration rate (GFR) which, in turn, stimulates baroreceptor-mediated AVP secretion and reduced water clearance with secondary water retention and hyponatremia *(19)*.

A unique form of hyponatremia due to primary renal sodium losses sometimes seen in critically ill patients with neurological lesions is cerebral salt wasting. This syndrome occurs following head injury or neurosurgical procedures. The initiating event is loss of sodium in the urine, which results in a decrease in intravascular volume leading to secondary water retention and hyponatremia because of a hypovolemic stimulus to AVP secretion. Superficially, cerebral salt wasting resembles syndrome of inappropriate antidiuretic hormone secretion (SIADH): both are hyponatremic disorders often seen after head injury with relatively high urine sodium excretion rates and urine osmolality along with plasma AVP levels that are inappropriately high in relation to serum osmolality. However, in patients who have cerebral salt wasting the increase in AVP is secondary to volume depletion, whereas a high AVP level is the primary etiologic event in patients with SIADH, who are euvolemic or have a modest increase in plasma volume from water retention. The relative distribution of cerebral salt wasting and SIADH among hyponatremic neurosurgery patients is unknown, and the etiology of cerebral salt wasting has not been definitively established. Abnormal sympathetic outflow to the kidney with a pressure natriuresis as well as abnormal secretion of atrial or brain natriuretic peptide (ANP, BNP) have been proposed as potential causes (20,21). Differentiation of cerebral salt wasting from SIADH hinges upon establishing that a period of urinary sodium loss and volume depletion preceded development of hyponatremia. Because infusion of isotonic saline into a euvolemic patient with SIADH results in a rapid excretion of the salt and fluid load to maintain balance, a high urine sodium concentration and urine flow rate alone do not establish that cerebral salt wasting is present. The patient's vital signs, weight, and input/output records should be reviewed carefully to determine what the patient's volume status and net fluid balance were just before and during the development of hyponatremia, and current physical findings and hemodynamic measures should also be taken into account (22).

In the acute care setting, depletional hyponatremia from decreased sodium ingestion rather than increased sodium loss can occur in patients on chronic enteral feedings, because many tube feed preparations are relatively low in sodium content (23). Elderly patients are at greater risk for hypovolemic hyponatremia from a variety of causes than are younger individuals (24).

EUVOLEMIC HYPOOSMOLAR HYPONATREMIA

Virtually any disease state causing hypoosmolality can present with what appears to be a normal hydration status based on the usual methods of ECF volume assessment. Clinical evaluation of volume status is not very sensitive, whereas laboratory measures such as normal or low blood urea nitrogen (BUN) and uric acid concentrations and an elevated U_{Na} are useful correlates of normal

ECF volume *(2,25)*. Many different disease states can present with euvolemic hyponatremia, and the largest subgroup of patients has presented with hypoosmolar hyponatremia across multiple studies over many years *(1,15,26)*.

Syndrome of inappropriate antidiuretic hormone secretion (SIADH). SIADH is the most common cause of euvolemic hyponatremia in acute illness. It is essential to recognize that hypoosmolality does not always imply that AVP secretion is inappropriate, especially in the hypovolemic patient. Diagnostic criteria for SIADH remain as defined in 1967 by Bartter and Schwartz (Table 2) *(27)*. First, ECF hypoosmolality must be present and hyponatremia secondary to pseudohyponatremia or hyperglycemia must be excluded. Second, urinary osmolality must be greater than maximally dilute urine (i.e., >100 mOsm/kg H_2O). However, urine osmolality must only be inappropriate at some plasma osmolality (i.e., <275 mOsm/kg H_2O), and not for all levels of plasma osmolality, as found in the *reset osmostat* variant of SIADH *(28)*. Third, clinical euvolemia must be present, since hypo- and hypervolemic states imply other causes of hyponatremia as described elsewhere in this article. A patient with SIADH may develop hyper- or hypovolemia for other reasons, but a diagnosis of SIADH

Table 2
Criteria for the Diagnosis of SIADH

ESSENTIAL:

1. Decreased effective osmolality of the extracellular fluid (P_{osm} < 275 mOsm/kg H_2O).
2. Inappropriate urinary concentration (U_{osm} >100 mOsm/kg H_2O with normal renal function) at some level of hypoosmolality.
3. Clinical euvolemia, as defined by the absence of signs of hypovolemia (orthostasis, tachycardia, decreased skin turgor, dry mucous membranes) or hypervolemia (subcutaneous edema, ascites).
4. Elevated urinary sodium excretion while on a normal salt and water intake.
5. Absence of other potential causes of euvolemic hypoosmolality: hypothyroidism, hypocortisolism (Addison's disease or pituitary ACTH insufficiency) and diuretic use.

SUPPLEMENTAL:

6. Abnormal water load test (inability to excrete at least 80% of a 20 ml/kg water load in 4 hours and/or failure to dilute U_{osm} to < 100 mOsm/kg H_2O).
7. Plasma AVP level inappropriately elevated relative to plasma osmolality.
8. No significant correction of plasma [Na^+] with volume expansion but improvement after fluid restriction.

cannot be made until euvolemia is restored. An increased U_{Na} (> 30 mmol/L) *(25)* is the fourth essential criterion, but patients with SIADH can have low U_{Na} if hypovolemia or solute depletion is present. Although increased natriuresis is primarily a manifestation of free water retention *(29)*, there may also be co-existing true sodium depletion secondarily *(30)*. Finally, SIADH is a diagnosis of exclusion, and can only be made in the setting of normal renal, thyroid, and adrenal function. Because up to 20% of patients who meet the above criteria for SIADH do not appear to have elevated AVP levels *(31)*, some have proposed renaming this entity the syndrome of inappropriate antidiuresis (SIAD) *(32)*.

It is always important to diagnose the underlying etiology of SIADH, as successful long-term correction of hyponatremia will also require treating the underlying disorder. The most common causes of SIADH in the acute care setting can be divided into five main categories: pulmonary disease, central nervous system disease, drug induced, tumors, and other etiologies (Table 3). Pulmonary infections common in the acute care setting such as viral, bacterial and tuberculous pneumonia, aspergillosis, and empyema can all cause hyponatremia, as can non-infectious pulmonary diseases such as asthma, atelectasis, pneumothorax, and acute respiratory failure. Some bacterial infections seem to be associated with a higher incidence of hyponatremia, particularly legionella pneumonia *(33,34)*. Both animal and human studies have demonstrated that hypoxia impairs free water diuresis via increased AVP secretion in the absence of decreased cardiac output, mean arterial pressure, or GFR *(35)*. Evidence suggests that hypercapnia also impairs free water excretion independent of the effect from hypoxia. In one prospective study of ventilated patients in the ICU, plasma AVP levels were significantly elevated in hypercapneic patients ($PaCO_2$ >45 mmHg) compared to the nonhypercapneic state *(36)*.

Glucocorticoid deficiency. Secondary adrenal insufficiency, or hypopituitarism, can also lead to hyponatremia but via a different mechanism than primary adrenal insufficiency. Secondary adrenal insufficiency causes a solute dilution via an increase in total body water rather than the solute depletion that characterizes primary adrenal insufficiency. The glucocorticoid deficiency that defines secondary adrenal insufficiency causes impaired free water clearance through both AVP-dependent and AVP-independent means *(37)*. Because the main regulator of aldosterone secretion is the RAAS and not ACTH secretion by the pituitary, hyponatremia is not a result of renal salt wasting from mineralocorticoid deficiency in secondary adrenal insufficiency, or relative adrenal insufficiency in septic shock. Nevertheless, glucocorticoid deficiency can result in a clinical picture almost identical to SIADH, because there is loss of hypoosmolar inhibition of osmoreceptor-mediated AVP release resulting in persistent nonosmotic AVP secretion *(38)*. This effect is further exacerbated in acute glucocorticoid deficiency by concomitant nausea, hypotension, and decreased GFR that

Table 3
Common Etiologies of SIADH

TUMORS

Pulmonary/mediastinal (bronchogenic carcinoma; mesothelioma; thymoma)
Non-chest (duodenal carcinoma; pancreatic carcinoma; ureteral/prostate
  carcinoma; uterine carcinoma; nasopharyngeal carcinoma; leukemia)

CENTRAL NERVOUS SYSTEM DISORDERS

Mass lesions (tumors; brain abscesses; subdural hematoma)
Inflammatory diseases (encephalitis; meningitis; systemic lupus; acute
  intermittent porphyria, multiple sclerosis)
Degenerative/demyelinative diseases (Guillan-Barré; spinal cord lesions)
Miscellaneous (subarachnoid hemorrhage; head trauma; acute psychosis;
  delirium tremens; pituitary stalk section; transphenoidal adenomectomy;
  hydrocephalus)

DRUG INDUCED

Stimulated AVP release (nicotine; phenothiazines; tricyclics)
Direct renal effects and/or potentiation of AVP antidiuretic effects
  (desmopressin; oxytocin; prostaglandin synthesis inhibitors)
Mixed or uncertain actions (angiotensin converting enzyme inhibitors;
  carbamazepine and oxcarbazepine; chlorpropamide; clofibrate; clozapine;
  cyclophosphamide; 3,4 methylenedioxymethamphetamine ['Ecstasy'];
  omeprazole; serotonin reuptake inhibitors; vincristine)

PULMONARY DISEASES

Infections (tuberculosis; acute bacterial and viral pneumonia; aspergillosis;
  empyema)
Mechanical/ventilatory (acute respiratory failure; COPD; positive pressure
  ventilation)

OTHER

Acquired immunodeficiency syndrome and AIDS-related complex
Prolonged strenuous exercise (marathon; triathalon; ultramarathon; hot-weather
  hiking)
Senile atrophy
Idiopathic

all further decrease free water clearance *(39)* and is particularly more marked in elderly patients *(40)*. With chronic glucocorticoid deficiency, impaired free water excretion also results from AVP-independent decreased cardiac output and renal perfusion, thereby reducing volume delivery to the distal diluting tubules of the nephron *(41)*.

Hypothyroidism. Hyponatremia can develop in hypothyroidism and in particular myxedematous states, although the mechanism by which hypothyroidism induces hyponatremia is not entirely understood. Patients with primary hypothyroidism have impaired free water excretion, which can be reversed by thyroid hormone replacement. It is well known that hypothyroidism is associated with low cardiac output, bradycardia, decreased in cardiac contractility, and reduced ventricular filling *(42–44)*. Low cardiac output stimulates baroreceptor-mediated activation of AVP secretion. It has been postulated that AVP secretion is inappropriately high in severe hypothyroidism therefore causing free water retention *(45)*, but recent studies have demonstrated that hyponatremia is more likely to be mediated by AVP-independent mechanisms. In a series of patients with untreated myxedema due to primary hypothyroidism, all of whom underwent hypertonic saline infusion and a subpopulation who subsequently underwent free-water loading, there was a significantly lower basal plasma AVP level in the study group (0.5 ± 0.1 pmol/L) when compared to normal controls (2.5 ± 0.5 pmol/L). In addition, the subsequent rise in plasma AVP levels following hypertonic saline infusion was not exaggerated in any patients and was reported to be normal or even below normal in all patients. Plasma AVP was appropriately suppressed in those hyponatremic myxedema patients who demonstrated a degree of impaired urinary dilution during free water loading, providing convincing evidence that decreased free water excretion in myxedema is not due to inappropriate plasma AVP elevation *(46)*.

Severe hypothyroidism is also associated with decreased renal function and impaired GFR. A study of patients with severe iatrogenic hypothyroidism demonstrated that approximately 90% of individuals had a significantly greater creatinine value in the hypothyroid as compared to the prior euthyroid state. Moreover, once thyroid hormone replacement was given and thyroid function normalized, creatinine values returned to their baseline euthyroid levels prior to the iatrogenically induced hypothyroid state *(47)*. Based on this combined evidence, the major cause of impaired water excretion in hypothyroidism appears to be an alteration in renal perfusion and GFR secondary to systemic effects of thyroid hormone deficiency on cardiac output and peripheral vascular resistance *(48–50)*.

HYPERVOLEMIC HYPOOSMOLAR HYPONATREMIA

In hypervolemic hyponatremia, there is an excess in both total body water and total body sodium, resulting in clinically evident edema and/or ascites. However, in many cases the increase in total body water is out of proportion to that of total body sodium, causing hyponatremia. Congestive heart failure, cirrhosis, and nephrotic syndrome all share this common pathophysiology, although the specific mechanisms vary among these disease states.

Congestive heart failure. Although clearly a condition of total body ECF overload, the decreased cardiac output in congestive heart failure causes a perceived intra-arteriolar volume depletion, best described as a decrease in the effective arterial blood volume at the level of the carotid artery and renal afferent arteriole baroreceptors *(51,52)*. Decreased renal perfusion activates both the RAAS and the sympathetic nervous system, resulting in increased sodium reabsorption and secondary passive free water reabsorption *(53)*. Decreased renal perfusion and subsequent increased baroreceptor firing also activates non-osmotic AVP secretion, resulting in increased free water reabsorption. The goal of these physiological mechanisms is to restore normal renal perfusion in a perceived state of intra-arteriolar volume depletion, but the net effect is to further exacerbate hypervolemia and progressive hyponatremia in the patient with heart failure.

In a study of over 200 patients with severe heart failure, those who were also hyponatremic were found to have a shorter median survival (164 versus 373 days). These patients were found to have elevated plasma renin activity, and there was a significant mortality benefit to treating this subgroup of patients with angotensin-converting enzyme inhibitors *(54)*. In addition, hyponatremia during the early-phase of acute myocardial infarction has been found to predict long-term mortality independently of left ventricular ejection fraction and other accepted predictors of cardiac outcome *(55)*.

Cirrhosis. Once ascites develops as a sequelae of chronic liver disease, approximately 30% of patients will manifest hyponatremia (serum $[Na^+]$ <130 mmol/L) *(56)*. Similar to the findings in congestive heart failure, there is impaired free water excretion in cirrhosis owing to the non-osmotic release of AVP *(57)*, but, in contrast to congestive heart failure, cirrhosis is characterized by a high cardiac output. Gastrointestinal endotoxin, which is less efficiently cleared due to portal-systemic shunting, stimulates nitric oxide production, and vasodilatation *(58)*. Arterial dilatation, particularly in the splanchnic vasculature, leads to arterial underfilling and the non-osmotic secretion of AVP *(51,52)*. Following disease progression with splanchnic vasodilatation, decreased mean arterial pressure, and reduced renal perfusion can lead to the hepatorenal syndrome *(59)*. The increase in AVP secretion and water retention is proportional to the severity of cirrhosis, such that the extent of hyponatremia reflects hepatic disease progression with serum $[Na^+]$ <125 mmol/L often indicative of end-stage disease *(60)*. In addition, diuretics commonly used to treat ascites often worsens hyponatremia by decreasing intravascular volume and renal perfusion, thereby increasing AVP levels and further compromising the kidney's ability to excrete free water *(61)*.

Advanced renal failure. Patients with mild-to-moderate renal dysfunction are generally able to excrete sufficient free water to maintain a normal serum [Na$^+$], whereas patients with end stage renal disease have impaired urinary dilution and free water excretion such that the minimum urine osmolality increases to 200–250 mOsm/kg H$_2$O, even though AVP secretion is appropriately suppressed. As a result, patients with advanced renal disease typically manifest hyponatremia as a result of water retention.

Treatment of Hyponatremia

The symptom severity of hyponatremia depends in large part upon the rapidity of the decrease in serum [Na$^+$]. Most patients are not symptomatic until serum [Na$^+$] decreases to <125 mmol/L *(62)*. Symptoms are predominantly neurologic in nature, including nausea, vomiting, headache, fatigue, irritability, and disorientation. Severe hyponatremia can progress to seizures, brain stem herniation, and death. Initial evaluation of patients in the acute care setting with hyponatremia includes a thorough history and physical exam, and careful evaluation of ECF volume status with assessment of orthostatic blood pressure and pulse. Initial laboratory evaluation should include serum electrolytes, glucose, evaluation of renal function with BUN and creatinine, serum osmolality, and urine osmolality and sodium. Treatment of hyponatremia must strike a balance between the risks of the hyponatremia itself and the risks of correction. The magnitude of these risks depends on the degree of brain volume regulation that has transpired as a result of intracranial fluid and solute shifts *(63)*. The treatment of some hyponatremia-associated disease states involves treating the underlying etiology such as steroids for adrenal insufficiency and thyroid hormone for hypothyroidism. However, in most cases the appropriate correction of serum [Na$^+$] relies on the identification of the underlying ECF volume status, the acuity with which the hyponatremia developed, and the severity of neurological symptoms present (Fig. 1) *(2)*.

───▶

Fig. 1. Algorithm for evaluation and therapy of hypoosmolar patients. *The dark grey arrow in the center emphasizes that the presence of central nervous system dysfunction due to hyponatremia should always be assessed immediately, so that appropriate therapy can be started as soon as possible in symptomatic patients even while the outlined diagnostic evaluation is proceeding.* Abbreviations: AVPR = arginine vasopressin receptor; D/C = discontinue; ECF = extracellular fluid volume; P$_{osm}$ = plasma osmolality; RX = treatment; SIADH = syndrome of inappropriate antidiuretic hormone secretion; 1° = primary; 2° = secondary; numbers referring to osmolality are in mOsm/kg H$_2$O, numbers referring to serum Na$^+$ concentration are in mmol/L.

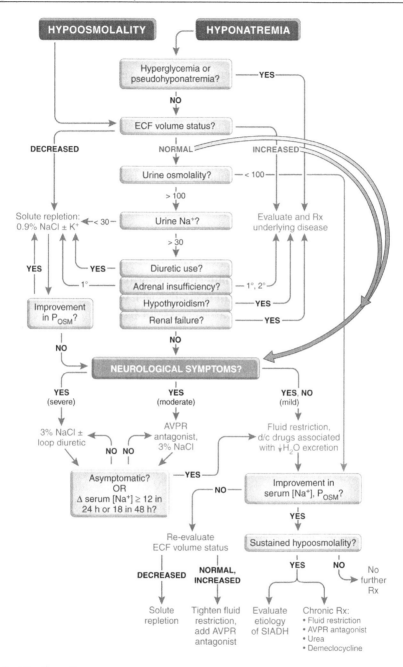

Fig. 1. (Continued)

Severe acute symptomatic hyponatremia. Acute hyponatremia (defined as <48 hours duration) with very low sodium values (<110–115 mmol/L) with seizures or coma is a medical emergency. The risk for neurological complications is high, because cerebral edema can evolve very quickly as a result of osmotic movement of water into the brain. In patients with severe acute hyponatremia, hypertonic (3%) NaCl should be infused at a rate to increase serum [Na$^+$] approximately 1–2 mmol/L/h until a less hyponatremic serum [Na$^+$] (i.e., 125–130 mmol/L) has been achieved. As a general rule, the infusion of 3% saline at a rate of 1 ml/kg body mass/hr raises serum sodium by approximately 1 mEq/hr. In comatose or seizing patients, a faster rate of sodium correction of 3–5 mmol/L/h for a short period of time may be warranted to avoid imminent brainstem herniation *(64)*. However, it is recommended that the total increase in serum [Na$^+$] over 24 hours is maintained at <10 mmol/L in 24 hours or <18 mmol/L in 48 hours as there is no evidence that a serum [Na$^+$] increase of greater magnitude improves outcomes *(65)*.

In hypovolemic states, including the majority of patients with U$_{Na}$ <30 mmol/L, fluid resuscitation with isotonic NaCl, with or without potassium, is appropriate with a goal serum [Na$^+$] increase of 0.5 mmol/L/h. Accumulated evidence in experimental humans and animals confirms that a slower rate of serum [Na$^+$] correction minimizes the risk of central pontine myelinolysis *(66)*. The serum [Na$^+$] should be measured every 2–4 hours during acute corrections of hyponatremia to ensure that the sodium correction is proceeding at the desired rate. Young pre-menopausal women appear to be at greater risk for neurological sequelae from hyponatremia with 75% of cases of brain damage occurring in this subpopulation in some studies *(67)*.

Treatment of hyponatremia in hypervolemic states includes free water restriction, diuresis with loop diuretics, and ACE inhibitors. Current clinical trials are underway investigating the use of AVP V$_2$ receptor antagonists for the treatment of euvolemic and hypervolemic hyponatremia, as will be described below.

Severe chronic symptomatic hyponatremia. In SIADH, fluid restriction is the mainstay of serum [Na$^+$] correction, with the goal of maintaining fluid intake 500 mL/d below urine output. However, this degree of fluid restriction is difficult to maintain in an intensive care setting where obligate fluid intakes for various therapies and parenteral nutrition often exceed this level. Furthermore, fluid restriction is not recommended to correct serum [Na$^+$] in hyponatremic patients with subarachnoid hemorrhage, because this patient subgroup has an increased risk of cerebral infarction that has been shown to be worsened by fluid restriction and lowered blood pressure *(68)*. Other therapies for chronic hyponatremia include demeclocycline (600–1200 mg/d), furosemide (20–40 mg/d), sodium tablets (3–18 g/d), and urea (30 g/d). Although these therapies are effective in some cases, in general they are suboptimal, and some patients, especially those with edema-forming states such as CHF and cirrhosis, are unable to tolerate the solute loads associated with these treatments.

AVP receptor antagonists are a novel therapeutic class known as the 'vaptans' (for *vas*opressin *an*tagonist*s*). These agents have been shown to be effective at preventing AVP-induced AQP2 membrane insertion in the renal collecting duct, causing the excretion of electrolyte-free water, termed *aquaresis (65,69)*. There are currently four non-peptide agents in various stages of clinical trials, and in December, 2005 the US Food and Drug Administration approved the use of intravenous conivaptan, a combined V1aR and V2R antagonist, for the treatment of euvolemic hyponatremia in hospitalized patients; this approval was subsequently extended to hypervolemic hyponatremia. A recent double-blind, multicenter, placebo-controlled study with euvolemic or hypervolemic hyponatremia (serum [Na$^+$] 115 to $<$ 130 mEq/L) randomized 84 patients to receive placebo or intravenous conivaptan administered as a 30-minute 20 mg bolus followed by 40 mg/d or 80 mg/d continuous infusion for 4 days. Conivaptan (both 40 mg/d and 80 mg/d) was significantly more effective than placebo in raising serum [Na$^+$] (measured as the change in serum [Na$^+$] area under the curve from baseline to end of the treatment period) during the first 2 days of treatment (p$<$0.001) and during the entire 4 day treatment (p$<$0.002). In addition, significantly more patients who received conivaptan demonstrated either a $\geq$ 6 mEq/L increase in serum [Na$^+$] over baseline or a normal serum [Na$^+$] $\geq$135 mEq/L as compared to placebo *(70)*. Conivaptan is a sensitive substrate and potent inhibitor of cytochrome P-450 3A4, and although oral conivaptan was demonstrated to raise serum sodium effectively in a placebo-controlled, randomized, double-blind study *(71)*, the FDA restricted its use to intravenous administration in order to minimize the risk of adverse drug interactions. Conivaptan is dosed as a 20 mg IV loading dose over 30 minutes followed by 20 mg as a continuous infusion over 24 hours for maximum of 4 days. The dose may be titrated to 40 mg/d continuous infusion if serum [Na$^+$] does not increase at the desired rate. Following initial administration of conivaptan, serum [Na$^+$] must be monitored closely during the acute phase of correction of hyponatremia (i.e., every 4–6 hrs) to prevent too rapid overcorrection. Evidence suggests that conivaptan may induce desirable changes in hemodynamics and urine output in patients with advanced (NYHA class II and IV) heart failure without adverse effects on blood pressure and heart rate *(72)*. Conivaptan is contraindicated in hypovolemic hyponatremia and hepatic cirrhosis, and infusion site reaction is the most commonly reported adverse event *(65,70)*.

Three oral agents with selective V2R antagonist activity currently in late development are lixivaptan, satavaptan, and tolvaptan. Studies have demonstrated that these agents increase serum [Na$^+$] by increasing aquaresis at a dose-dependent rate in both euvolemic and hypervolemic hyponatremia *(73,74)*. The Study of Ascending Levels of Tolvaptan in Hyponatremia (SALT-1 and SALT-2) trials were multicenter, international, randomized, double-blind, placebo-controlled studies that investigated the efficacy of tolvaptan in 448 adults with chronic hypervolemic or euvolemic hyponatremia of diverse origin including CHF, cirrhosis, and SIADH. Fluid restriction was permitted at the physician's discretion but was not mandated and patients were randomized to receive placebo or tolvaptan 15 mg titrated to 30 mg or 60 mg if needed. Results demonstrated the following: (1) serum [Na$^+$] increased more on tolvaptan than placebo during 4 days (P<0.001) and 30 days (P<0.001) of therapy, (2) patients on tolvaptan showed significant improvements in mentation, and (3) during the week after discontinuation of tolvaptan, hyponatremia recurred. Side effects associated with tolvaptan included increased thirst, dry mouth, and increased urination *(75)*. In another prospective, multicenter, randomized trial, tolvaptan was compared to fluid restriction in raising serum [Na$^+$] in hospitalized patients with serum [Na$^+$] <135 mmol/L during 27 days of treatment and 65 days of follow-up. Whereas fluid restriction and placebo raised serum [Na$^+$] by 1.0 +/– 4/7 mmol/L, tolvaptan increased serum [Na$^+$] by 5.7 +/– 3.2 mmol/L (p = 0.0065), and there was no difference in adverse events between the two groups *(76)*. The Efficacy of Vasopressin Antagonism in Heart Failure Outcome Study with Tolvaptan (EVEREST) investigators conducted two short-term randomized, double-blind, placebo-controlled studies in 4,133 patients hospitalized with heart failure in North American, South American, and European sites. Patients with heart failure were randomized to receive either tolvaptan 30 mg/d or placebo for 60 days along with standard therapy. Tolvaptan had no effect on long term mortality or heart function related morbidity during the mean follow up of 9.9 months *(77)*. In a second study by the EVEREST investigators, those patients receiving tolvaptan 30 mg/d along with standard therapy for heart failure including diuretics demonstrated some improvement in the signs and symptoms of heart failure including improvement in dyspnea and decrease in body weight at day 1 as compared to placebo *(78)*.

In patients with SIADH, the oral agent satavaptan has been investigated in a two-part study for both efficacy and safety during 1 and 12 month periods. Mean baseline serum [Na$^+$] levels were 125–127 mmol/L, and 79% of those on 25 mg daily and 83% of those on 50 mg daily were found to increase their serum [Na$^+$] levels by at least 5 mmol/L as compared to only 13% of those on placebo. In the subsequent open-label long-term phase of the study, serum [Na$^+$] was maintained in 12 of 18 patients over 6 months and 10 of 18 patients over 12 months, and although some patients experienced increased thirst and orthostatic hypotension, no serious adverse events related to satavaptan were noted during this period *(79)*. Lixivaptan has been primarily studied in cirrhotic patients and has been demonstrated to increase serum [Na^+] level compared to placebo in a placebo-controlled, randomized, multicenter 7-day study in hospitalized patients with stable hyponatremia (< 130 mEq/L for 3 days). Patients were administered lixivaptan 25, 125, or 250 mg twice daily or placebo, and lixivaptan showed dose related increases in serum [Na^+] and free water clearance. However, 50% of patients on 250 mg twice daily had to have medication withheld on multiple occasions due to excessive thirst and dehydration reflected by substantial rises in serum [Na^+] *(80)*. Another study with lixivaptan 100 mg or 200 mg daily in hyponatremic patients (baseline serum [Na^+] 127–128 mEq/L) with cirrhosis demonstrated that 27% of those receiving 100 mg/d and 50% of those receiving 200 mg/d achieved normal serum [Na^+] compared to 0% of those receiving placebo *(81)*. These agents are generally well-tolerated and show great promise for the treatment of both euvolemic and hypervolemic hyponatremia *(65)*.

HYPERNATREMIA

Similar to hyponatremia, hypernatremia can be induced by a number of illnesses in the acute care setting. The underlying etiology of hypernatremia can be frequently ascertained after a thorough history. Hypernatremia is generally categorized according to the causal factors involved: hypervolemic, hypodipsic, and increased free water losses (Table 4).

Hypervolemic Hypernatremia

Hypervolemic hypernatremia can result from the infusion of hypertonic fluids (i.e., $NaHCO_3$ or total parenteral nutrition) or from enteral feedings with inadequate free water administration.

Hypodipsic Hypernatremia

Decreased water intake, or hypodipsia, probably represents the leading cause of hyperosmolality encountered in acute care settings. One prospective cohort study of found that 86% of patients who developed hypernatremia (serum [Na^+] ≥150 mEq/L) while hospitalized did not have access to water, 74% had daily enteral water intake of less than 1 L, and 94% were administered less than 1 L of intravenous free water daily *(82)*. Hypodipsic hypernatremia is particularly prevalent among patients who have altered mental status who do not respond appropriately to physiologic stimuli that signal increased thirst and among the elderly *(83)*. One small series investigating age-related thirst changes found elderly individuals to have a lower thirst sensitivity to hypertonicity as manifest by both decreased thirst and decreased water consumption of elderly

Table 4
Pathogenesis of Hyperosmolar Disorders

WATER DEPLETION (DECREASES IN TOTAL BODY WATER IN EXCESS OF BODY SOLUTE):

1. INSUFFICIENT WATER INTAKE

Unavailability of water
Hypodipsia (osmoreceptor dysfunction, age)
Neurological deficits (cognitive dysfunction, motor impairments)

2. HYPOTONIC FLUID LOSS*

A. RENAL: DIABETES INSIPIDUS
Insufficient AVP secretion (central DI, osmoreceptor dysfunction)
Insufficient AVP effect (nephrogenic DI)

B. RENAL: OTHER FLUID LOSS
Osmotic diuresis (hyperglycemia, mannitol)
Diuretic drugs (furosemide, ethacrynic acid, thiazides)
Post-obstructive diuresis
Diuretic phase of acute tubular necrosis

C. NON-RENAL FLUID LOSS
Gastrointestinal (vomiting, diarrhea, nasogastric suction)
Cutaneous (sweating, burns)
Pulmonary (hyperventilation)
Peritoneal dialysis

SOLUTE EXCESS (INCREASES IN TOTAL BODY SOLUTE IN EXCESS OF BODY WATER):

1. SODIUM

Excess Na^+ administration (NaCl, $NaHCO_3$)
Sea water drowning

2. OTHER SOLUTES

Hyperalimentation (intravenous, parenteral)

* Most hypotonic fluid losses will not produce hyperosmolality unless insufficient free water is ingested or infused to replace the ongoing losses, so these disorders also usually involve some component of insufficient water intake.

(age 65–78 years) compared to young (20–32 years) individuals despite similar serum $[Na^+]$ increases. The investigators also concluded that there may be an increased thirst threshold in elderly individuals such that thirst is stimulated at higher levels of tonicity than in younger individuals *(84)*.

Hypernatremia from Increased Water Losses

A variety of diseases can cause increased free water losses in the acute care setting, including gastrointestinal water losses, intrinsic renal disease, hypercalcemia, hypokalemia, and solute diuresis, which is most commonly a result of hyperglycemia and glucosuria. Although these etiologies represent the most frequent causes of hypernatremia in the acute care setting, they must be differentiated from diabetes insipidus, which represents the quintessential clinical cause of hypernatremia. Generally, a urine osmolality <800 mOsm/kg H_2O in the setting of elevated serum osmolality is indicative of a renal concentrating defect. In the absence of glucosuria or other causes of osmotic diuresis, this generally reflects the presence of diabetes insipidus *(2)*. However, diabetes insipidus must be distinguished from other causes of polyuria, which is generally defined as a urine output of approximately >3 L/d. The most common cause of polyuria not related to diabetes insipidus is primary polydipsia. Individuals with primary polydipsia, also known as psychogenic polydipsia, retain normal pituitary function and hence AVP secretion, normal nephrogenic response to AVP, and normal renal concentrating ability, although there may be a decreased renal concentrating gradient induced by excessive water intake. Plasma AVP levels will likely be suppressed, but may increase following water deprivation (Table 5). Primary polydipsia is associated with psychiatric disorders and medications that cause dry mouth such as phenothiazines. Rarely, infiltrative diseases affecting the hypothalamic thirst center such as sarcoidosis may be the underlying etiology of primary polydipsia *(85)*. Depending on the amount of water ingested, serum osmolality may be low, which is helpful in distinguishing primary polydipsia from diabetes insipidus. Diabetes insipidus is generally subdivided into central diabetes insipidus, nephrogenic diabetes insipidus, and gestational diabetes insipidus.

CENTRAL DIABETES INSIPIDUS

Central diabetes insipidus is caused by a deficiency of AVP secretion from the posterior pituitary, but does not fully manifest itself until >85% of magnocellular neurons are damaged *(86)*. Central diabetes insipidus is quite rare, with a prevalence of 1:25,000. The majority of cases (40–50%) are secondary to a hypothalamic lesion such as a tumor or infiltrative diseases such as sarcoidosis and histiocytosis. Approximately 20–30% of central diabetes insipidus is categorized as idiopathic, but most of these patients likely have underlying autoimmune disorder. Lymphocytic infundibuloneurohypophysitis is the foremost cause of spontaneous diabetes insipidus without prior head trauma or neurosurgery, accounting for as many as 50% of cases *(87,88)*. A small fraction of cases (5%) are genetic, often with a delayed-onset. Sellar lesions and pituitary

Table 5
Water Deprivation Test

PROCEDURE

1. Initiation of the deprivation period depends on the severity of the DI; in routine cases the patient should be made NPO after dinner, while in cases with more severe polyuria and polydipsia this may be too long a period without fluids and the water deprivation should be begun early in the morning of the test (e.g., 6 AM).
2. Stop the test when body weight decreases by 3%, the patient develops orthostatic blood pressure changes, the urine osmolality reaches a plateau (i.e., less than 10% change over 3 consecutive measurements), or the serum sodium is > 145 mmol/L.
3. Obtain a plasma AVP level at the end of the test when the plasma osmolality is elevated, preferably above 300 mOsm/kg H_2O.
4. If the serum sodium concentration is <146 mmol/L or the plasma osmolality is <300 mOsm/kg H_2O, then consider infusion of hypertonic saline (3% NaCl at a rate of 0.1 ml/kg/min for 1–2 h) to reach these endpoints.
5. Administer AVP (5 U) or desmopressin (1 μg) sc and continue following urine osmolality and volume for an additional 2 hours.

INTERPRETATION

1. An unequivocal urine concentration after AVP/desmopressin (>50% increase) indicates neurogenic DI and an unequivocal absence of urine concentration (<10%) strongly suggests nephrogenic DI (NDI) or primary polydipsia (PP).
2. Differentiating between NDI and PP as well as for cases in which the increase in urine osmolality after AVP administration is more equivocal (e.g., 10–50%) is best done using the plasma AVP levels obtained at the end of the dehydration period and/or hypertonic saline infusion and the relation between plasma AVP levels and urine osmolality under basal conditions.

adenomas are not a common cause of diabetes insipidus, because, over time, the secretion of AVP from magnocellular neurons can shift to regions higher in the hypothalamus. Because these lesions are typically slow-growing, if a sellar lesion is detected within the context of new-onset diabetes insipidus, this suggests the presence of a rapidly enlarging sellar mass such as metastatic disease. The presence of the posterior pituitary bright spot on sagittal views of precontrast magnetic resonance imaging can be useful in determining the presence of central diabetes insipidus, but with two caveats: (1) there is an age-associated loss of the posterior pituitary bright spot, and (2) the posterior pituitary bright spot may still be apparent in a patient with central diabetes insipidus secondary to the persistence of oxytocin also stored in the posterior pituitary *(5)*. It is important to note that individuals with diabetes insipidus with an intact thirst mechanism, access to water, and an appropriate level of alertness may not be hypernatremic because they may be able to consume enough fluid to keep up with free water losses. However, if a central lesion impairs the thirst mechanism, if fluids are not accessible, or if the mental state is impaired, severe hypernatremia may result.

Post-operative diabetes insipidus occurs in up to 18–31% of patients following trans-sphenoidal surgery *(89,90)*. In the majority of patients with this complication, diabetes insipidus is transient with only 2–10% experiencing prolonged polyuria *(89,90)*. The classic post-operative triple phase response consists of diabetes insipidus followed by the syndrome of inappropriate antidiuresis and then subsequent diabetes insipidus. The first phase of diabetes insipidus occurs after damage to the pituitary stalk disrupts the axonal connections between magnocellular cell bodies in the hypothalamus and nerve terminals in the posterior pituitary, therefore preventing AVP release. After several days, the second phase of inappropriate antidiuresis develops and is caused by leakage of AVP into the bloodstream from the damaged and degenerating nerve terminals in the posterior pituitary. After AVP stores are exhausted, the third phase of diabetes insipidus follows if 15% or fewer functional AVP-secreting hypothalamic neuronal cell bodies remain *(91)*.

NEPHROGENIC DIABETES INSIPIDUS

Nephrogenic diabetes insipidus is caused by end-organ resistance of the kidney to the antidiuretic effects of AVP. Whereas familial or hereditary nephrogenic diabetes insipidus is secondary to X-linked inherited mutations of the AVP V_2 receptor or autosomal recessive mutations of the AQP2 water channel, acquired nephrogenic diabetes insipidus can be caused by hypercalcemia (serum $[Ca^{++}] > 13$), hypokalemia (serum $[K^+] < 2.5$), or medications such as lithium and demeclocycline. A recent review of 155 published studies of nephrogenic diabetes insipidus found the most reported risk factors to be medications including lithium, antibiotics, antifungal agents, antineoplastic agents, and antiviral agents followed by metabolic disturbances. The authors concluded that while most reported cases of reversible nephrogenic diabetes insipidus were due to medications, long-term lithium administration seemed to result in irreversible nephrogenic diabetes insipidus *(92)*. A plasma AVP level is useful to distinguish central diabetes insipidus from nephrogenic diabetes insipidus; however, to differentiate definitively nephrogenic diabetes insipidus from central diabetes insipidus, and from normal individuals with primary polydipsia as described above, a water deprivation test is often necessary (Table 5).

GESTATIONAL DIABETES INSIPIDUS

During pregnancy, the threshold for thirst and for release of AVP is decreased compared to the non-pregnant state. Although subclinical forms of diabetes insipidus unrecognized pre-partum may be unmasked during pregnancy, gestational diabetes insipidus most commonly presents in the 3rd trimester and is mediated by trophoblast derived vasopressinase, a cystine aminopeptidase which degrades both AVP and oxytocin. Normal vasopressinase activity increases by 1000-fold between 4 and 38 weeks of gestation and decreases by approximately 25% per day following delivery of the placenta such that there is virtually no vasopressinase activity 12 days post-partum *(93,94)*. Gestational diabetes inisipidus results when the degradation of vasopressinase itself is reduced such that vasopressinase activity is prolonged and AVP degradation is increased. Vasopressinase activity seems to be proportional to the weight of the placenta, and vasopressinase catabolism may be hepatically mediated since vasopressinase activity increases in the setting of hepatic dysfunction such as fatty liver of pregnancy, hepatitis, and pre-eclampsia *(93)*. Gestational diabetes insipidus may be treated with desmopressin, since unlike AVP this agent is not degraded by vasopressinase, and there are no known fetal adverse reactions. Gestational diabetes insipidus is typically transient and carries only a small risk of recurrence in subsequent pregnancies. Gestational diabetes insipdus, the onset of which is during pregnancy as discussed above, must be distinguished from diabetes insipidus occurring shortly after delivery caused by Sheehan syndrome *(95)*.

Treatment of Hypernatremia

Treatment goals of hypernatremia include correcting the established water deficit and reducing the ongoing excessive urinary water losses. Patients in the intensive care setting are typically unable to drink in response to thirst, and progressive hypertonicity from untreated diabetes insipidus can be associated with grave consequences unless appropriately treated. The following formula may be used to estimate the pre-existing water deficit *(96)*:

$$\text{Water deficit} = 0.6 \times \text{premorbid weight} \times [1-140/(\text{serum } [Na^+] \text{ mmol/L})]$$

This formula assumes that total body water is 60% of body weight, that no body solute is lost as hypertonicity developed, and that the premorbid serum $[Na^+]$ is 140 mmol/L, but the formula does not take into account ongoing water losses. Serum $[Na^+]$ should be lowered to approximately 330 mOsm/kg H_2O within the first 24 hours of correction in order to reduce the risk of exposure to the CNS of ongoing hypertonicity.

The treatment of central diabetes insipidus with desmopressin is an effective means of improving polyuria and hypernatremia with an initial dose in the acute setting of 1 to 2 micrograms (intravenous, intramuscular, or subcutaneous). If hypernatremia is present, free water should also be given in an effort to correct serum sodium, with 5% dextrose in water as the preferred intravenous replacement fluid. desmopressin is preferred over AVP as the former has a longer duration of action, avoids the vasopressor effects of AVP at V_{1a} receptors, and is available in both intranasal and oral preparations. The dose equivalency of desmopressin is 1 mcg intravenous, intramuscular, or subcutaneous = 10 mcg intranasal = 100 mcg oral. Although some cases of nephrogenic diabetes insipidus respond to large doses of desmopressin, traditionally nephrogenic diabetes insipidus is treated with sodium restriction and thiazide diuretics (any drug in this class may be used with equal potential for benefit), which block sodium absorption and act to decrease renal diluting capacity and free water clearance. Amiloride may be used to prevent or treat mild to moderate, potentially reversible lithium-induced nephrogenic diabetes insipidus. Lithium gains entry into collecting duct cells via luminal membrane sodium channels prior to inducing AVP resistance. Because amiloride closes these particular sodium channels, it can decrease entry and intracellular accumulation of lithium thereby improving renal concentrating ability (97,98). Prostaglandins increase renal blood flow and decrease medullary solute concentration, resulting in a small decrease in the interstitial gradient for water reabsorption. Therefore, prostaglandin synthase inhibitors such as indomethacin promote water reabsorption and impair urinary dilution, thereby reducing free water clearance, and urine output. These agents may be helpful as adjunctive therapy in the treatment of nephrogenic diabetes insipidus.

SUMMARY

Disorders of sodium and water metabolism are commonly encountered in the intensive care setting. This is predominantly due to the large number of varied disease states that can disrupt the balanced mechanisms that control the intake and output of water and solute. Disorders of body water homeostasis can be divided into hypoosmolar disorders, in which there is an excess of body water relative to body solute, and hyperosmolar disorders, in which there is a deficit of body water relative to body solute. Prompt identification and appropriate intervention of these disturbances are important to prevent the increase morbidity and mortality that accompanies disorders of body fluid homeostasis in patients in the acute care setting.

REFERENCES

1. Anderson RJ, Chung HM, Kluge R, Schrier RW. Hyponatremia: a prospective analysis of its epidemiology and the pathogenetic role of vasopressin. *Ann Int Med* 1985; 102: 164–168.
2. Verbalis JG. Disorders of body water homeostasis. *Best Pract Res Clin Endocrinol Metab* 2003; 17(4): 471–503.
3. Upadhyay A, Jaber BL, Madias NE. Incidence and prevalence of hyponatremia. *Am J Med* 2006; 119(7 Suppl 1):S30–S35.
4. Subramanian S, Ziedalski TM. Oliguria, volume overload, Na+ balance, and diuretics. *Crit Care Clin* 2005; 21(2): 291–303.
5. Robinson AG, Verbalis JG. The posterior pituitary. In: Larsen PR, Kronenberg HM, Melmed S, Polonsky KS, editors. Williams Textbook of Endocrinology, 10th edition. Philadelphia: W.B. Saunders, 2003; 281–329.
6. Knepper MA. Molecular physiology of urinary concentrating mechanism: regulation of aquaporin water channels by vasopressin. *Am J Physiol* 1997; 272(1 Pt 2):F3–12.
7. Knepper MA. Long-term regulation of urinary concentrating capacity. *Am J Physiol* 1998; 275(3 Pt 2):F332–F333.
8. Sladek CD. Regulation of vasopressin release by neurotransmitters, neuropeptides and osmotic stimuli. *Prog Brain Res* 1983; 60: 71–90.
9. Sklar AH, Schrier RW. Central nervous system mediators of vasopressin release. *Physiol Rev* 1983; 63(4): 1243–1280.
10. Baylis PH. Regulation of vasopressin secretion. *Baillieres Clin Endocrinol Metab* 1989; 3(2): 313–330.
11. Holmes CL, Patel BM, Russell JA, Walley KR. Physiology of vasopressin relevant to management of septic shock. *Chest* 2001; 120(3): 989–1002.
12. Leng G, Brown CH, Russell JA. Physiological pathways regulating the activity of magnocellular neurosecretory cells. *Prog Neurobiol* 1999; 57(6): 625–655.
13. Boscoe A, Paramore C, Verbalis JG. Cost of illness of hyponatremia in the United States. *Cost Eff Resour Alloc* 2006; 4(1):10.
14. DeVita MV, Gardenswartz MH, Konecky A, Zabetakis PM. Incidence and etiology of hyponatremia in an intensive care unit. *Clin Nephrol* 1990; 34: 163–166.
15. Bennani SL, Abouqal R, Zeggwagh AA, Madani N, Abidi K, Zekraoui A et al. [Incidence, causes and prognostic factors of hyponatremia in intensive care]. *Rev Med Interne* 2003; 24(4): 224–229.
16. Fried LF, Palevsky PM. Hyponatremia and hypernatremia. *Med Clin North Am* 1997; 81(3): 585–609.
17. Hillier TA, Abbott RD, Barrett EJ. Hyponatremia: evaluating the correction factor for hyperglycemia. *Am J Med* 1999; 106(4): 399–403.
18. Spital A. Diuretic-induced hyponatremia. *Am J Nephrol* 1999; 19(4): 447–452.
19. Vachharajani TJ, Zaman F, Abreo KD. Hyponatremia in critically ill patients. *J Intensive Care Med* 2003; 18(1): 3–8.
20. Damaraju SC, Rajshekhar V, Chandy MJ. Validation study of a central venous pressure-based protocol for the management of neurosurgical patients with hyponatremia and natriuresis. *Neurosurgery* 1997; 40(2): 312–316; discussion 316–317.
21. Palmer BF. Hyponatraemia in a neurosurgical patient: syndrome of inappropriate antidiuretic hormone secretion versus cerebral salt wasting. *Nephrol Dial Transplant* 2000; 15(2): 262–268.

22. Palmer BF. Hyponatremia in patients with central nervous system disease: SIADH versus CSW. *Trends Endocrinol Metab* 2003; 14(4): 182–187.

23. Rudman D, Racette D, Rudman IW, Mattson DE, Erve PR. Hyponatremia in tube-fed elderly men. *J Chronic Dis* 1986; 39(2): 73–80.

24. Hodak SP, Verbalis JG. Abnormalities of water homeostasis in aging. *Endocrinol Metab Clin North Am* 2005; 34(4): 1031–1046, xi.

25. Chung HM, Kluge R, Schrier RW, Anderson RJ. Clinical assessment of extracellular fluid volume in hyponatremia. *Am J Med* 1987; 83: 905–908.

26. Gross PA, Pehrisch H, Rascher W, Schomig A, Hackenthal E, Ritz E. Pathogenesis of clinical hyponatremia: observations of vasopressin and fluid intake in 100 hyponatremic medical patients. *Eur J Clin Invest* 1987; 17: 123–129.

27. Bartter FC, Schwartz WB. The syndrome of inappropriate secretion of antidiuretic hormone. *Am J Med* 1967; 42: 790–806.

28. Michelis MF, Fusco RD, Bragdon RW, Davis BB. Reset of osmoreceptors in association with normovolemic hyponatremia. *Am J Med Sci* 1974; 267: 267–273.

29. Leaf A, Bartter FC, Santos RF, Wrong O. Evidence in man that urinary electrolyte loss induced by pitressin is a function of water retention. *J Clin Invest* 1953; 32: 868–878.

30. Verbalis JG. Whole-body volume regulation and escape from antidiuresis. *Am J Med* 2006; 119(7 Suppl 1):S21–S29.

31. Zerbe R, Stropes L, Robertson G. Vasopressin function in the syndrome of inappropriate antidiuresis. *Annu Rev Med* 1980; 31: 315–327.

32. Robertson GL, Aycinena P, Zerbe RL. Neurogenic disorders of osmoregulation. *Am J Med* 1982; 72: 339–353.

33. Sabria M, Campins M. Legionnaires' disease: update on epidemiology and management options. *Am J Resp Med* 2003; 2: 235–243.

34. Sopena N, Sabria-Leal M, Pedro-Botet ML, et al. Comparative study of the clinical presentation of Legionella pneumonia and other community-acquired pneumonias. *Chest* 1998; 113: 1195–1200.

35. Anderson RJ, Pluss RG, Berns AS, Jackson JT, Arnold PE, Schrier RW et al. Mechanism of effect of hypoxia on renal water excretion. *J Clin Invest* 1978; 62(4): 769–777.

36. Leach RM, Forsling ML. The effect of changes in arterial PCO2 on neuroendocrine function in man. *Exp Physiol* 2004; 89(3): 287–292.

37. Verbalis JG. SIADH and Other Hypoosmolar Disorders. In: Schrier RW, editor. Diseases of the Kidney and Urinary Tract. Philadelphia: Lippincott Williams & Wilkins, 2001: 2511–2548.

38. Oelkers W. Hyponatremia and inappropriate secretion of vasopressin (antidiuretic hormone) in patients with hypopituitarism. *N Eng J Med* 1989; 321: 492–496.

39. Kamoi K, Tamura T, Tanaka K, Ishibashi M, Yamaji T. Hyponatremia and osmoregulation of thirst and vasopressin secretion in patients with adrenal insufficiency. *J Clin Endocrinol Metab* 1993; 77(6): 1584–1588.

40. Yatagai T, Kusaka I, Nakamura T, Nagasaka S, Honda K, Ishibashi S et al. Close association of severe hyponatremia with exaggerated release of arginine vasopressin in elderly subjects with secondary adrenal insufficiency. *Eur J Endocrinol* 2003; 148(2): 221–226.

41. Ishikawa S, Schrier RW. Effect of arginine vasopressin antagonist on renal water excretion in glucocorticoid and mineralocorticoid deficient rats. *Kidney Int* 1982; 22: 587–593.

42. Klein I, Ojamaa K. Thyroid hormone and the cardiovascular system. *N Engl J Med* 2001; 344(7): 501–509.

43. Crowley WF, Jr., Ridgway EC, Bough EW, Francis GS, Daniels GH, Kourides IA et al. Noninvasive evaluation of cardiac function in hypothyroidism. Response to gradual thyroxine replacement. *N Engl J Med* 1977; 296(1): 1–6.

44. Wieshammer S, Keck FS, Waitzinger J, Henze E, Loos U, Hombach V et al. Acute hypothyroidism slows the rate of left ventricular diastolic relaxation. *Can J Physiol Pharmacol* 1989; 67(9): 1007–1010.

45. Skowsky WR, Kikuchi TA. The role of vasopressin in the impaired water excretion of myxedema. *Am J Med* 1978; 64: 613–621.

46. Iwasaki Y, Oiso Y, Yamauchi K, Takatsuki K, Kondo K, Hasegawa H et al. Osmoregulation of plasma vasopressin in myxedema. *J Clin Endocrinol Metab* 1990; 70: 534–539.

47. Kreisman SH, Hennessey JV. Consistent reversible elevations of serum creatinine levels in severe hypothyroidism. *Arch Intern Med* 1999; 159(1): 79–82.

48. Derubertis FR, Jr., Michelis MF, Bloom ME, Mintz DH, Field JB, Davis BB. Impaired water excretion in myxedema. *Am J Med* 1971; 51: 41–53.

49. Schmitz PH, de Meijer PH, Meinders AE. Hyponatremia due to hypothyroidism: a pure renal mechanism. *Neth J Med* 2001; 58(3): 143–149.

50. Hanna FW, Scanlon MF. Hyponatraemia, hypothyroidism, and role of arginine-vasopressin. *Lancet* 1997; 350(9080): 755–756.

51. Schrier RW. Pathogenesis of sodium and water retention in high-output and low-output cardiac failure, nephrotic syndrome, cirrhosis, and pregnancy (2). *N Eng J Med* 1988; 319: 1127–1134.

52. Schrier RW. Pathogenesis of sodium and water retention in high-output and low-output cardiac failure, nephrotic syndrome, cirrhosis, and pregnancy (1). *N Eng J Med* 1988; 319: 1065–1072.

53. Oren RM. Hyponatremia in congestive heart failure. *Am J Cardiol* 2005; 95(9A): 2B–7B.

54. Lee WH, Packer M. Prognostic importance of serum sodium concentration and its modification by converting-enzyme inhibition in patients with severe chronic heart failure. *Circulation* 1986; 73(2): 257–267.

55. Goldberg A, Hammerman H, Petcherski S, Nassar M, Zdorovyak A, Yalonetsky S et al. Hyponatremia and long-term mortality in survivors of acute ST-elevation myocardial infarction. *Arch Intern Med* 2006; 166(7): 781–786.

56. Arroyo V, Rodes J, Gutierrez-Lizarraga MA, Revert L. Prognostic value of spontaneous hyponatremia in cirrhosis with ascites. *Am J Dig Dis* 1976; 21: 249–256.

57. Bichet D, Szatalowicz V, Chaimovitz C, Schrier RW. Role of vasopressin in abnormal water excretion in cirrhotic patients. *Ann Int Med* 1982; 96: 413–417.

58. Guarner C, Soriano G, Tomas A, Bulbena O, Novella MT, Balanzo J et al. Increased serum nitrite and nitrate levels in patients with cirrhosis: relationship to endotoxemia. *Hepatology* 1993; 18(5): 1139–1143.

59. Fernandez-Seara J, Prieto J, Quiroga J, Zozaya JM, Cobos MA, Rodriguez-Eire JL et al. Systemic and regional hemodynamics in patients with liver cirrhosis and ascites with and without functional renal failure. *Gastroenterology* 1989; 97(5): 1304–1312.

60. Papadakis MA, Fraser CL, Arieff AI. Hyponatraemia in patients with cirrhosis. *Q J Med* 1990; 76(279): 675–688.

61. Sherlock S, Senewiratne B, Scott A, Walker JG. Complications of diuretic therapy in hepatic cirrhosis. *Lancet* 1966; 1(7446): 1049–1052.

62. Arieff AI, Llach F, Massry SG. Neurological manifestations and morbidity of hyponatremia: correlation with brain water and electrolytes. *Medicine* 1976; 55: 121–129.

63. Verbalis JG. The syndrome of inappropriate antidiuretic hormone secretion and other hypoosmolar disorders. In: Schrier RW, editor. Diseases of the Kidney and Urinary Tract. Philadelphia: Lippincott Williams & Wilkins, 2001: 2511–2548.

64. Gross P, Reimann D, Neidel J, Doke C, Prospert F, Decaux G et al. The treatment of severe hyponatremia. *Kidney Int Suppl* 1998; 64:S6–11.

65. Verbalis JG, Goldsmith SR, Greenberg A, Schrier RW, Sterns RH. Hyponatremia Treatment Guidelines 2007: Expert Panel Recommendations. *Am J Med* 2007; 120(11A):S1–S21.

66. Sterns RH, Riggs JE, Schochet SS, Jr. Osmotic demyelination syndrome following correction of hyponatremia. *N Eng J Med* 1986; 314: 1535–1542.

67. Ayus JC, Wheeler JM, Arieff AI. Postoperative hyponatremic encephalopathy in menstruant women. *Ann Int Med* 1992; 117: 891–897.

68. Wijdicks EF, Vermeulen M, Hijdra A, van Gijn J. Hyponatremia and cerebral infarction in patients with ruptured intracranial aneurysms: is fluid restriction harmful? *Ann Neurol* 1985; 17: 137–140.

69. Verbalis JG. Vasopressin V2 receptor antagonists. *J Mol Endocrinol* 2002; 29(1): 1–9.

70. Zeltser D, Rosansky S, van Rensburg H, Verbalis JG, Smith N. Assessment of the efficacy and safety of intravenous conivaptan in euvolemic and hypervolemic hyponatremia. *Am J Nephrol* 2007; 27(5): 447–457.

71. Ghali JK, Koren MJ, Taylor JR, et al. Efficacy and safety of oral conivaptan: a V1A/V2 vasopressin receptor antagonist, assessed in a randomized, placebo-controlled trial in patients with euvolemic or hypervolemic hyponatremia. *J Clin Endocrinol Metab* 2006; 91: 2145–2152.

72. Udelson JE, Smith WB, Hendrix GH, et al. Acute hemodynamic effects of conivaptan, a dual V(1A) and V(2) vasopressin receptor antagonist, in patients with advanced heart failure. *Circulation* 2001; 104: 2417–2423.

73. Greenberg A, Verbalis JG. Vasopressin receptor antagonists. *Kidney Int* 2006; 69(12): 2124–2130.

74. Palm C, Pistrosch F, Herbrig K, Gross P. Vasopressin antagonists as aquaretic agents for the treatment of hyponatremia. *Am J Med* 2006; 119(7 Suppl 1):S87–S92.

75. Schrier RW, Gross P, Gheorghiade M, Berl T, Verbalis JG, Czerwiec FS et al. Tolvaptan, a selective oral vasopressin V2-receptor antagonist, for hyponatremia. *N Engl J Med* 2006; 355(20): 2099–2112.

76. Gheorghiade M, Gottlieb SS, Udelson JE, et al. Vasopressin V2 receptor blockade with tolvaptan versus fluid restriction in the treatment of hyponatermia. *Am J Cardiol* 2006; 97: 1064–1067.

77. Konstam MA, Gheorghiade M, Burnett JC. Effects of Oral Tolvaptan in Patients Hospitalized for Worsening Heart Failure: The EVEREST Outcome Trial. *JAMA* 2007; 297: 1319–1331.

78. Gheorghiade M, Konstam MA, Burnett JC, et al. Short-term Clinical Effects of Tolvaptan, an Oral Vasopressin Antagonist, in Patients Hospitalized for Heart Failure: The EVEREST Clinical Status Trials. *JAMA* 2007; 297: 1332–1343.

79. Soupart A, Gross P, Legros JJ, et al. Successful long-term treatment of hyponatermia in syndrome of inappropriate antidiuretic hormone secretion with satavaptan (SR121463B), an orally active nonpeptide vasopressin V2-receptor antagonist. *Clin J Am Soc Nephrol* 2006; 1: 1154–1160.

80. Wong F, Blei AT, Blendis LM, Thuluvath PJ. A vasopressin receptor antagonist (VPA-985) improves serum sodium concentration in patients with hyponatremia: a multicenter, randomized, placebo-controlled trial. *Hepatology* 2003; 37: 182–191.

81. Gerbes AL, Gulberg V, Gines P, et al. Therapy of hyponatremia in cirrhosis with a vaso-pressin receptor antagonist: a randomized double-blind multicenter trial. *Gastroenterology* 2003; 124: 933–999.

82. Palevsky PM, Bhagrath R, Greenberg A. Hypernatremia in hospitalized patients. *Ann Intern Med* 1996; 124: 197–203.

83. Phillips PA, Rolls BJ, Ledingham JG, Forsling ML, Morton JJ, Crowe MJ et al. Reduced thirst after water deprivation in healthy elderly men. *N Engl J Med* 1984; 311(12): 753–759.

84. Phillips PA, Bretherton M, Johnston CI, Gray L. Reduced osmotic thirst in healthy elderly men. *Am J Physiol* 1991; 261:R166–171.

85. Rose BD, Post TW. Clinical Physiology of Acid-Base and Electrolyte Disorders. [5th ed], 748–772. 2001. New York, Mc-Graw Hill.

86. Heinbecker P, White HL. Hypothalamico-hypophyseal system and its relation to water balance in the dog. *Am J Physiol* 1941; 133: 582–593.

87. Huang CH, Chou KJ, Lee PT, Chen CL, Chung HM, Fang HC. A case of lymphocytic hypophysitis with masked diabetes insipidus unveiled by glucocorticoid replacement. *Am J Kidney Dis* 2005; 45(1): 197–200.

88. Imura H, Nakao K, Shimatsu A, Ogawa Y, Sando T, Fujisawa I et al. Lymphocytic infundibu-loneurohypophysitis as a cause of central diabetes insipidus. *N Engl J Med* 1993; 329(10): 683–689.

89. Hensen J, Henig A, Fahlbusch R, et al. Prevalence, predictors and patterns of postopera-tive polyuria and hyponatraemia in the immediate course after transsphenoidal surgery for pituitary adenomas. *Clin Endocrinol* 1999; 50: 431–439.

90. Nemergut EC, Zuo Z, Jane.J.A. Jr., Laws ERJr. Predictors of diabetes insipidus after transsphenoidal surgery: a review of 881 patients. *J Neurosurg* 1995; 103: 448–454.

91. Loh JA, Verbalis JG. Diabetes insipidus as a complication after pituitary surgery. *Nat Clin Pract Endocrinol Metab* 2007; 3(6): 489–494.

92. Garofeanu CG, Weir M, Rosas-Arellano MP, et al. Causes of reversible nephrogenic diabetes insipidus: a systematic review. *Am J Kidney Dis* 2005; 45: 626–637.

93. Barbey F, Bonny O, Rothuizen L. A pregnant woman with *de novo* polyuria-polydipsia and elevated liver enzymes. *Nephrol Dial Transplant* 2003; 18: 2193–2196.

94. Lindheimer MD, Davison JM. Osmoregulation, the secretion of arginine vasopressin and its metabolism during pregnancy. *Eur J Endocrinol* 1995; 132: 133–143.

95. Molitch ME. Pituitary disease in pregnancy. *Semin Perinatol* 1998; 22: 457–470.

96. Robinson AG, Verbalis JG. Diabetes insipidus. *Curr Ther Endocrinol Metab* 1997; 6: 1–7.

97. Boton R, Gaviria M, Batlle DC. Prevalence, pathogenesis, and treatment of renal dysfunction associated with chronic lithium therapy. *A J Kidney Dis* 1987; 10(5): 329–345.

98. Batlle DC, von Riotte AB, Gaviria M, Grupp M. Amelioration of polyuria by amiloride in patients receiving long-term lithium therapy. *N Engl J Med* 1985; 312(7): 408–414.

Index

CPSIA information can be obtained at www.ICGtesting.com
Printed in the USA
LVOW01*1153230214

374819LV00006B/341/P

PTU dose during thyroid storm